P9-BAU-247

Eating Expectantly

A Practical and Tasty Guide to Prenatal Nutrition

Bridget Swinney, M.S., R.D.

with

Tracey Anderson, R.N., B.S., F.A.C.C.E.

 **Meadowbrook Press**

Distributed by Simon & Schuster
New York

Library of Congress Cataloging-in-Publication Data
Swinney, Bridget, 1960-
      Eating expectantly: a practical and tasty approach to prenatal nutrition / by Bridget Swinney and
      Tracey Anderson.
            p. cm.
      Includes bibliographical references and index.
      ISBN 0-88166-371-9 (Meadowbrook)–ISBN 0-671-31820-9 (Simon & Schuster)
         1. Pregnancy–Nutritional aspects. 2. Mothers–Nutrition. 3. Prenatal care. I. Anderson, Tracey.
      II.Title.

   RG559 .S949 2000
   618.2'4–dc21

                                            00-028403

Managing Editor: Christine Zuchora-Walske
Proofreaders: Joseph Gredler, Megan McGinnis
Production Manager: Paul Woods
Desktop Publishing: Danielle White
Cover and Interior Art: Jone Hallmark

Text © 2000 by Bridget Swinney

All rights reserved. No part of this book may be reproduced or transmitted in any form or by any means,
electronic or mechanical, including photocopying, recording, or using any information storage and
retrieval system, without written permission from the publisher, except in the case of brief quotations
embodied in critical articles and reviews.

Published by Meadowbrook Press, 5451 Smetana Drive, Minnetonka, MN 55343

www.meadowbrookpress.com

BOOK TRADE DISTRIBUTION by Simon & Schuster, a division of Simon and Schuster, Inc.,
1230 Avenue of the Americas, New York, NY 10020

The contents of this book have been reviewed and checked for accuracy and appropriateness by professionals in the field of nutrition. However, the authors, editors, reviewers, and publisher disclaim all
responsibility arising from any adverse effects or results that occur or might occur as a result of the inap-
propriate application of any of the information contained in this book. If you have a question or concern
about any of the information in this book, consult your health-care professional.

04 03 02 01 00   10 9 8 7 6 5 4 3 2 1

Printed in the United States of America

Dedication

This book is dedicated to the memory of two people:
my mother, Marjorie Morgan Swinney,
and my friend and mentor, Robert Chambers.
It is also dedicated to the three special men
in my life: Frank, Nicolas, and Robert.

Acknowledgments

Thanks to my family for sticking by me through yet another revision: to Robert and Nicolas for late-night hugs and help around the house and to my personal MIS consultant (and husband), Frank, for helping me through major techno-problems and for being Mr. Mom when I was doing "book stuff." Thanks to colleagues Cathy Fagen, M.S., R.D., at the California Diabetes and Pregnancy Program; Dr. Barbara Luke at the University of Michigan Multiples Clinic; and Sandy Eardley for their assistance and kind words. Thanks to my writer friends who are always willing to lend an ear or give advice: Connie Evers, Amy Tracy, and Brenda Ponichtera. Thanks to my friends who offered meals, helped with the kids, and provided encouragement: Alicia and John Barrera, Leo and Wanda Melendez, Debbie and Bert Navar, and Beatrice and Jose Leyba. Thanks to my dad and my sisters Judy and Colleen for their continued support.

Thank you to all the past readers of *Eating Expectantly* for making a third edition possible.

Thanks to Bruce Lansky for *still* believing in this book as much as I do.

Special kudos to one awesome editor, Christine Zuchora-Walske, whose skillful editing of this edition was outstanding. (And I'm not just saying that because she extended my deadlines!)

Thanks to Danielle White for the easy-to-read typesetting and to Jone Hallmark for another beautiful cover.

Thanks to Steve Linders and Phil Theibert from the Meadowbrook PR department for their enthusiastic promotion of *Eating Expectantly*. And thanks to all the other folks at Meadowbrook Press for helping this book to be.

Contents

Foreword . . . . **x**

Introduction: *Why You Need This Book* . . . . **xi**

Section I

Nutrition Needs, Challenges, and Eating Tips

Chapter One: Contemplating Pregnancy **3**
- Why Prepregnancy Planning Is Best 3
- Who Should Have Genetic Counseling? 4
- The Importance of Good Nutrition before and during Pregnancy 4
- A Few Words about Infertility 8
- Planning a Healthy Pregnancy 11
- Focus on Folate 13

Chapter Two: The Knowledgeable Pregnancy **17**
- Ten Steps to a Healthy Diet 18
- Everything You Ever Wanted to Know about Weight Gain during Pregnancy 20
- All about Fat 25
- Changing Your Mindset for Pregnancy 28
- The Essential Guide to Vitamins and Minerals 28
- Vitamin Supplements: You May Need Them 36
- Keeping Your Baby's Environment Safe 39
- Traveling during Pregnancy 45
- The Positives of Pregnancy 46

Chapter Three: The First Trimester **49**
- How Baby Is Growing 49
- Weight Gain and Energy Needs 50
- Protein Needs 50
- Other Nutrient Needs 52
- Focus on Fiber 53
- The Eating Expectantly Eating Plan 55
- Morning Sickness 56
- Other First-Trimester Challenges 58
- Food Planning for the First Trimester 61

Chapter Four: The Second Trimester **63**

- How Baby Is Growing 63
- Weight Gain and Energy Needs 64
- How's Your Diet? 64
- Protein Needs 66
- Other Nutrient Needs 66
- The Power of Soy 68
- Focus on Calcium 68
- Focus on Iron 72
- "Thrive on Five" 74
- Smart Snacking 75
- Second-Trimester Challenges 77
- Food Planning for the Second Trimester 79

Chapter Five: The Third Trimester **81**

- How Baby Is Growing 81
- Weight Gain and Energy Needs 82
- Other Nutrient Needs 83
- Focus on Vitamin B_6 and Zinc 84
- What about Sugar? 85
- Tips for Keeping Your Energy Up 86
- Third-Trimester Challenges 87
- Food Planning for the Third Trimester 89

Chapter Six: Vegetarian Eating **91**

- Vegetarians: The Healthy Minority 92
- The Pregnant Vegetarian 92
- Nutrients of Special Concern 93
- The Eating Expectantly Vegetarian Eating Plan 96
- Vegetarian Shopping List 98
- Vegetarian Food Planning 100
- Eating Out Vegetarian-Style 100
- Vegetarian Convenience-Food Choices 102
- Eating after Delivery 104

Chapter Seven: Special Care for High-Risk Pregnancies **107**
- Expect the Unexpected 107
- Dealing with Your Emotions 107
- Preexisting Diabetes 108
- Gestational Diabetes 115
- The Diabetic Eating and Exercise Plan 118
- High Blood Pressure 128
- Multiple Births 133
- Coping with Bed Rest 140
- Older Moms 144
- Teen Pregnancy 145

Chapter Eight: Considering Breastfeeding **151**
- My Experiences with Breastfeeding 151
- The Feeding Decision: It's Up to You 152
- Why You Should Consider Breastfeeding 153
- Possible Obstacles 154
- A Note to Dad 157
- Preparing for Breastfeeding 158
- Nutrition during Breastfeeding 161
- Nutrients of Special Concern 164
- Drugs and Breastfeeding 165
- Breastfeeding for Special Groups 165
- Tips for Formula Feeding 173
- About Bonding 174

Chapter Nine: The First Weeks with Baby **175**
- What to Expect after Delivery 175
- Menus for the First Week with Baby 176
- Going Back to Work 177
- Your Body Is Changing 178
- Losing that Baby Fat Sensibly 179
- Weight-Loss Plans 181
- Preparing for Your Next Pregnancy 186

Chapter Ten: Fitting Fitness In **187**
- Benefits of Exercise 187
- What Every Pregnant Woman Should Know about Exercise 188
- Fitting Fitness into Your Busy Lifestyle 191
- Exercise after Pregnancy 192
- Tips for Getting with the Program after Your Baby Is Born 193

Section II

Shopping, Cooking, and Eating Out

Chapter Eleven: Stocking the Pregnant Kitchen **199**
- Check Out Your Kitchen 199
- A Peek in My Kitchen 200
- Reading Food Labels 201
- Eating on a Budget 205
- Stocking the Kitchen Toolbox 208
- Keeping the Vitamins in Your Vegetables 209
- The Essential Guide to Food Safety 210
- How to Lower Your Risk 215
- Food Safety Reports: Whom to Believe? 229
- Food Safety in a Nutshell 230

Chapter Twelve: Fast Foods: Eating In and Eating Out **235**
- Tips for Choosing Convenience Foods 235
- Complete, Convenient Meals for One 236
- Convenience Foods for the Whole Family 238
- Healthy Convenience-Food Menus 239
- Last-Minute Meals from the Cupboard 242
- Fifty Quick-and-Easy Meals or Snacks 242
- Choosing Wisely at Restaurants 246
- Choosing Nutritious Fast Foods 249
- Healthy Fast-Food Menus for Pregnancy 250

Chapter Thirteen: Menus and Recipes for the First Trimester **257**
- About the Eating Expectantly Menus 257
- About the Eating Expectantly Recipes 258
- First-Trimester Menus 259
  - Don't Feel Like Eating Menus 259
  - Don't Feel Like Cooking Menus 259
  - Don't Feel Like Cooking or Eating Menu 260
  - Feel Like Staying in Bed but Can't Menu 260
  - Feel Great Menu 261
  - Blender Breakfasts (or Snacks to Go) 261
  - Snack Ideas 261
  - High-Energy Snack Ideas 263
- First-Trimester Recipes 265

Chapter Fourteen: Menus and Recipes for the Second Trimester **291**

   • Second-Trimester Menus 291
     A Month of Breakfast Ideas 291
     Menus for a Hungry Appetite 292
     I Could Cook All Day Menus 293
     Company's Coming! Menus 293
   • Second-Trimester Recipes 295

Chapter Fifteen: Menus and Recipes for The Third Trimester **323**

   • Third-Trimester Menus 323
     Using Leftovers with Flair 323
     Meals in Minutes 325
     Feel Full Menus 326
     Best Bite Snacks 327
     Vegetarian Budget Menus 327
   • The Bean Routine 332
   • Third-Trimester Recipes 333

References **371**

Recommended Resources **383**

Index **387**

Recipe Index **396**

Foreword

Eating Expectantly effectively informs expectant parents of the value (for both mother and baby) of optimal maternal nutrition during pregnancy. The 1990 report of the Food and Nutrition Board of the National Academy of Sciences entitled "Nutrition during Pregnancy" played a special role in focusing our attention on nutrition during pregnancy and provided a thorough review of the major issues.

This report came exactly twenty years after the Food and Nutrition Board's 1970 report on "Maternal Nutrition and the Course of Pregnancy." The convening of an expert committee, including leaders in the field of nutrition and obstetrics, to write this report reflects the substantial advances in our knowledge during the intervening years and the need to apply recent findings to prenatal care.

Of the many conclusions reached by this expert committee, two are especially noteworthy. The first is the recommendation for greater maternal weight gain than previously recommended. This recognizes the association between maternal weight gain during the second and third trimesters and the growth of the baby prior to birth. The committee recommends a minimum weight gain of twenty-five pounds, unless the mother is overweight prior to pregnancy. For mothers who are underweight prior to pregnancy, even greater weight gain is recommended.

The second recommendation of particular note is that routine micronutrient supplements be limited to a daily iron supplement of 30 milligrams. While other specific micronutrient supplements are advised in a number of special circumstances, a routine prenatal vitamin/mineral supplement is not recommended. Rather, the emphasis is on an optimal diet as the source of micronutrients.

The reasons for emphasizing the foods we eat reach far beyond the simple fact that we don't need to take supplements if we consume an adequate, nutritionally well-balanced diet. One important reason is the very real risk that we will consciously or subconsciously pay less attention to an optimal diet if we take our daily multivitamin/mineral pill. Shortcomings of the latter approach include the risk of nutrient/nutrient interactions and imbalances, an area about which we continue to learn more. "New" micronutrients that are important for human health continue to be discovered. Not surprisingly, regular consumption of fruits and vegetables results in health benefits far greater than those obtained by vitamin supplements.

One of the most important reasons for selecting an optimal diet rather than a substitute pill is the fact that prenatal vitamins are not prescribed until the first prenatal visit to an obstetrician. This visit usually does not occur prior to conception or prior to the critical early development of the baby during the first four to six weeks of pregnancy. We now know, for example, that an adequate intake of folate, one of the B vitamins, in the preconceptional period will greatly reduce the risk of spina bifida and other neural tube defects. To be protective, however, adequate folate must be taken prior to conception and in those first few weeks of pregnancy. The bottom-line message is that the emphasis on an optimal diet being important to all women of childbearing age at all times—not only during pregnancy—has been confirmed.

I commend Bridget Swinney for her timely and informative guide. You should get your copy now and not wait until you are pregnant.

Michael Hambidge, M.D., Sc.D., Professor of Pediatrics, Director of the Center for Human Nutrition, University of Colorado Health Sciences Center.

Introduction
Why You Need This Book

When a woman became pregnant years go, she didn't change her lifestyle very much. The baby's health was thought to depend mostly on chance, and the placenta was thought to protect the fetus from all dangerous substances. Things are different today. We have an abundance of knowledge about pregnancy and nutrition, and the amount of research on the subject grows daily. Now we know that the placenta only acts as a screen, and many toxic substances can still get through to the baby. We've learned that mom is the true gatekeeper.

You will probably find pregnancy more high-tech than it was as recently as ten years ago. But even with all the diagnostic tests and fancy equipment now available, good nutrition is still the most important factor in giving your baby a healthy start in life.

Eating Expectantly puts nutrition and health during pregnancy into perspective. It gives you answers to questions you may want to ask but are not quite sure whom to ask. This book is based on a realistic and practical approach to eating, instead of one that relies on theoretical advice that doesn't work in the real world.

Eating Expectantly not only gives you guidance on what to eat, it provides over 100 delicious recipes developed specifically for each stage of pregnancy. In addition, it has over 300 menus to meet different needs; you'll find Don't Feel Like Cooking Menus, Meals in Minutes, I Could Cook All Day Menus, Healthy Fast-Food Menus, Company's Coming! Menus, and much more.

If you are vegetarian or trying to eat meatless meals more often, you'll find the vegetarian chapter helpful. If you experience one of the unexpected challenges of pregnancy, such as gestational diabetes, high blood pressure, or bed rest, *Eating Expectantly* will explain the facts and provide tips

for eating and food preparation.

If you're not pregnant yet, you will benefit even more from this book. You'll know what your eating habits should be and you'll know what to expect during pregnancy. I suggest that you read the entire book, skipping the chapter on high-risk pregnancies (unless you already have a chronic disease such as diabetes). Then, start using the menus and recipes now! This will get you used to eating right, and healthy eating will be easy to keep up when you're pregnant. Just keep in mind that you won't need to increase your calories until you are pregnant.

Eating Expectantly answers the following questions and more:

- What can I do before I get pregnant to help ensure a healthy baby?
- Will pesticides and preservatives in foods affect my baby?
- What if I can't drink milk? Do I really need a lot of calcium?
- I'm vegetarian. How can I meet my nutrient needs?
- Help! I was just diagnosed with gestational diabetes. What do I do?
- Should I take a vitamin supplement?
- How much weight should I gain?
- How effective is my current eating plan?
- Do I need to reduce salt intake if I start to have high blood pressure?
- How can I eat right when I'm on bed rest?
- I don't feel like cooking. Help!
- What are the best fast-food and restaurant choices for me while I'm pregnant?
- Should I exercise?

This book uses knowledge and experience gathered from hundreds of pregnant women and mothers, including myself. I've also collected answers from scientific experts: those who do nutrition research and who work with pregnant and breast-feeding women daily.

If you have any questions or concerns about what to eat, how much to eat, or how to practice good nutrition—before, during, and after your pregnancy—this book is a must! I hope you enjoy reading it as much as I enjoyed writing it. More importantly, I hope that by reading and following the advice in *Eating Expectantly,* you will give your baby and yourself the gift of good nutrition and good health!

Bridget Swinney

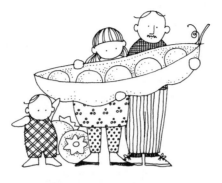

Section I

Nutrition Needs, Challenges, and Eating Tips

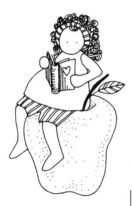

CHAPTER ONE

Contemplating Pregnancy

What you will find in this chapter:

• Why Prepregnancy Planning Is Best
• Who Should Have Genetic Counseling?
• The Importance of Good Nutrition before and during Pregnancy
• A Few Words about Infertility
• Planning a Healthy Pregnancy
• Focus on Folate

This chapter answers such questions as:

• How can I cut down on caffeine?
• How will I know if I'm healthy enough to have a baby?
• How can I stop eating junk food?

Why Prepregnancy Planning Is Best

Thinking about having a baby? If you're thinking about starting a family or having another child and are seeking information about pregnancy, you're making a smart move. In addition to reading about pregnancy on your own, you may also want to visit with your health-care provider when you decide you're ready to become pregnant. Prepregnancy counseling is recommended for several reasons:

1. It provides the information you need to change lifestyle habits that may affect your pregnancy, especially smoking, drinking, caffeine intake, and eating habits.

2. It gives you time to start eating a well-balanced diet, build up nutrient stores, start exercising regularly, and lose or gain weight, if needed.

3. It can teach you about fetal development and help you understand the importance of changing your habits before the first weeks of pregnancy. Much critical development takes place during the first weeks after conception, and this is when poor diet or lifestyle habits can damage the fetus the most. Most of a fetus's brain cell division, for example, occurs before most women know they're pregnant.

4. If you have a chronic medical condition, such as high blood pressure, diabetes, or kidney disease, prepregnancy counseling can help you get it under control before you become pregnant. This is vital to having the healthiest baby possible!

5. If you have had a miscarriage or have delivered a baby with birth defects, prepregnancy counseling can teach you how to improve your chances of having a healthier baby next time.

6. If this is your first pregnancy and you have a history of genetic defects in your family, or if you have a genetic condition that you could pass on to your children, prepregnancy counseling will give you time to seek genetic counseling.

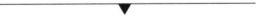

Who Should Have Genetic Counseling?

According to the March of Dimes, anyone who has unanswered questions about diseases in the family or who is concerned about being at increased risk for having a child with a birth defect or inherited disorder should consider genetic counseling. It is also suitable for:

Couples who . . .

- already have a child with mental retardation, an inherited disorder, or a birth defect.
- have or are concerned that they might have an inherited disorder or birth defect.
- have an infant who has a genetic disease diagnosed by routine newborn screening.
- are concerned that their jobs, lifestyles, or medical histories may pose a risk to pregnancy because of exposure to radiation, medications, chemicals, infections, or drugs.
- would like testing or more information about genetic defects that occur frequently in their ethnic group (such as Tay-Sachs disease, thalassemia, and sickle cell anemia).
- are first cousins or other close blood relatives.

Women who . . .

- will be thirty-four years old or older at the time of pregnancy.
- have had two or more miscarriages or babies who died in infancy.
- based on tests such as ultrasound or alpha-fetoprotein, have been told that they may be at increased risk for pregnancy complications or birth defects.

If you would like more information on genetic counseling and other helpful information about pregnancy, contact your local chapter of the March of Dimes Birth Defects Foundation.

The Importance of Good Nutrition before and during Pregnancy

The following examples illustrate the importance of good nutrition and early prenatal care for a healthy pregnancy:

- Folic acid is critical before and during the first trimester of pregnancy for the prevention of neural tube defects

(defects of the formation of the spinal column) such as spina bifida. Up to 70 percent of neural tube defects could be prevented by consuming adequate folate before and during the first trimester. The Institute of Medicine recommends that all women of childbearing potential consume 400 micrograms of folic acid daily from fortified foods or a supplement in addition to the folic acid found in a healthy diet. (An intake of 600 micrograms is recommended during pregnancy.) However, only 7 percent of women are aware of this recommendation.[1] To reduce your risk for birth defects, you should consider taking a multivitamin containing folic acid.[2] Women who have had a child with a neural tube defect are much more likely to have another child with the same problem; these women should talk to their health-care providers about a larger supplement of folic acid. (See page 28 to learn more about the key nutrients for pregnancy.)

- According to certain studies, your child's health as an adult could be affected by your eating habits during pregnancy. Recent research shows that babies who are born small for their gestational age and who are small during their first year are at higher risk later in life for insulin resistance (which could lead to diabetes), elevated triglycerides, lower HDL cholesterol levels, and heart disease.[3]
- Another study showed that women's lower weight gain between fifteen and thirty-five weeks gestation was related to

higher blood pressure when their children were ten to twelve years old. It was also found that the thinner a mother's triceps skinfold (a measure of nutritional status), the greater the chance of her child having higher blood pressure.[4]

- Women with preexisting diabetes are several times more likely to have a baby with birth defects than nondiabetic women. This fact may be related to glucose control before conception and in the very early weeks of pregnancy.[5] However, this increased risk can be reduced significantly with good control of blood sugars and early prenatal counseling.
- Research shows that iron and folic acid intake are related to increased infant body weight and length—another reason to make sure your diet includes adequate iron and folate during pregnancy.[6]
- Anyone who is unknowingly pregnant might drink alcohol or take medication that could harm the fetus. Excessive alcohol intake can cause birth defects and long-lasting problems such as mental and physical retardation, hyperactivity, and smaller birth weight. Because researchers aren't sure what small amounts of alcohol could do to a fetus, the safest strategy is to avoid alcohol during prepregnancy and pregnancy.
- According to researcher Michael Crawford of the Institute of Brain Chemistry and Human Nutrition in London, "The individual responsibility for the development of the brain rests with the mother. Some 70 percent of the total number of brain cells to last an

The Prepregnancy Quiz

The following quiz will help you and your partner determine whether your diet and lifestyle are ready for pregnancy. Circle "Yes" or "No" after each statement; then follow the scoring directions on the next page.

1. I eat at least three servings of fruit and three servings of vegetables on most days. **Yes** **No**

2. I eat a vitamin-C-rich food daily. (Examples include citrus fruit or juice, berries, papaya, mango, pineapple, melon, broccoli, cauliflower, tomato, and vegetable juice.) **Yes** **No**

3. I eat a wide variety of foods, including many types of protein foods. **Yes** **No**

4. I do some form of aerobic exercise at least twice each week. **Yes** **No**

5. I don't smoke and I avoid secondhand smoke. **Yes** **No**

6. I consume one or fewer caffeinated beverages a day. **Yes** **No**

7. I avoid taking drugs of any kind: prescription drugs, over-the-counter drugs, herbal preparations, or "street drugs." **Yes** **No**

8. I am at or close to my desirable body weight. **Yes** **No**

9. I avoid exposure to radiation, pesticides, herbicides, solvents, PCBs, and other chemicals. **Yes** **No**

10. I limit my consumption of shark, swordfish, or lake whitefish to once a month or less. **Yes** **No**

11. I usually eat three balanced meals a day and watch my saturated fat intake. **Yes** **No**

12. I eat three servings of calcium-rich foods daily. (Examples include milk, yogurt, cheese, high-calcium vegetables, tofu made with calcium, and juice fortified with calcium.) **Yes** **No**

13. I take a multivitamin/mineral supplement containing 400 micrograms of folic acid daily. **Yes** **No**

14. I avoid taking any single vitamin supplements (such as vitamin A) without my physician's approval. **Yes** **No**

15. I avoid drinking alcohol. **Yes** **No**

16. I avoid eating raw milk, eggs, shellfish, or foods that are made with these. (Examples include caesar salad dressing, mousse with uncooked egg, and sushi.) **Yes** **No**

17. I eat three servings of whole-grain breads, cereals, or other whole-grain products on most days. **Yes** **No**

	The Prepregnancy Quiz		
18.	I live a moderately paced lifestyle, get eight hours of sleep most nights, and feel generally happy.	**Yes**	**No**
19.	I have not followed any severe diets or had an eating disorder in the last three months.	**Yes**	**No**
20.	I am a vegetarian who eats no animal products, though I do take vitamin B_{12} and calcium supplements if recommended by my physician.	**Yes**	**No**
21.	I have visited my physician and discussed a future pregnancy.	**Yes**	**No**

How Did You Do?

Count your "Yes" answers and see how you scored below.

17-21: Congratulations! Your body is ready for pregnancy!

13-16: You're doing pretty well; you have just a few things to work on for the healthiest pregnancy possible.

9-12: Start working; you may need a few months to make the changes necessary to have the healthiest pregnancy possible.

9 or fewer: Oops! Your lifestyle may need an overhaul! Talk to your health-care provider before beginning a pregnancy.

individual's lifetime have divided before birth." Crawford also proposes that developmental disorders common to low-birth-weight infants (such as mental retardation, cerebral palsy, and blindness) are the result of poor maternal nutrition before and during the first trimester.[7]

- Children of women who have had gestational diabetes are at greater risk for obesity and impaired glucose tolerance. However, by starting pregnancy close to ideal body weight and exercising regularly, a woman can prevent gestational diabetes.[8]

- Evidence shows that smoking during pregnancy is not only related to lower birth weight, but may also affect neuro-logical development and behavior.[9] Also, smoking by either parent during pregnancy is related to a higher risk of childhood cancer.[10]

- According to a recent government survey, women's diets need some work. In 1994, only 55 percent of women ate a fruit or drank juice daily. Soft drink consumption for women has surpassed milk consumption. Women are not meeting the Dietary Reference Intakes (DRI) for iron, zinc, calcium, magnesium, and vitamin E. Average fiber intake is 10 grams short of the recommendation, and 44 percent of women report consuming 15 teaspoons of sugar daily.[11] One out of four adults skips breakfast—a significant source of nutrients, especially folic acid.[12]

Based on this information, it could be concluded that many women start their pregnancies a bit malnourished.

- An overweight woman is more likely to lose her fetus late in pregnancy than a woman of normal weight.[13] Also, two studies have recently shown that obese women are two to four times more likely to have a baby with a neural tube defect than women who are not significantly overweight.[14] The solution? If you are overweight, and especially if you are 20 percent or more over your ideal weight, lose weight before you conceive. (See Recommended Resources for weight-control resources.)

A few words of advice: Make sure that you don't become pregnant while you are on a weight-loss diet; your intake of certain vitamins may not be enough for the important stages of early fetal development. Taking a vitamin/mineral supplement during the weight-loss period is advisable. (See page 36.)

Eating at least the number of servings of each food listed in the Before-Baby Eating Plan will help you become a healthy future mom. As soon as you find out you're pregnant, you can switch over to the Eating Expectantly Eating Plan on page 55. The two diets are not very different, so your transition will be easy. (If you're wondering how to begin eating a healthy diet, see Chapter Eleven: Stocking the Pregnant Kitchen.)

▼

A Few Words about Infertility

Infertility, defined as not conceiving after one year of unprotected intercourse, affects about one in ten people of reproductive age. Some of these numbers may be a result of delaying pregnancy. Generally, the older we are, the longer we take to conceive. Seeking assistance for infertility can be an emotionally charged venture, to say the least.

Nutrition can and does play a role in fertility. If you are seeking help for infertility, please make sure you are not underweight. If you are underweight when you become pregnant, your chances of having a low-birth-weight infant are much higher. Some fertility treatments greatly increase your chances for having twins or more, and this further increases your chances for having low-birth-weight infants.

Here is an overview of some of the effects body weight, smoking, nutrition, and activity level have on fertility.

The Before-Baby Eating Plan	
Food	**Daily Servings**
Grains/starches	6 or more
Fruits	3 or more
Vegetables Be sure to include at least 1 vitamin-C- and 1 vitamin-A-rich fruit or vegetable daily.	3 or more
Protein or equivalent	4–6 ounces
Dairy or calcium-rich foods	3 or more

Body Weight

The female body appears to be very protective of an unborn baby. Conceiving is more difficult if you are underweight or overweight. Body fat seems to be the synchronizing factor (or the conductor, if you will) for the harmonious hormonal symphony that must take place for pregnancy to occur and be carried to term. Being close to your ideal body weight before you become pregnant can help you conceive and can reduce your risk of complications and of having a low-birth-weight or premature baby.

Overweight

Having too much body fat can affect fertility because part of the body's estrogen is made in the fat of the breasts and abdomen. Excess body fat can affect the amount and types of circulating hormones that influence fertility. Obesity is also related to polycystic ovarian disease, a cause of infertility. Studies show that overweight women have great success in conceiving once they have gotten closer to their ideal body weight.[15]

Underweight

Regular function of ovulation and menstrual cycles requires a minimum weight for height. In fact, body weight changes of just 10 to 15 percent can disrupt menstrual cycles. A maternal body weight closer to ideal weight is best for conceiving and for carrying a healthy baby to term. It may also help the health of future generations: Women born with low birth weights are more likely to have poor pregnancy outcomes than women with higher birth weights.[16]

Smoking

Smoking is related to decreased sperm quality and infertility in men as well as oxidative damage to sperm, which could be responsible for birth defects and other diseases.[17] Smoking can also deplete antioxidants (especially vitamins C and E), which can result in DNA damage to sperm.[18] It appears that women who smoke also have a higher risk of infertility and other problems associated with pregnancy.[19]

Nutrition

Caffeine

In a large multicountry study, it was found that women who consumed over 500 milligrams of caffeine (the equivalant of about 4 cups of coffee) took 11 percent longer to become pregnant. The effect was even stronger in women who also smoked.[20]

Vegetarian Diet

A meatless eating plan can be very healthy. (See Chapter Six for more information.) However, one study showed that a low-calorie vegetarian weight-loss diet caused seven out of nine women in the study to stop ovulating. The same study related an abrupt switch to a vegetarian diet to lack of ovulation.[21] If you are vegetarian and are having trouble conceiving, take a very close look at your diet to make sure you are not lacking any nutrients. Compare your diet to the recommended diet in Chapter Six. You may also want to take a multivitamin supplement.

Eating Disorders

Amenorrhea (lack of menstrual periods) and oligomenorrhea (infrequent periods) often occur in women with anorexia nervosa and are also seen in about 50 percent of women with bulimia. Reproductive hormones are also reduced in women who maintain a lower-than-normal body weight.[22] An increase in body weight and a balanced food intake will help restore normal reproductive functions.

If you have an eating disorder, you should try to resolve the underlying causes of the disorder for a permanent recovery. The eating habits and health problems associated with some eating disorders can put your baby at risk for birth defects, low birth weight, or prematurity. So, it is best to normalize your eating habits and make sure you are not below your ideal body weight prior to pregnancy.[23] Comprehensive programs that involve a psychologist, physician, and dietitian are most helpful.

Depleted Iron Stores

Women whose depleted iron stores were supplemented with iron and vitamin C had increased chances of conception.[24] So, make sure your diet includes ample iron from food or a supplement.

Alcohol

For couples trying to conceive, both men and women should avoid alcohol. Even moderate alcohol intake by women (less than five drinks per week) can affect fertility.[25] It has been suggested that alcohol intake by men can affect fertility as well as pregnancy outcome.[26]

Vitamin C

Two different studies demonstrated that vitamin C supplements of 200 milligrams improved fertility in men, in both heavy smokers as well as in nonsmokers.[27] Vitamin C may also protect against DNA damage to sperm—all the more reason to make sure both partners follow the Before-Baby Eating Plan. Men may especially want to increase intake of vitamin C foods or take a supplement.

Zinc

Zinc is important in the male and female reproductive systems. A zinc deficiency in men is related to decreased sperm count, decreased sperm motility, and decreased serum testosterone (a sex hormone) levels.[28] All of these factors could have a large impact on fertility. (See page 33 for food sources of zinc.)

Selenium

Inadequate and excess selenium are both related to male fertility. To make sure both partners' intake of selenium is adequate, eat plenty of seafood and whole grains.

Too Many Carrots

Women who ate no red meat and who supplemented their diet of mostly vegetables and salads with up to a pound of carrots a day had stopped ovulating. After reducing carrot intake, most women's menstrual function improved, which points to the conclusion that their infertility problem could be completely diet related.[29] Although this conclusion is speculative, it does draw attention to the important concept of moderation.

Activity Level

Women involved in competitive sports some-times reduce their body fat so much that they stop menstruating. Strenuous exercise and decreased body weight and body fat are related to reproductive problems, including infertility. Regular exercise is important for good health. However, if you take exercise to the extreme and are having trouble con-ceiving, you may need to slow down.

▼

Planning a Healthy Pregnancy

Several months before you become preg-nant, both you and your partner should fol-low the advice below. Men are often left out of pregnancy planning–but they must also take good care of themselves, since sperm is affected by diet and the environment.

▶ **Don't drink alcohol or take drugs.**

That includes aspirin! If you take a pre-scription medication, ask your doctor if it is safe to take during pregnancy. If your med-icine is not safe, your doctor may substitute one that is. Find out from your health-care provider which over-the-counter medica-tions are safe during pregnancy, especially during the first trimester.

▶ **Make a prepregnancy visit to your health-care provider.**

During this visit you can discuss your cur-rent health as well as your immunity to dis-eases such as chickenpox and rubella. These diseases are fairly harmless most of the time, but if you contract them during pregnancy, they could cause serious problems to the fetus. You may want to get immunized.

▶ **Both you and your partner should follow the Before-Baby Eating Plan.**

Since one cycle of sperm production takes ten weeks, you should both follow the Before-Baby Plan for three months prior to pregnancy.[30] When couples discuss preg-nancy, they often ignore the father's diet. However, research shows that the father's diet *can* affect his sperm and, ultimately, the fetus. A joint project at the University of California-Berkeley and the U.S. Department of Agriculture (USDA) Western Human Nutrition Research Center has linked low dietary intakes of vitamin C to increased genetic damage in sperm, which presum-ably translates into a higher risk for birth defects and genetic disease.[31] (See page 33 for good food sources of vitamin C.)

Study leader Dr. Bruce Ames says, "All we know now is that if your dietary intake of vitamin C gets below a certain level– about 60 milligrams per day, which is the Recommended Daily Allowance–you get into trouble. This strongly indicates that vit-amin C protects against DNA damage."

▶ **Keep your environment safe.**

For both partners, this means avoiding expo-sure to pesticides, herbicides, radiation (x-rays), and fumes from paint, extermination chemicals, and glue. Avoid exposure to lead, which can cause premature birth, brain damage, learning disabilities, and kidney and liver damage. More than forty million people have too much lead in their drinking water.[32] (See page 40 for the important details.)

If you smoke, try to quit or reduce your smoking. Avoid or limit exposure to second-hand smoke.

▶ Avoid or limit caffeine.

The pendulum seems to swing back and forth on caffeine and its effects on fertility and other reproductive issues. Low birth weight and birth defects don't seem to be related to caffeine consumption. On the other hand, caffeine intake may be linked to infertility and miscarriage. Common sense says to avoid caffeine or limit your intake to one serving per day.

▶ Take a multivitamin supplement containing 400 micrograms of folic acid and no more than 100 percent of the RDA of other nutrients...

...recommends the March of Dimes. The main reason is to prevent neural tube defects such as spina bifida. Some evidence shows that vitamin supplementation may also prevent other birth defects, such as heart and limb defects and oral cleft problems. On the other hand, avoid taking supplements of individual vitamins, especially vitamin A; as mentioned earlier, extreme doses of certain vitamins may produce unwanted results.

▶ Reduce stress or learn how to cope with it effectively.

Extreme stress is thought to affect fertility. However, stress is hard to measure because people perceive it differently. Exercise is a good stress reliever.

▶ Avoid exposure to high temperatures.

Sperm production is reduced in men who weld inside storage tanks, who drive a truck and literally sit on a hot seat for hours, and who regularly sit in a hot tub. Tight briefs or pants can also reduce sperm production. However, most experts believe that to have a real effect on fertility, a man's exposure to high temperatures would have to be continuous over a long period of time.[33]

Also, a woman who takes long hot baths or sits in a hot tub or sauna can actually damage her embryo's nervous system during the first thirty days after conception.

▶ Analyze your workplace for reproductive hazards.

Many occupations use chemicals or energy that is dangerous to unborn children. Much controversy surrounded a lawsuit that addressed removing women from jobs involving exposure to lead because of the reproductive hazard. However, your baby or your ability to become pregnant could be affected by what you and your partner are exposed to at work (and in other places, too). One study showed that the wives of men exposed to ethylene oxide, rubber chemicals, solvents used in refineries, and solvents used in the manufacturing of rubber products had increased risk of miscarriage.[34] Other known hazards include exposure to radiation, lead, solvents, paints, anesthetic gases, glues, copper, arsenic, cadmium, solder fumes, polyvinyl chloride, aerosol sprays, and dyes.[35]

Employers are required to provide a Material Safety Data Sheet (MSDS) for any hazardous material used in the workplace.

Read the MSDS to make sure you are not exposed to any materials that would pose reproductive hazards. For more information, contact the National Institute for Occupational Safety and Health (NIOSH) at 800-35-NIOSH or www.cdc.gov/niosh. NIOSH produces a brochure titled *Workplace Hazards for Female Reproductive Health* (DHHS [NIOSH] publication #99-104) and one titled *Workplace Hazards for Male Reproductive Health* (DHHS [NIOSH] publication #96-132). These publications can also be found on-line. For information on the safety of art materials, request a brochure titled *Safety Alert on Art Materials* from the Consumer Product Safety Commission (CPSC), Washington, DC 20207, 800-638-CPSC.

▶ **Be safe at the plate.**

Food safety is essential for the health of the unborn fetus. For example, a food-borne illness caused by the organism *Listeria monocytogenes* can cause miscarriage or stillbirth. Listeriosis has been associated with eating soft white cheeses, prepared meats, hot dogs, and unpasteurized milk. Toxoplasmosis is a parasitic infection that can cause mental retardation and blindness. It has been found in uncooked and undercooked meat, unwashed fruits and vegetables, and cat feces.[36] For more information on food safety, see page 210.

▼

Focus on Folate

Folate, also called folic acid or folacin, is a B vitamin that is very important during pregnancy; it plays a critical role in making new cells and in making hemoglobin in red blood cells. Folacin is water-soluble and can be destroyed by cooking, so when you cook vegetables, cook in as little water as possible for as short a time as possible.

People who may need more folacin in their diet are those who have been on such medications as anticonvulsants and some birth control pills. The U.S. Public Health Service now recommends that all women of childbearing age who are capable of becoming pregnant should consume 400 micrograms of folic acid per day.[37] If you have had a child with a neural tube defect, you will need to take a much higher dose—check with your health-care provider.

? Questions You May Have

Q: I drink about 4 cups of coffee every day. Any advice on cutting down?

A: Caffeine is a stimulant, and as most people know, it is habit-forming. In addition, caffeine is a diuretic: It causes your body to lose fluid, and during pregnancy your need for fluid increases. Substances found in coffee and tea also interfere with the absorption of iron. All of the above are good

Best Sources of Folate

The DRI* for folate is 400 micrograms during pregnancy; 500 micrograms for breastfeeding.

Food	Serving Sizes	Folate (micrograms†)
Lentils	1 cup	358
Sunflower seeds	1 cup	317
Pinto beans	1 cup	294
Asparagus	1 cup	262
Navy beans	1 cup	255
Spinach, frozen, drained	1 cup	204
Sunflower seeds, roasted	3 ounces	201
Soybean nuts, roasted	½ cup	181
Turnip greens, fresh	1 cup	171
Black beans, canned	1 cup	158
Artichoke	1	153
Hummus	1 cup	146
Split peas	1 cup	127
Black-eyed peas, canned	1 cup	123
Pistachios or peanuts, dry roasted	3 ounces	123
Baked beans, homemade	1 cup	122
Papaya	1 medium	116
Avacado, California	1 meduim	113
Orange juice, from concentrate	1 cup	109
Broccoli, frozen	1 cup	104
Peas, frozen	1 cup	94
Tempeh	1 cup	86
Boysenberries, frozen	1 cup	84
Romaine lettuce, shredded	1 cup	76
Creamed corn	1 cup	74
Beets, canned Harvard	1 cup	73
Arby's Ham and Cheese Sandwich	1	71
Trail mix	3 ounces	60
Wakame (seaweed), raw	1 ounce	55
Kombu (seaweed), raw	1 ounce	51
Vegetable juice	1 cup	51
Blackberries, frozen	1 cup	49
Refried beans, canned	1 cup	28

*Formerly known as RDA

†Numbers are rounded to nearest whole number; numbers are for cooked foods, as applicable.

Sources: Pennington, J. *Bowes and Church's Food Values of Portions Commonly Used*, 17th edition. Philadelphia: Lippincott Williams and Wilkins, 1998.

U.S. Department of Agriculture. USDA Nutrient Database for Standard Reference, Release 13, 1999.

reasons for reducing coffee, caffeinated soda, and tea intake. Cut down gradually to avoid such side effects as headaches. You may want to substitute low-caffeine drinks such as "half the caffeine" coffee, decaffeinated tea or coffee, or hot cocoa.

Q: Help! I'm a junk-food junkie! I eat fast food every day and actually crave it. How can I improve my diet?

A: Fast food can fit into a balanced diet if done right. However, if you eat fast food often (and you're not making healthy choices), you are likely to have decreased intakes of vitamin A, vitamin B$_6$, vitamin C, and calcium, which are all important nutrients during pregnancy.[38] The other problem is that most restaurant meals are higher in fat and calories than those eaten at home.

Try switching to healthier choices, such as bean burritos, grilled chicken sandwiches, or salads with low-fat meats. Add a salad bar or side salad with lots of fruits and vegetables, drink low-fat or skim milk with your meal, and bring along a fruit for dessert. Be sure to eat more fruits, vegetables, and whole grains at other meals to reach your totals. (See page 250 for more information and suggested menus from fast-food restaurants.)

Q: I've been taking birth control pills for five years. Is there anything special I should do before I become pregnant?

A: Physicians usually recommend that you have at least two periods off the pill to make sure your hormone levels are back to normal. However, the American College of Obstetricians and Gynecologists no longer has a recommendation regarding this. They state, "Using birth control pills before you become pregnant does not cause birth defects, no matter how close to conception you stop using them."[39] However, your periods may be irregular at first, which makes it difficult to determine your fertile times or to calculate your due date when you become pregnant. If you had painful or heavy periods before you started taking the pill, you may experience those types of menstrual cycles again.

Nutritionally, you should make sure your diet is better than average, since any medication taken over a long period of time can affect your nutritional status. Oral contraceptives can increase your need for B vitamins, including folic acid, so be sure to take a multivitamin/mineral supplement containing folic acid.

Q: I am diabetic and always thought trying to have a baby would be dangerous, but I hear things are different now.

A: You're right! The important thing is for your diabetes to be under control before you get pregnant, because high blood sugar could cause birth defects in the first few weeks of pregnancy. Also, during pregnancy your insulin needs will change often, and you will need close monitoring. Visit your primary physician and talk about your plan.

Your physician will probably refer you to an obstetrician who specializes in taking care of diabetic moms. You may also want to see an eye doctor. (See page 108 for more advice for diabetic moms-to-be.)

Q: I'm thirty-eight, and my biological clock just went off. Anything I can do before pregnancy to ensure the health of my baby?

A: Visit your health-care provider to get a checkup and a clean bill of health. Older women who are in good health and who receive early and regular prenatal care can have perfectly healthy babies. Preparing for your pregnancy and establishing good lifestyle habits can start your baby out right. However, older moms do face increased risks during pregnancy. This is mostly because as women get older, conditions such as diabetes and high blood pressure are more common. (See page 144 for more information.)

Q: Before I realized I was pregnant, I drank too much at a party. What should I do?

A: Your situation is not uncommon; many pregnancies are a surprise. The best thing to do is stay calm. Start following all the advice above and don't think about what you've done in the past. Discuss your concerns with your health-care provider, who will help you put them in perspective.

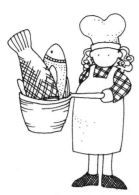

CHAPTER TWO

The Knowledgeable Pregnancy

What Every Woman Needs to Know

What you will find in this chapter:

• *Ten Steps to a Healthy Diet*
• *Everything You Ever Wanted to Know about Weight Gain during Pregnancy*
• *All about Fat*
• *Changing Your Mindset for Pregnancy*
• *The Essential Guide to Vitamins and Minerals*
• *Vitamin Supplements: You May Need Them*
• *Keeping Your Baby's Environment Safe*
• *Traveling during Pregnancy*
• *The Positives of Pregnancy*

This chapter answers such questions as:

• *Should I take a vitamin supplement?*
• *What if I'm not gaining enough weight?*
• *How often should I weigh?*
• *How much caffeine is okay during pregnancy?*
• *How can I reduce my exposure to lead?*
• *Should I take individual vitamin supplements?*
• *How much caffeine is in hot chocolate?*

So you're pregnant—or planning to be. Congratulations! You are about to begin the most exhilarating, exhausting, challenging, and special time of your life. No doubt you will find yourself daydreaming in the months to come: "What will my baby look like? How will I be as a first-time (or second- or third-time) mom? What will my baby grow up to do—discover the cure for cancer or become President?" And your thoughts will inevitably drift back to one important question: "Will my baby be healthy?"

Fortunately, the answer to that question depends mostly on you. Although genetics and pure chance can affect your baby's health, taking good care of yourself gives your baby the best possible odds of being born healthy.

If you are just considering pregnancy, you are one step ahead of the game and have time to get your body and personal habits into great shape. (See Chapter One: Contemplating Pregnancy.) Prepregnancy counseling is a popular buzzword among hopeful moms-to-be, and with good reason. Prepregnancy counseling allows your health-care provider to give you important advice on eating, exercise, alcohol, and so on. If you are diabetic or have another medical condition, counseling is an especially good idea.

As a pregnant or soon-to-be-pregnant woman, you have a unique opportunity to make your health the best it can be. The good habits you start now can be with you and your family for life! In fact, exciting research shows that your diet and nutritional status before and during pregnancy and your baby's birth weight can have an effect on your baby's risk of chronic diseases like diabetes, high blood pressure, and cardiovascular disease. Apparently, a poor diet before and during pregnancy leads to lower birth weight and so "programs" your baby to have health problems as an adult. (See Chapter One for more specifics.)

Good nutrition is not something you should worry about only during pregnancy. I've seen many a fifty-year-old who needed to change his or her eating habits to lose weight, reduce blood sugar, or lower cholesterol. But it's tough to teach an old dog new tricks. If your children learn good eating habits from the start, they will never have to worry about changing them!

▼

Ten Steps to a Healthy Diet

Because so much conflicting advice is available on nutrition today, I've put together ten easy eating tips to follow, now and after your pregnancy.

1. *Variety provides good balance.* We all know people who eat a tuna sandwich and an apple for lunch day in and day out. What's missing is variety. Variety not only is the spice of life, it also helps provide the right balance of nutrients, vitamins, and minerals you need. Not that a tuna sandwich is a bad lunch. But just think of all the other foods and nutrients you'd miss if you ate one for lunch every day! Variety and balance are especially important during pregnancy to

ensure that you don't get too much of certain vitamins or additives and that you get the right mix of vitamins and minerals for your baby's growth and development.

2. *Moderation is the key* to an enjoyable life, and it's also the key to good health. In a survey of fourth- to eighth-graders, 85 percent of the students said that you should avoid all high-fat foods, and 77 percent thought that you should never eat foods that have a lot of sugar.[1] Wrong! There is no food that you should *never* eat, unless you are a diabetic who must strictly control your blood sugar. (The occasional sweet is probably okay, but you should discuss this with your health-care provider or diabetes educator first.) For most people, high-fat and high-sugar foods are harmless in small amounts.

3. *Follow the Food Guide Pyramid.* This is a wonderful visual representation of how our diet should be built. Below is a food pyramid designed especially for pregnancy. Start with

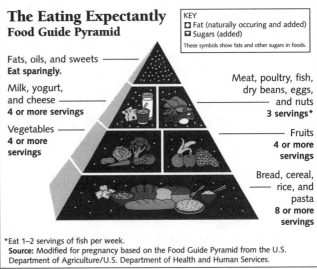

The Eating Expectantly Food Guide Pyramid

KEY
☐ Fat (naturally occuring and added)
☑ Sugars (added)
These symbols show fats and other sugars in foods.

Fats, oils, and sweets — **Eat sparingly.**

Milk, yogurt, and cheese — **4 or more servings**

Vegetables — **4 or more servings**

Meat, poultry, fish, dry beans, eggs, and nuts — **3 servings***

Fruits — **4 or more servings**

Bread, cereal, rice, and pasta — **8 or more servings**

*Eat 1–2 servings of fish per week.
Source: Modified for pregnancy based on the Food Guide Pyramid from the U.S. Department of Agriculture/U.S. Department of Health and Human Services.

a base of whole grains and cereals and add fruits, vegetables, protein, milk, and tiny amounts of sugar and fat. If your grocery cart doesn't reflect the food pyramid, you should reconsider your shopping list.

4. *Bone up on calcium.* Calcium has never been more important in the diet. In fact, a National Institutes of Health panel recommended calcium intakes above the Dietary Reference Intakes (DRI) for all age and sex groups. During pregnancy, supplemental calcium has been shown to lower blood pressure and reduce the risk of preeclampsia (a form of hypertension occurring in pregnancy).[2] But even after pregnancy, you should try to have two or three servings of calcium-rich food every day (more if you're breast-feeding). Research on calcium is promising–higher calcium intake is linked to lower blood pressure and is also related to a lower risk of colon cancer.[3]

Of course, calcium is well known for building bones to their maximum strength and keeping them that way, thus helping to prevent osteoporosis. You start losing bone mass in your thirties, so be sure to consume adequate calcium either in your diet or in supplements throughout your lifetime.

5. *Don't skimp on iron.* Getting enough iron in your diet may be a real challenge: Women need more iron than men, yet we generally eat much fewer calories. Factor in nutritionally unbalanced diets and too many meals eaten on the run, and the result is often iron-deficiency anemia. One study showed that anemia during early pregnancy results in a three-times-higher risk of delivering a low-birth-weight baby and a double risk of having a premature infant.[4] (See page 33 to learn more about the importance of iron.)

6. *Go for whole grains.* Three are key. Women often shy away from foods like bread, pasta, and corn, which are seen as fattening. But, because of their nutritional punch, such foods should be the foundation of every meal. They provide energy, fiber, vitamins, and minerals. Recent research links eating more fiber from whole grains with reduced risk of fatal colon cancer, breast cancer, and endometrial cancer. Examples of whole grains are whole-grain (such as whole-wheat) breads and cereals, brown rice, and whole-grain pastas.[5]

Whole grains also contain trace minerals that are important for chronic disease prevention, but are in short supply in the American diet. Some of these minerals are chromium, selenium, zinc, copper, manganese, and magnesium.

7. *Don't forget the exercise.* We've become a nation of couch potatoes, and as the saying goes: Couch potatoes have tater tots! This is changing as people realize the many benefits of exercise: stress reduction, improved endurance, lowered resting heart rate, blood pressure control, cardiovascular efficiency, improved self-esteem and body image, better sleep habits, and lowered risk of heart attack, stroke, diabetes, and even some types of cancer. During pregnancy, staying limber can ease aches and pains, help reduce fatigue, and get you ready for the "mother's marathon"–labor and delivery. However, you should take care to exercise appropriately

during pregnancy. (See Chapter Ten: Fitting Fitness In.)

8. *Get your fill of fluids.* The human body is composed of about 60 percent water, so drinking plenty of water is common sense. Thirst is the first sign of dehydration, but it lags behind actual need. By the time you feel thirsty, you are already behind in your fluid intake. Eight to ten glasses per day are recommended during pregnancy. With your increased blood supply, amniotic fluid, and extra tissue to support, the more fluids you have, the better. You can drink fluid in the form of juice and decaffeinated tea and soda, but try to drink most of it as clear, clean water.

9. *Focus on fiber.* The National Cancer Institute recommends consuming 20 to 35 grams of fiber per day,[6] but most of us don't get enough. During pregnancy, you'll find yourself trying to eat more high-fiber foods to combat constipation. Adequate fiber in the diet may reduce risk of colon cancer and breast cancer, and during pregnancy fiber can prevent constipation and hemorrhoids. (See page 53 for more fiber facts.)

10. *Take it easy on the extras.* As mentioned before, no food should be totally off-limits. However, you can easily go overboard with fat, sugar, and even artificial sweeteners if you let your taste buds rule. You should eat extras like candy, junk food, and ice cream as treats only after you have eaten all the "must" foods. With all the extra nutrients you need during pregnancy, you can't afford to eat many empty-calorie foods.

Everything You Ever Wanted to Know about Weight Gain during Pregnancy

Putting on pounds may be a woman's nightmare, but during pregnancy the amount of weight you gain and how you gain it may make the difference between a healthy, full-term baby and one that is born small and premature.

A review of thirteen studies shows that inadequate weight gain and a low rate of weight gain in the latter part of pregnancy are both associated with preterm delivery.[7] Happily watching yourself gain weight may be tough, but try to get used to it.

Suggested Weight Gain	
Prepregnancy Weight	**Suggested Weight Gain**
Underweight (10% below ideal body weight)	28–40 pounds
Normal weight (Average weight for height)	25–35 pounds
Overweight (20% or more over ideal body weight)	15–25 pounds

Teens and African-American women should strive for gains at the upper end of the range. Women under 5'3" should gain an amount of weight at the lower end of the range.

Source: *Nutrition during Pregnancy: Part I, Weight Gain; Part II, Nutrient Supplements,* Subcommittee on Nutritional Status and Weight Gain during Pregnancy, National Academy of Sciences.

Where the Weight Goes	
Tissue	**Pounds**
Breast	1–2
Placenta	1½
Enlarged uterus	2
Increased blood and fluids	8½
Baby	7½
Fat stores	4–14
Total gained	**25–35**

Where the Weight Goes

You have probably seen a life-size picture of a fetus no bigger than a spoon that weighs less than an ounce. So why have you gained 5 pounds? Since the average birth weight is about 7 pounds and the average weight gain is 30 pounds, pregnancy weight gain is obviously more than just baby. During pregnancy your blood supply increases, your breasts and uterus enlarge, you acquire miscellaneous extra fluids, and–you guessed it– you put on FAT! The fat provides additional calories for breastfeeding. During pregnancy, your body also builds additional muscle to carry the extra weight. The chart above shows where your weight goes.

Weight gain recommendations have changed dramatically over the years. Once, pregnant women were told to gain as little weight as possible and were sometimes reprimanded for gaining weight! Now we know that good nutrition and a specific pattern of weight gain are the keys to having healthier babies.

According to University of California-Berkeley nutritional epidemiologist Barbara Abrams, coauthor of a large study that looked at weight gain in pregnant women, "Our study shows that maternal weight gain is an important factor in pregnancy outcome, especially the baby's birth weight. Since low birth weight is the major cause of infant mortality and mental and physical disability, it can be dangerous to restrict a pregnant woman's weight gains."[8]

The recommended weight gain for the average woman is 25 to 35 pounds, but many don't fit the average mold. The amount of weight you should gain depends on your weight before you were pregnant and on whether you are having twins or more. (See

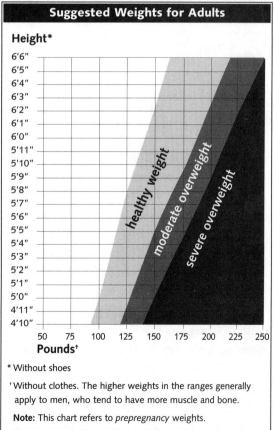

Suggested Weights for Adults

Height*

6'6" 6'5" 6'4" 6'3" 6'2" 6'1" 6'0" 5'11" 5'10" 5'9" 5'8" 5'7" 5'6" 5'5" 5'4" 5'3" 5'2" 5'1" 5'0" 4'11" 4'10"

healthy weight *moderate overweight* *severe overweight*

50 75 100 125 150 175 200 225 250

Pounds†

* Without shoes

† Without clothes. The higher weights in the ranges generally apply to men, who tend to have more muscle and bone.

Note: This chart refers to *prepregnancy* weights.

Source: *Report of the Dietary Guidelines Advisory Committee on the Dietary Guidelines for Americans,* 1995, pages 23–24.

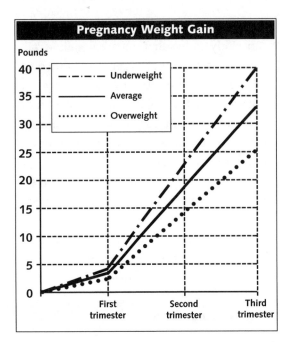

Pregnancy Weight Gain

Pounds

- — · — · — Underweight
- ———— Average
- ·············· Overweight

| 40 | 35 | 30 | 25 | 20 | 15 | 10 | 5 | 0 |

First trimester · Second trimester · Third trimester

page 133 for information on multiple births.) Refer to the chart above to see how much you should gain.

What's "Ideal Weight"?

Ideal weight has different definitions. Some health professionals use insurance weight charts, some use the "rule of five," and others use the Suggested Weights for Adults from the U.S. Department of Agriculture and U.S. Department of Health and Human Services. You could also define ideal body weight as the weight at which you feel best.

To use the "rule of five"(for women), start with 100 pounds for 5 feet of height. Add 5 pounds for every inch over 5 feet you are. Keep in mind a 10 percent variance to account for body build and so on.

Monitoring Your Weight Gain

Remember that your *pattern* of weight gain is just as important as the *amount* of weight you gain. Your weight gain should be gradual and should roughly follow the Pregnancy Weight Gain chart at left. You should gain approximately 2 to 4 pounds during the first trimester and close to a pound per week during the second and third trimesters, when the baby grows the most. If your goal is more or less than average, adapt these numbers accordingly.

If you are eating healthy foods with just a few splurges, your weight gain will follow the right pattern for you. Remember that women have fluctuating weights, which vary even more during pregnancy. A few tips for weighing yourself are listed below.

▶ **Always weigh yourself at the same time of day and under the same conditions.**

For example, you might weigh yourself first thing in the morning after you use the restroom, wearing the same nightgown.

▶ **Weigh yourself weekly, not daily.**

Weighing yourself daily could drive you nuts! Since your weight depends on what you've had to eat and drink, the amount of sodium you've consumed, and your bowel habits, you could show a 3-pound "weight gain" on Monday and a 4-pound "weight loss" on Wednesday.

▶ **Compare only weights from the same scale.**

If your health-care provider's scale shows a 4-pound weight gain compared to your home scale, don't panic! Scales are often different, so compare only weights from the same scale.

Gaining Too Fast or Too Much

Most women fear gaining too much, because they think the weight will be difficult to take off. Also, gaining too much weight can cause excessive infant size and increased risk of a cesarean section. Regardless of how much you gain, pregnancy is never the time to try to lose weight. If you have reached your goal of a 30-pound weight gain by week thirty-five, don't think you should not gain any more for the remaining five weeks!

Here are several explanations for gaining too much weight or gaining weight too fast:

- You may be overeating or eating too many high-fat, high-calorie foods. Are you trying to eat for two? See the quiz below to evaluate the extras in your diet.
- You may be carrying multiple fetuses. If you don't feel that your weight gain is related to eating, consult your health-care provider about the possibility of multiple births.
- Inaccurate weighing or weighing after eating or drinking. (Weighing after drinking a quart of water, for example, will add 2 pounds to your weight!)
- Preeclampsia/high blood pressure. If you gain 3 or more pounds per week in the second or third trimester of pregnancy, and you also experience swelling of feet and/or hands, severe headaches, or vision problems, contact your health-care provider immediately! These could be the first signs of preeclampsia, a potentially serious problem. (See page 128 for more information.)

Will You Gain Too Much Weight?

1. Do you eat sweets four times a week or more?
2. Do you snack on foods like chips, nuts, nachos, or French fries four times a week or more?
3. Do you use a lot of margarine, salad dressing, sour cream, or cheese?
4. When you cook, do you pour more than 1 teaspoon of oil per serving into the pan?
5. Do you regularly eat the skin on chicken, fat on steak, and so on?
6. Do you eat typical fast food or fried food more than once a week?
7. Do you often eat when you're bored, depressed, angry, or happy—but not hungry?
8. Do you usually eat while doing something else, such as reading or watching TV?
9. Do you eat snacks like regular ice cream and regular cheese?

If you answered "yes" to three or more of the above questions, you have a good chance of gaining too much weight (or too much fat) during your pregnancy. Keeping an eye on fat intake will help you now—and later, when you are trying to lose your "baby fat."

How to Avoid Gaining Too Much Weight

Now that the recommended weight gain is higher than it was a few years ago, you will definitely look pregnant! However, three factors control your weight gain and how it looks on you: your genes, your activity level, and your diet.

The distribution of pregnancy weight varies among women. You will hear myths about your weight gain. Some people will tell you that if you're having a boy, the weight will be all in your abdomen. And if your weight gain is spread out all over, many will predict a girl. The truth is, your genes control where the weight goes.

If you start a low-impact exercise program approved by your health-care provider (such as swimming or walking) or continue an established exercise program, you will be well toned and will look and feel better. Being in good overall physical shape will help you feel good about your expanding waistline. Having more lean muscle tissue will also help you lose weight after you have your baby.

One mother of two says: "I lost all my weight within a few months after having Brian. I swam regularly right up to delivery. However, with Emily, I was very sick with bronchitis the last six weeks of pregnancy and spent a lot of time in bed. Overall, I was much less active when I was pregnant with Emily, and it took me much longer to take the weight off after Emily was born."

Of course, your diet may need critical analysis. If you follow the Eating Expectantly Eating Plan (see Chapter Three), you shouldn't have any problem with excess weight gain. The quiz on page 23 may shed some light on your eating habits.

Not Gaining Enough

There are as many reasons for not gaining enough weight as there are for gaining too much. Though not gaining enough weight may seem like a blessing, the lack can cause major problems for your baby. Women who don't gain enough are more likely to deliver premature babies, and their babies are likely to be smaller. Newborn death is more related to prematurity and low birth weight than to any other cause.[9] So, if you are having problems gaining enough weight, be sure to find the reason below and do something about it.

- You have fast metabolism. Women who were underweight before pregnancy may simply burn calories more quickly. You may need help from a registered dietitian, who can closely analyze your diet for ways to increase calories.
- You can't eat much because of nausea, heartburn, stress, or other problems. First, you need to get to the root of the problem. Nausea usually goes away after the first trimester. The other problems may have simple solutions. Psychosocial stress has been known to decrease weight gain, and you may need help from a counselor or social worker. Ask your health-care provider for assistance.
- You go a mile a minute. Some moms-to-be have very active lifestyles and don't slow down for pregnancy. This could result in burning too many calories or not taking the time to eat enough. Either

scenario leaves fewer calories for baby to grow on. If your lifestyle is interfering with your weight gain, you may need to look at reducing your activities or exercise and/or increasing your calories.

• Psychological factors are interfering. If you have ever had a weight problem or an eating disorder, you might find gaining weight psychologically difficult. Your overall psychosocial well-being may also have an effect on your weight status. Depression, anxiety, low self-esteem, and lack of social support may all affect your weight gain.[10] You may need help from your health-care provider or a psychotherapist.

• You smoke. Smoking is associated with reduced weight gain, sudden infant death syndrome (SIDS), fetal death, and placenta previa (an abnormal placement of the placenta that may cause complications during delivery).[11] Do your best to quit or cut down.

What to Do If You Aren't Gaining Enough Weight

▶ **Make sure your diet is similar to the Eating Expectantly Eating Plan on page 55.**

▶ **Slow down!**

▶ **Increase the amount of food you eat.**

If you are having trouble eating more, increase fat intake–the easiest way to increase calories without increasing bulk. To increase fat intake, the best foods to add are those rich in unsaturated fats, such as vegetable oils, salad dressings, wheat germ, nuts, seeds, avocado, peanut butter, and margarine with liquid oil or water as the first ingredient.

▶ **Don't forget the snacks.**

If you're eating only three meals a day, you're probably not eating enough. Most pregnant women need a few additional snacks to fit in all the nutrients and calories they need. (See page 263 for snack ideas for high-energy moms.)

▶ **Increase what I call "healthy splurges" —foods that have some nutritive value, but have extra calories, too— such as milk shakes, frozen yogurt, breads made with fruits or vegetables (like banana bread or zucchini bread), sweet potato or pumpkin pie, pudding, and egg custard.**

To add calories, you may also want to add a food supplement such as Carnation Instant Breakfast to your milk.

All about Fat

Watching the types and amounts of fat you eat is important–for the short and long term–for several reasons:

• Ounce per ounce, fat has more than twice as many calories as carbohydrate or protein.

• Some types of fat are absolutely essential for humans because the body cannot make them. Eicosapenaenoic acid (EPA) and docosahexanenoic acid (DHA), two omega-3 oils found in fish, are important for the building of fetal brain tissue (which is 60 percent fat) and eye tissue. The body can convert alpha-linolenic acid found in polyunsaturated vegetable oils into EPA and DHA, but not very efficiently. Sources of alpha-linolenic acid include flaxseed and linseed oil, canola oil, soybean oil and soy products, walnut oil and walnuts, and wheat germ oil.

Another essential fat that can't be made in your body is linoleic acid (omega-6). All vegetable oils contain linoleic acid, but safflower oil is richest. Most people's diets contain too much omega-6 and not enough omega-3. Omega-6 and omega-3 oils form biologically active compounds that affect body functions such as blood pressure, blood clotting, and immune response, so the right balance could make a profound difference in overall health. To get enough of these essential fats in your diet, try to have a balance of oils rich in omega-6 and omega-3. Eating fish (especially fatty fish) a few times per week can help ensure adequate omega-3 intake. (See page 223 for "The Facts on Fish.")

- Fat calories are stored easier than calories from other sources. The more fat you eat, the more fat you wear.
- A high-fat intake is implicated in heart disease and certain types of cancer, especially breast, prostate, and colon cancer.[12]
- A high-fat diet from eating fried foods can aggravate the nausea of early pregnancy and heartburn later in pregnancy.

- Types of fat called trans-fatty acids (also called trans fat) are made when liquid oils are hydrogenated for storage or cooking—for example, when oil is made into shortening or stick margarine. These types of fat appear worse than saturated fat regarding heart disease and may have widespread implications for other diseases. Research also shows that trans fat gets into the fetal bloodstream in proportion to the mother's consumption; trans fat could restrict birth weight.[13] Trans fat is mostly found in margarine, shortening, and products made from these, such as bakery goods, commercially fried foods, and snack foods. You may want to avoid margarine or use as little as possible and keep processed, high-fat foods to a minimum. Look at the label of several margarines and choose a tub product that has liquid oil as the first ingredient. Currently, the amount of trans fat is not listed on food labels. It has been proposed that the amount of trans fat per serving be added to the amount of saturated fat per serving, so that the resulting amount and percent of Daily Value (%DV) per serving on Nutrition Facts panels will be based on the sum of both types of fat.

Most health organizations recommend that we eat 30 percent or less of our calories from fat. A specific guideline for pregnancy hasn't been established, but somewhere around 30 percent fat is a prudent recommendation. Sonja Connor, M.S., R.D., research associate professor in the Department of Medicine at Oregon Health Science Center, says that a case can be made for watching fat intake during pregnancy, but she cautions intake below 20 percent, saying, "You may have trouble gaining weight and not laying down the fat you need to support lactation." If you are having difficulty gaining weight, you may need to increase your fat intake, but try to get the extra fat from vegetable sources such as avocado, nuts, peanut butter, and vegetable oils.

The average pregnant woman needs 2,200 to 2,400 calories, and 30 percent of those calories would be about 70 to 90 grams of fat. This may sound like a lot. Are you savvy about fat? Look at the following diet and guess how much fat it contains.

How Much Fat?

Breakfast
  Cereal with 1 cup 2% milk
  2 slices toast with 2 teaspoons margarine
  Fresh fruit
Snack
  1 ounce cheese
  10 wheat crackers
Lunch
  Deluxe cheeseburger
  Fries
  Side salad with 2 tablespoons dressing
Snack
  2 tablespoons peanut butter on Melba toast
  1½ cups 2% milk

Dinner
  6 ounces fish sautéed in safflower oil
  Baked potato with 2 tablespoons sour cream and 2 teaspoons margarine
  Fresh, steamed spinach
  Tomatoes and cucumbers with 2 tablespoons vinaigrette dressing
Snack
  Ice cream
  Chocolate-chip cookie

Believe it or not, the above menu has 160 grams of fat, or double the amount recommended. Let's change a few things and see how the fat adds up in our modified menu.

Breakfast
  Cereal with 1 cup skim milk
  2 slices toast with 1 teaspoon margarine and 2 teaspoons fruit spread
  Banana
Snack
  1 ounce low-fat cheese
  8 wheat crackers
Lunch
  Grilled chicken sandwich
  Side salad with pasta salad and light vinaigrette dressing
  Peaches and pineapple
  1 cup 2% milk
Snack
  2 tablespoons peanut butter
  ½ bagel
  Vegetable juice
Dinner
  6 ounces fish baked with a crumb topping of Parmesan cheese and 1 teaspoon margarine
  Boiled new potatoes with 2 teaspoons margarine

Steamed fresh spinach
Melon balls
Skim milk
Snack
Frozen yogurt
Graham crackers

We've cut the fat in half with just a few changes! The menu now has under 80 grams of fat, a much better number. You can check the vitamin and mineral aspects of your diet by taking the nutrition quiz on page 64.

Changing Your Mindset for Pregnancy

Up to now you've been the perfect model of health. You don't eat eggs, you work out five times a week, and you haven't eaten red meat in years. Now you're craving a steak, don't feel like exercising (or doing much of anything, for that matter), and eggs seem to go down really well. What's a woman to do? First, let's set a few things straight.

The average American diet does contain too much protein, but eating lean red meat in moderation is fine. You just need to choose lean cuts like top round, eye of round, and flank steak. Red meat is rich in iron, and small amounts of red meat can help your body absorb iron from nonmeat sources. It is also a good source of zinc, an important nutrient during pregnancy.

Eggs are a great source of protein, and eating them in moderation is not a problem for most people. Even the American Heart Association allows three to four egg yolks a week in its Eating Plan for Healthy Americans.[14] Sometimes eggs are easier to get down, so don't feel guilty about eating extra eggs. Just take it easy on the bacon, sausage, biscuits, hash browns, cheese, and so on.

Your body is going through a tremendous amount of change (no kidding!), and not feeling quite as energetic as you used to is normal. You may also feel uncomfortable about the size or look of your "body with baby," which may make you squeamish about getting into an exercise outfit or swimsuit. Try to get some exercise, even if it's just walking around the neighborhood. Exercise will help maintain muscle tone and will make you feel good mentally and physically. (See Chapter Ten for more on exercise.) And remember that pregnancy doesn't last forever, even though sometimes it feels as if it might!

The Essential Guide to Vitamins and Minerals

The body needs many different nutrients every day. Every vitamin and mineral plays a small but important role in the making of a healthy baby.

New Terminology: Dietary Reference Intakes

Since 1943, the Recommended Daily Allowance (RDA) has been the standard for suggested nutrient intake. However, expanded knowledge about nutrient needs made it necessary for the Food and Nutrition Board to coin a new term, Dietary Reference Intake (DRI). Dietary Reference Intake is based on four different ways of estimating nutrient needs. If you'd like to learn more about the development of and rationale behind DRIs, visit the Food and Nutrition Board's website at www.nas.edu/iom/fnb.

The Energy-Releasing Nutrients

You have probably heard people say, "Vitamins give me more energy." Actually, vitamins have no calories, but you need them to be able to use the energy in your food. Because of this, the nutrients listed below are needed in amounts relative to the amount and type of food you eat.

Thiamin (Vitamin B₁)

DRI for pregnancy: 1.4 milligrams; for breastfeeding: 1.5 milligrams.

Functions: Releases energy from carbohydrate. Used in appetite and nervous-system function.

Sources: Brewer's yeast, enriched cereals and breads, pork, sunflower seeds, oatmeal, wheat germ, dried beans, and peas.

Note: Thiamin is unstable in heat and light. Vegetables high in thiamin and other water-soluble vitamins should be cooked minimally, with as little water as possible.

Riboflavin (Vitamin B₂)

DRI for pregnancy: 1.4 milligrams; for breastfeeding: 1.6 milligrams.

Functions: Helps release energy from all foods. Maintains normal vision and skin health.

Sources: Fortified cereals, milk, yogurt, and cheese.

Niacin (Vitamin B₃)

DRI for pregnancy: 1.8 milligrams; for breastfeeding: 1.7 milligrams.

Functions: Helps release energy from food. Supports health of skin, nervous system, and digestive system.

Sources: Fortified cereals, poultry, fish, meat, legumes, and nuts.

Pantothenic Acid

DRI for pregnancy: 6 milligrams; for breastfeeding: 7 milligrams.

Functions: Helps release energy from food. Involved in antibody production.

Sources: Widespread in many foods. Salmon, trout, and avocado are good sources.

Biotin

DRI for pregnancy: 30 micrograms; for breastfeeding: 35 micrograms.

Functions: Helps release energy from food. Assists in fat synthesis and carbohydrate storage.

Sources: Widespread in many foods. Oatmeal, hazelnuts, and peanuts are good sources.

The Building Nutrients

These nutrients are responsible for helping build bone, muscle tissue, hormones, and other tissues.

Calcium

DRI for pregnancy and breastfeeding: 1,000 milligrams. The National Institutes of Health Consensus Conference on Optimal Calcium Intake recommends an intake of 1,200 to 1,500 milligrams of calcium daily for pregnant and nursing women.[15]

Functions: Principal ingredient in bones and teeth; vital in muscle contraction, nerve function, blood clotting, blood pressure, and immune defense. Research shows a possible relationship between adequate calcium in the diet and reduced risk of hypertension and colon cancer.[16] Adequate calcium over the lifespan protects against osteoporosis.

Sources: Milk and milk products, small fish with bones, blackstrap molasses, calcium-fortified tofu, broccoli, greens, legumes, some seaweed, and sea vegetables.

Choline

A DRI has been established recently for choline. DRI for pregnancy: 450 milligrams; for breastfeeding: 550 milligrams.

Functions: As a component of lecithin, choline is important in the structure of all cell membranes, lipoproteins, and pulmonary surfactant.

Sources: Eggs, soybeans, cauliflower, and lettuce.

Vitamin B$_{12}$ (Cobalamin)

DRI for pregnancy: 2.6 micrograms; for breastfeeding: 2.8 micrograms.

Functions: Helps in new red blood cell production; helps maintain health of nerve cells.

Sources: Muscle meats, fish, eggs, milk and milk products, and fortified foods.

Note: Only foods of animal origin and certain fortified foods contain Vitamin B$_{12}$. Check food labels to see whether B$_{12}$ is added. (See page 94 for more information.)

Phosphorus

DRI for pregnancy and breastfeeding: 700 milligrams.

Calcium and phosphorus make up three-fourths of the total weight of minerals found in the body. Unlike calcium, a deficiency of phosphorus is rare.

Functions: Used in building bones and teeth. Needed in every cell membrane, in genetic material, as part of energy production, and in the body's buffering system.

Sources: Primary sources of phosphorus in the American diet are animal protein and carbonated sodas.

Note: Excess phosphorus may draw calcium out of the body.

Magnesium

DRI for pregnancy: 350 milligrams; for breastfeeding: 310 milligrams.

Functions: Used in bone mineralization, protein building, enzyme action, muscle contraction, transmission of nerve impulses, and maintenance of teeth. Also helps in the regulation of blood sugar and insulin. Low intakes of magnesium have been implicated in increased risk of heart disease.

Sources: Nuts, legumes, whole grains, dark green vegetables, and seafood.

Vitamin A

DRI for pregnancy: 800 retinol equivalents; for breastfeeding, first six months: 1,300 retinol equivalents, for second six months: 1,200 retinol equivalents. One retinol equivalent is equal to 1 microgram of vitamin A or 6 micrograms of beta-carotene. The body converts beta-carotene into vitamin A.

Functions: Helps in cell growth and development and in formation of bones and teeth. Needed for healthy skin, mucous membranes, cornea of the eye, and reproductive health. Diets rich in beta-carotene, an antioxidant, have been shown to be related to decreased risk of heart disease and cancer.

Sources: Fortified milk, cheese, and eggs.

Warning: Excess vitamin A is very toxic to the fetus, so if you are taking an individual supplement of vitamin A, a high-potency multivitamin containing several times the DRI for vitamin A, or medication containing vitamin A (such as Retin-A), STOP IMMEDIATELY and consult your healthcare provider. Recent research shows that women who took a supplement of just four times the DRI for vitamin A were nearly five times more likely to have a baby with a birth defect.[17] You should also avoid all types of liver and fish liver oils while you are pregnant, because liver is a very concentrated source of vitamin A.

Beta-Carotene

The body converts beta-carotene to vitamin A as needed, so don't worry about consuming too much beta-carotene. However, people who have consumed large amounts of carrots or carrot juice have had their skin turn orange! The skin returns to normal after the person resumes a moderate diet.

Sources: Spinach and other dark leafy greens; broccoli; deep-orange fruits like apricots, peaches, and cantaloupe; and orange vegetables like squash, carrots, sweet potatoes, and pumpkin.

Vitamin K

DRI for pregnancy and breastfeeding: 65 micrograms.

Vitamin K is made in the digestive tract. Infants are given a dose at birth before their own vitamin K production starts.

Functions: Needed in the synthesis of blood-clotting proteins.

Sources: Seaweed (dulse and rockweed), green tea, soybean oil, turnip greens, and lettuce.

Vitamin D

DRI for pregnancy and breastfeeding: 5 micrograms or 400 International Units (IU).

Functions: Used in bone mineralization through control of calcium and phosphorus in the body.

Sources: Sunshine, fortified milk, fortified cereals, and egg yolks.

Note: The best source of vitamin D is sunlight! Your skin produces its own vitamin D when exposed to sufficient sunlight. Women who develop deficiencies generally avoid dairy products, have very dark skin, or usually protect their skin from the sun with clothes or sunscreen. Women who live in northern latitudes (such as Boston, Massachusetts) or possibly southern latitudes (such as Christchurch, New Zealand) are also at risk for vitamin D deficiency because those areas don't get sufficient sunshine in the winter.[18] If any of the above risk factors apply to you, you should eat more foods fortified with vitamin D, spend more time in the sun, or ask your health-care provider about taking a supplement. (Use caution in supplementing vitamin D on your own; it is toxic in large doses.)

Exposing your hands and face to sunshine ten to fifteen minutes per day, two to three times per week in the summer is enough to produce adequate vitamin D levels. (Sunscreen and air pollution can block vitamin D synthesis.) If you do not get this much unprotected exposure or you have dark skin, make sure you have a dietary source of vitamin D. The DRI for vitamin D can be obtained from 2 cups of milk.

Another good reason to make sure your body makes enough vitamin D: Studies show that reduced circulating vitamin D may lead to increased risk for breast, colon, and prostate cancer.[19]

Vitamin B_6 (Pyridoxine)

DRI for pregnancy: 1.9 milligrams; for breastfeeding: 2.0 milligrams.

Functions: Used in amino acid and fatty acid metabolism; helps make red blood cells. Vitamin B_6 is needed in amounts proportional to the amount of protein in the diet.

Sources: Green and leafy vegetables, meats, fish, poultry, shellfish, legumes, fruits, and whole grains.

Note: Women—pregnant or not—don't seem to have enough vitamin B_6 in their diets. Some women who take birth control pills may have a slightly increased need for vitamin B_6. Deficiency can cause anemia, irritability, and abnormal brain wave pattern.

Vitamin B_6 and Morning Sickness: Vitamin B_6 appears to be useful in treating morning sickness. However, large amounts of B_6 can be neurotoxic, so please discuss B_6 supplements with your health-care provider before self-prescribing.

Folate (Folacin, Folic Acid)

DRI for pregnancy: 600 micrograms; for breastfeeding: 500 micrograms.

Functions: Needed for all new cell production and use of amino acids. Also needed for some enzymes.

Sources: Spinach, leafy green vegetables, black-eyed peas, lentils, red kidney beans, broccoli, Brussels sprouts, beets, okra, green peas, asparagus, legumes, orange and grapefruit juice, and fortified cereals.

Note: The need for folacin more than doubles during pregnancy due to vast increases in the number of new cells being made. Folate can be easily destroyed in cooking. Certain medications, such as oral contraceptives, anticonvulsants, aspirin, chemotherapy drugs, and antacids, can affect your folate status. Alcohol and smoking can also increase the need for folate.[20] If you take any of the above medications, smoke, or drink regularly, or if you did just prior to pregnancy, your need for folate is probably greater than average. You will need to choose your diet more carefully and may want to discuss folacin supplementation with your health-care provider.

Folacin and Birth Defects: A landmark study done in several countries showed that folacin supplementation around the time of conception could prevent about 70 percent of recurrent neural tube defects. It is thought that folacin supplementation can also prevent first-time occurrences. The Institute of Medicine recommends that all women of childbearing potential consume 400 micrograms of folic acid per day from fortified foods or a supplement in addition to the folic acid found in a healthy diet. (An intake of 600 micrograms is recommended during pregnancy).[21]

Iron

DRI for pregnancy: 30 milligrams; for breastfeeding: 15 milligrams.

Functions: Plays a very important role in pregnancy. Part of the blood protein hemoglobin, which carries oxygen in the body. Part of muscle protein. Necessary for the use of energy in the body.

Sources: Clams, fortified cereals, tofu, lentils, eggs, chicken, legumes, and dried fruit.

Note: Iron-deficiency anemia is still a public health problem in the U. S. Pregnant women with iron-deficiency anemia are more likely to have a premature or low-birth-weight baby. In the 1985 Continuing Surveys of Food Intakes of Individuals (CSFII), only 4 percent of women met or exceeded the DRI for iron.[22]

Zinc

DRI for pregnancy: 15 milligrams; for breastfeeding, first six months: 19 milligrams, for second six months: 16 milligrams.

Functions: Promotes normal growth of tissues and bones; needed for the normal development of a fetus; involved in making genetic material, in immune reactions, in taste and smell, and in wound healing. Zinc is also required for sperm production.

Sources: Oysters, turkey, lean pork, wheat germ, whole grains, lima beans, and almonds.

Note: Zinc deficiency during pregnancy can cause low birth weight, increased pregnancy complications, and premature births. A zinc deficiency during fetal brain development could cause fetal brain injury.[23]

Vitamin C (Ascorbic Acid)

DRI for pregnancy: 70 milligrams; for breastfeeding, first six months: 95 milligrams; for second six months: 90 milligrams.

Functions: Needed for thyroid hormone, collagen synthesis, and production of amino acids. Strengthens resistance to infection, helps absorption of iron, and acts as an antioxidant, meaning it breaks down oxidants, or free radicals, which can be destructive to cell membranes.

Sources: Kiwi, mango, papaya, citrus fruits, melons, peppers, berries, leafy green vegetables, tomatoes, broccoli, cauliflower, and cabbage.

The Support Nutrients

These nutrients help all the other nutrients with their functions.

Vitamin E (Tocopherol)

DRI for pregnancy: 10 milligrams; for breastfeeding, first six months: 12 milligrams, for second six months: 11 milligrams (all based on alpha-tocopherol equivalents).

Functions: Strong antioxidant. Works together with other antioxidants, vitamin C, and beta-carotene. There is some evidence that vitamin E intake above the DRI may be associated with decreased risk of heart disease and certain cancers. Research continues. If you followed a low-fat diet or took cholesterol-lowering drugs before your pregnancy, your body may be partially depleted of vitamin E.

Sources: Wheat germ and wheat germ oil, sunflower oil, safflower oil, almond oil and almonds, hazelnuts, and mayonnaise and salad dressings made with the above oils.

Sodium

There is no DRI for sodium; estimated minimum requirement for pregnancy: 570 milligrams; for breastfeeding: 635 milligrams.

Functions: Maintains normal fluid balance. Needed for nerve impulse transmission.

Note: Historically, women lowered their salt and sodium intake during pregnancy to reduce water retention and sometimes to prevent preeclampsia. Now, moderation rather than restriction is the key for pregnant women.

Potassium

There is no DRI for potassium; estimated minimum requirement for pregnancy: 2,000 milligrams; for breastfeeding: 2,500 milligrams.

Functions: Maintains fluid balance and helps maintain normal blood pressure. Helps with nerve impulses and muscle contractions.

Sources: Bananas, oranges and orange juice, watermelon, cantaloupe, vegetables, meats, milk, grains, and legumes.

Note: A high potassium intake has been linked to a reduced incidence of high blood pressure in certain populations.[24] In the 1985 CSFII, women's potassium intakes were well below the estimated safe and adequate daily dietary intake.[25]

Other Trace Elements

Zinc and iron are considered trace elements, but they are so important during pregnancy that I included them in the section above. Other trace elements are copper, iodine, selenium, fluoride, manganese, chromium, and molybdenum. According to the Subcommittee on Dietary Intake and Nutrient Supplements, routine supplementation of trace elements (with the exception of iron) during pregnancy does not seem to be necessary.

Copper

The estimated DRI for adults is 1.5 to 3 milligrams.

Functions: Helps in red blood cell production; is found in nerve coverings and connective tissue. Also assists in energy production and in respiration. Copper deficiency during pregnancy is unknown.

Sources: Whole grains, shellfish, kidney, raisins, nuts, peas, and beans.

Iodine

DRI for pregnancy: 175 micrograms; for breastfeeding: 200 micrograms.

Functions: An essential component of the thyroid hormone thyroxine, which is responsible for regulating the basal metabolic rate (the amount of energy the body needs at rest). Iodine deficiency during pregnancy can cause fetal disorders such as stillbirth, birth defects, and neurological impairment. However, there is no evidence of iodine deficiency in the U.S.

Sources: Seafood, iodized salt, and food grown in ocean areas that contain iodine-rich soil.

Selenium

DRI for pregnancy: 65 micrograms; for breastfeeding: 75 micrograms.

Functions: As an antioxidant, selenium works to protect body compounds from oxidation. Research links selenium and other antioxidants with reduced cancer risk.

Sources: Seafood, meats, and grains.

Fluoride

The estimated safe and adequate daily dietary intake for adults is 1.5 to 4 milligrams.

Functions: Bonds calcium and phosphorus in bones and teeth; prevents cavities in teeth.

Sources: Water that naturally contains fluoride or water that has fluoride added. If you are not sure whether your water contains fluoride, you might want to have it tested.

"The bottom-line message: The emphasis on optimal diet is of the greatest importance to all women of the childbearing age at all times—not only when pregnancy has been confirmed."

– *Michael Hambidge, M.D., Sc.D., Director of the Center for Human Nutrition, University of Colorado Health Sciences Center*

Manganese

The estimated safe and adequate daily dietary intake for adults is 2 to 5 milligrams.

Functions: Part of enzymes that are active in many cell processes and a component of an important antioxidant.

Sources: Whole grains, beans, peas, and nuts.

Chromium

The estimated safe and adequate daily dietary intake for adults is 50 to 200 micrograms.

Functions: Associated with insulin; needed for the release of energy from glucose. Inability to use glucose results in diabetes-like deficiency symptoms. There is some concern that increased refinement of foods such as whole grains could lead to decreased intake of this trace mineral.

Sources: Whole grains, meat, mushrooms, asparagus, and brewer's yeast.

Molybdenum

The estimated safe and adequate daily dietary intake for adults is 75 to 250 micrograms.

Functions: A component of enzymes used in many body processes.

Sources: Legumes, cereals, and organ meats.

Nutrient Content of Protein Foods								
Food	Fat (grams)	Protein (% DRI)	Thiamin (% DRI)	Iron (% DRI)	Zinc (% DRI)	Vitamin B_6 (% DRI)	Vitamin B_{12} (% DRI)	Niacin (% DRI)
Beef top sirloin, fat trimmed off (3.5 ounces)	10	40	7	9	35	19	91	19
Beef arm chuck roast, trimmed to ⅛ inch fat (3.5 ounces)	19	40	3	9	40	13	98	15
Ground beef, extra lean (3.5 ounces)	13	40	3	8	36	14	83	28
Leg of lamb, lean (3.5 ounces)	6	40	6	6	28	8	88	30
Pork top loin, lean (3.5 ounces)	7	44	54	2	13	18	23	25
Chicken breast (3.5 ounces)	3	44	3	3	6	27	11	65
Salmon (3.5 ounces)	7	34	6	1	3	25	103	35
Tuna (3.5 ounces)	1	36	1	4	2	15	98	62
Shrimp (3.5 ounces)	1	29	1	9	9	6	48	12
Clams, steamed (3.5 ounces)	2	36	9	79	15	5	3200	16
Tofu, firm (3.5 ounces)	2	10	6	3	3	0.5	0	1
Pinto beans (1 cup)	1	23	22	15	12	14	0	4

Source: U.S. Department of Agriculture. USDA Nutrient Database for Standard Reference, Release 13, 1999.

Of Special Concern

Studies of pregnant women's diets have shown that intakes of folate, iron, calcium, zinc, magnesium, and vitamins B_6, D, and E were below the DRIs. Check the preceding pages to see if you have sources of these nutrients in your diet.

Selected Nutrients in Various Cuts of Meat

All animal proteins are not equal; they provide varying amounts of zinc, iron, and vitamins B_6 and B_{12}. The graph above shows why you should eat a variety of meats.

▼

Vitamin Supplements: You May Need Them

The general need for vitamin/mineral supplements has been debated for years, and so has their use during pregnancy.

Prenatal vitamins have been prescribed across the board for most pregnant women. However, a National Academy of Sciences subcommittee recommends in its report *Nutrition during Pregnancy* that prenatal vitamin supplements should be prescribed on an individual basis, based on each woman's current nutritional status.[26]

The reason for the concern is that large doses of certain nutrients—including iron, zinc, selenium, and vitamins A, B₆, C, and D—can be toxic to the fetus. Moreover, an increase in the amount of one nutrient may negatively affect how other nutrients are absorbed and used.[27]

Because of the evidence about folic acid and neural tube defects, several organizations have come out in favor of taking either a folic acid supplement or a multivitamin supplement containing folic acid before conception. For example, the March of Dimes Foundation recommends that all women capable of becoming pregnant take a daily multivitamin supplement that contains 400 micrograms of folic acid. The Institute of Medicine recommends women consume 400 micrograms of folic acid from fortified foods or a supplement in addition to the folic acid found in a healthy diet. A federal regulation mandates that any grain products calling themselves fortified must be fortified with folic acid.

Even if you eat fortified grains, you must still eat other foods containing folic acid to meet the recommended intake.

Since up to 60 percent of pregnancies in the U.S. may be unplanned, it makes sense to have the proper mix of nutrients in your body before conception to prevent birth defects.

If You Take Supplements

Here are some words of advice about taking vitamin supplements:

▶ **DO NOT TAKE INDIVIDUAL SUPPLEMENTS, except for calcium or vitamin C.**

Large amounts of certain vitamins can be toxic to the fetus, causing birth defects, or can create imbalances, with certain nutrients competing with other nutrients for absorption. Recent research shows that women who took more than 10,000 IU of vitamin A—just four times the DRI—had five times the risk of birth defects compared to women who consumed 5,000 IU or less.[28]

▶ **Three months before you are pregnant and during the first months of pregnancy, it is important to take a multivitamin/mineral supplement that contains 400 micrograms of folic acid and no more than 100 percent of the DRI for all nutrients. It may also be advisable for men to take a multivitamin/mineral supplement three months prior to conception.**

You can find this information on the label. When you confirm your pregnancy, your health-care provider will probably suggest that you take a prenatal vitamin. Remember that a vitamin/mineral supplement is no substitute for a healthy diet!

▶ **Remember that vitamin supplements are not the only sources of substantial amounts of vitamins.**

Fortified cereals such as Total also provide 100 percent of the DRI for many nutrients. If you were to take a multivitamin in addition to several servings of fortified food, you could potentially get too many vitamins, and the excess could be toxic.

▶ **If your health-care provider suggests a supplement that is nauseating you, consider taking the supplement with a light snack before you go to bed.**

Calcium Supplements

Calcium is vital during pregnancy for your baby's health and especially for your future bone health. Research also shows some correlation between increased calcium in the diet and reduced incidence of high blood pressure during pregnancy.[29]

Yet many women, both pregnant and not, do not have enough calcium in their diet. Women often start thinking about osteoporosis around the time of menopause, but they should actually consider their bone health all their lives. Bone continues to grow until age twenty-five and gradually starts losing mass after age thirty-five. (See page 68 for information on how to sneak calcium into your diet.)

Recent research shows another good reason to have enough calcium in your diet: As your bones lose calcium to make up for calcium missing from your diet, lead stored in your bones is released. You are exposed to small amounts of lead over a lifetime from drinking water and other sources, and it is stored in your bones. During times when bones lose calcium (during pregnancy and lactation and after menopause, in women), lead is released into the bloodstream.

Adequate dietary calcium is essential in preventing, or at least minimizing, the turnover of bone. If you have had substantial lead exposure (by living in a house with lead pipes or eating leaded paint chips as a child), adequate calcium is even more important to prevent lead poisoning of yourself and your unborn child.[30]

The National Institutes of Health recommend 1,200 to 1,500 milligrams of calcium per day for pregnant and breast-feeding women. They suggest you try to get your calcium from food first. If you can't, then take a supplement.

If you are currently taking a calcium or iron supplement, you should consider a few things about the way you take them:

Type of Calcium

Calcium is best absorbed from calcium citrate and calcium carbonate. Calcium carbonate is the most concentrated and economical form of calcium. Many women take Tums because it contains calcium carbonate. If you take too much calcium carbonate at one time, it can cause "rebound hyperacidity"–excess stomach acid. If this becomes a problem, consider taking the calcium supplement in several doses during the day, since it is absorbed better that way. Avoid oyster shell calcium and dolomite due to possible lead and heavy metal contamination.

What You Take with It

Calcium is best absorbed when taken with food; iron is best absorbed on an empty stomach. If you take an iron supplement along with calcium citrate or calcium phosphate on an empty stomach, the amount of iron you absorb may be decreased.[31]

The Solution

If you take both iron and calcium, take them at different times. Take your iron supplement on an empty stomach or with a light snack that does not include a dairy product. Take your calcium supplement with a light snack. Registered pharmacist Nellie Whaley suggests that if you take both calcium and iron, take the calcium at least two hours after or one hour before you take the iron.

Some women find that iron or prenatal vitamin supplements nauseate them. Taking supplements right before bedtime or with a snack usually helps. Whenever you decide to take your supplements, make it a ritual; calcium or iron left in the bottle won't bring you any benefit!

▼

Keeping Your Baby's Environment Safe

The "don'ts"—you knew they were coming. A physician who specializes in high-risk pregnancies once told me, "You have only one chance to give your baby what it needs. Why not do everything you can to help your baby along? It's only nine months." Giving advice is easy, but following it may not be so easy. If you are having problems with your health habits, talk to your health-care provider.

Smoking

The first trimester—and before pregnancy if possible—is a good time to kick some bad habits and pick up some good ones. Kiss your cigarettes good-bye, because babies of smokers weigh an average of ½ pound less

than those of nonsmokers. Research shows that quiting smoking is the single most important thing you can do to improve the growth and long-term health of your baby.

Other adverse affects of smoking while pregnant include higher risk of preterm delivery, early infant death, and possible problems with long-term growth, intellectual performance, and behavioral development. Babies of mothers who smoked during pregnancy were found to have a greater risk of obstructive sleep apnea, a disorder that causes infants to stop breathing while sleeping.[32] Smoking while you are pregnant may also affect your baby's neurological development.[33] Recent research has shown that the chemicals to which a fetus is exposed when a mother smokes can affect the brain in various ways. Girls are more likely to smoke and are five times more likely to be addicted to drugs in adolescence. Boys are more likely to have conduct disorders as adolescents and to be involved in criminal behavior as adults.[34] And after your baby is born, he or she will also suffer the ill effects of secondhand smoke: higher risk of lower respiratory infections, middle ear infections, sudden infant death syndrome, and asthma.[35]

Smokers may need extra nutrients, such as vitamins B_{12} and C, amino acids, folate, and zinc, so a multivitamin/mineral supplement may be necessary.[36]

Quitting smoking has many benefits—but it may be easier said than done. For help, call the Cancer Information Service at 800-4CANCER.

Lead Exposure

Although lead isn't something you consume consciously, you may receive a regular dose of it from your drinking water. According to the Environmental Protection Agency (EPA), as many as forty million people may have too much lead in their drinking water. Pregnant women and children run the highest risk of problems from lead exposure because of increased absorption. Lead exposure can cause increased rates of miscarriage and stillbirth and may lead to such long-term effects as learning disability, brain damage, hyperactivity, high blood pressure, and kidney disease.[37] You may have too much lead exposure if:

- Your home was built in the last five years. The use of copper pipes with lead solder is widespread. As time passes, mineral deposits form a coating on the inside of the pipes that insulates the water from the solder. But during the first five years (before the coating forms), water is in direct contact with the lead.
- Your home was built before 1930. These homes often used lead pipes instead of copper ones. Also, water companies installed lead pipes underground to bring water to homes built during the first part of the century.
- You have "soft" or acidic water. Soft or acidic water can strip away the mineral coating on water pipes and thus expose lead solder. Soft water is not dangerous if no lead was used either in your pipes or in the service pipes carrying water to your home.

- Your home has faucets or fittings made of brass, which contains some lead.

To be safe, you should have your water tested. To find a reliable laboratory, contact your local health department or call the EPA Safe Drinking Water Hotline. (See phone numbers on page 41.) Avoid do-it-yourself tests—they are often inaccurate. Beware of scam artists who provide free lead testing and then sell you a treatment system you don't really need. The EPA action level for lead is fifteen parts per billion. You should take action to decrease the lead in your water if it has fifteen parts per billion in the "first draw" or five parts per billion after you have let the water run for a minute or more.[38]

To decrease the lead in your water until you can do further testing or treatment, run cold water for several minutes before using for drinking or cooking. (Instead of wasting the water, consider saving it to water plants or wash windows.) If you usually use hot water to make coffee, tea, or for cooking, use cold water instead.

Inexpensive faucet-mounted and carafe water filtration systems are now available. Top-rated for lead removal by *Consumer Reports Magazine* are the Culligan and Pur Plus faucet-mounted filters and the Brita and Pur carafe filters. Filtered water is also available for purchase in most grocery stores. Keep in mind that water filters may filter out fluoride; if yours does, check with your dentist to see if you should have supplemental fluoride.

Other possible sources of lead exposure include leaded crystal, pottery with leaded glaze (especially imported pottery), and lead-based paint that is chipping or being removed. Paint applied before 1978 contains lead.

Stripping lead paint from your home should be done only by a professional who is certified or licensed in lead safety. If not removed properly, fine lead particles can circulate throughout the home and cause even more problems.

Hot, acidic drinks like coffee can cause lead to leach from lead-glazed mugs. Similarly, fruit juice and acidic foods can cause lead to leach from leaded crystal. If you eat canned imported foods regularly, be aware that the cans may contain lead solder.[39]

For More Information, Contact:
National Lead Information Center
800-424-LEAD
www.epa.gov/lead/nlic.htm
Call the phone number above to request a lead information packet.

National Sanitation Foundation International
P.O. Box 130140
Ann Arbor, MI 48113-0140
800-NSF-MARK or 734-769-8010
www.nsf.org
This nonprofit organization certifies and sets standards for water filtration systems.

EPA Safe Drinking Water Hotline
800-426-4791
www.epa.gov/safewater/
The EPA can give you a list of state-certified testing labs and can answer questions about the water supply.

Coalition to End Childhood Lead Poisoning
800-370-5323
www.leadsafe.org
This nonprofit group offers an educational website and encourages legislative action.

If you think your job exposes you to dangerous amounts of lead, contact the nearest office of the Occupational Safety and Health Administration (OSHA). Look for OSHA in the phone book under U.S. Department of Labor or call OSHA's Office of Information and Consumer Affairs at 202-523-8151.

Illness during Pregnancy

Though no one plans to get sick or to be exposed to illness during pregnancy, knowing the facts can help. Some illnesses can affect your risk of miscarriage or low birth weight, and some can cause birth defects.

Immunization against the diseases listed below is often recommended before pregnancy. Ask your health-care provider for information.

Chickenpox (varicella): Can cause birth defects and low birth weight.

Hepatitis B: Can cause low birth weight.

Rubella (German measles): Can cause birth defects and low birth weight.

Practicing good hygiene, such as frequent hand washing, can prevent the spread of infectious diseases like the ones below.

Cytomegalovirus (CMV): Can cause birth defects, low birth weight, and developmental disorders.

Human immunodeficiency virus (HIV): Can cause low birth weight and cancer.

Human parvovirus B19: Can cause miscarriage.

Toxoplasmosis: Can cause miscarriage, birth defects, and developmental disorders. This parasite is passed in cat feces and can also be transmitted by uncooked and undercooked meats and unwashed fruits and vegetables.

Women with immunity through vaccinations or earlier exposures are not generally at risk from hepatitis B, human parvovirus B19, German measles, or chickenpox. But pregnant women without prior immunity should avoid contact with infected children or adults.

Warning: Alcohol Can Cause Birth Defects

"Think before you drink" is a slogan that the March of Dimes has used to remind women of the risk of drinking alcohol when pregnant. Fetal Alcohol Syndrome (FAS) and a variation, Fetal Alcohol Effect (FAE), can scar children whose mothers drink during pregnancy. FAS occurs in as many as three out of every thousand births, making it the leading cause of mental retardation in the United States. FAS can also cause permanent damage to growth and the central nervous system.[40] Mild cases of FAE can cause irritability, impulsiveness, and learning disabilities and may go undiagnosed for years. Many kids affected by FAE end up dropping out of school.

Alcohol is now recognized as a potent teratogen (a substance capable of causing birth defects) that can cause growth retardation (both in the womb and after birth) and facial abnormalities. Chronic alcohol abuse has been defined as more than two drinks per day. One drink per day has been shown to decrease birth weight.[42] Since alcohol freely crosses the placenta, the fetus's blood alcohol level is equal to the mother's. So one drink in a day might not be risky, but a drinking binge on a critical day of development could damage the fetus.

According to the Public Health Service, as many as 86 percent of women drink once during pregnancy; women with a higher level of education appear to drink more. In the past twenty years, there has been a fourfold increase in FAS in the United States.[43]

The good news is that if you are a drinker, whenever you stop, you increase your chances of having a healthy baby. Women who stopped drinking before their seventh month of pregnancy had healthy babies with no symptoms of FAS.[44]

What about an occasional drink? Research concerning low levels of alcohol consumption is limited and inconsistent. "Because there is no level of drinking that is known to be safe, it is best to completely avoid alcohol during pregnancy," says March of Dimes Medical Director Richard B. Johnston, M.D. If you have other concerns about alcohol, discuss them with your health-care provider.

Caffeine

You may be one of those people who "aren't worth a darn" before their first cup of coffee. The bulk of the research about caffeine and pregnancy shows that moderate consumption (one cup of coffee per day, for example)

Caffeine Content of Your Favorite Beverages and Foods

Beverage or Food	Caffeine (milligrams)	Beverage or Food	Caffeine (milligrams)
Soft Drinks (12 ounces)		**Tea*(continued)**	
Mountain Dew	55	8 ounces green	8–16
Mello Yello	35	8 ounces herbal	0
Coke, Cherry Coke, Diet Coke	31	Instant (1 teaspoon)	31
Tab	31	16 ounces Snapple, all flavors	48
Pepsi	37	Arizona Iced Tea	15–30
Diet Pepsi	36	**Cocoa Drinks**	
Sprite, 7-Up, Slice (regular or diet)	0	Chocolate powder in milk (2–3 heaping teaspoons)	8
Any decaffeinated sodas	0	Hot cocoa (1-ounce packet)	5
Coffee		**Foods**	
Brewed (8 ounces)	135	1 ounce milk chocolate	11
Instant (8 ounces)	95	¼ cup chocolate chips (semisweet)	26
Instant, decaffeinated (1 rounded teaspoon)	2	½ cup Jell-O chocolate pudding	5
Starbucks espresso (1 ounce)	90	Jell-O chocolate pudding pop with chocolate coating	3
Starbucks drip (8 ounces)	200	8 ounces Dannon coffee yogurt	45
Coffee Drinks (2 teaspoons, rounded)		6 ounces Yoplait Cafe au Lait Yogurt	5
Café Amaretto	60	1 cup Ben and Jerry's No Fat Coffee Fudge Ice Cream	85
Suisse Mocha	40		
Dutch Chocolate Mint	30	1 cup Häagen-Dazs Fat-Free Coffee Frozen Yogurt	40
Tea*			
8 ounces black (Ceylon, Darjeeling, English breakfast, Earl Grey)	25–110		
8 ounces oolong	12–55		

*Caffeine content varies with tea type, leaf size, and steeping time.

Sources: *Food Values of Portions Commonly Used*, 17th edition, by Jean Pennington; General Foods; Starbucks; Center for Science in the Public Interest, *Caffeine Content of Food and Drugs.*

is probably safe, yet there is some conflicting research. Heavy caffeine consumption of 300 milligrams per day has been shown to cause small reductions in birth weight, which could be detrimental to low-birth-weight or premature babies. Several studies have also suggested an association between caffeine and miscarriage.[45]

The Food and Drug Administration continues to advise pregnant women to consume caffeine in moderation. Caffeine stimulates the central nervous system, is addictive, acts as a diuretic, and interferes with mineral absorption. The best advice: Instead of relying on caffeine, get more sleep and take a brisk afternoon walk for a pick-me-up. If you must have some caffeine, switch to lower-caffeine products and consume as little as possible.

Herbal Preparations and Teas

Many people turn to herbal teas to cut their caffeine intake. However, you should stay away from teas containing coltsfoot, sassafras, calamus, or comfrey, all of which are carcinogenic.[46] Many herbal preparations, whether sold as teas or quasi medications, can act as drugs because they contain natural active chemicals. Some of these chemicals can be harmful to a fetus. Dr. Varro Tyler, Professor of Pharmacognosy at Purdue University and author of *The Honest Herbal,* advises, "It is best to avoid herbal supplements during pregnancy unless you have expert knowledge about herbs or you are under the care of a physician who does. Because they aren't approved as drugs, herbs don't undergo long-term toxicity testing."

Remember that many of the drugs we use today first came from herbs, flowers, and trees. Exceptions are teas accepted as harmless, such as peppermint and chamomile. You should be safe if you stay with name-brand herbal and decaffeinated teas.

Drugs

All drugs, legal and illegal—even those as seemingly harmless as aspirin—have the potential to seriously harm your baby. So, let your health-care provider know if you are regularly taking any kind of drug. Also, ask what is safe to take for a cold, flu, or bad headache. Avoiding all medications is best when you're pregnant, especially during the first trimester. However, if you must take something, have your health-care provider approve it first.

When you are pregnant, you'll still be susceptible to headaches, colds, flu, and other problems for which you might ordinarily take medication. You may be on vacation and suddenly have a bad case of hay fever. For these times, have a list of over-the-counter medications approved by your health-care provider.

Cocaine

It has been estimated that over half the people addicted to crack cocaine are women.[47] Three studies done in urban areas showed that between 10 and 17 percent of women registered for prenatal care showed evidence of cocaine use.[48]

Cocaine addiction is, of course, harmful to the mother, but it can also have lifelong effects on a baby. Cocaine may take up to six days to leave the fetal blood supply. This increased exposure to the drug can result in premature separation of the placenta, fetal growth retardation, premature delivery, and decreased birth weight, length, and head circumference. Cocaine may also cause miscarriages, birth defects, and increased neurological and behavioral problems that may last a lifetime.[49]

If you are addicted to cocaine or any other drug, seek help through your local health department or drug treatment center. If you'd like to read more about drugs and pregnancy, I recommend an excellent handbook titled *Drugs, Vitamins, and Minerals in Pregnancy* by Ann Karen Henry, Pharm. D., and Jil Feldhausen, M.S., R.D., Fisher Books, 1989.

▼

Traveling during Pregnancy

Chances are that during the nine months of pregnancy, you will travel somewhere. Traveling while pregnant may be "business as usual," but it could also be challenging. Traveling can affect your exercise schedule and the types and amounts of food that you eat.

In the Plane

▶ **Find out whether a meal will be served.**

If you'd like a bit more control over your food on the flight, call the airline at least twenty-four hours before your flight to request a special meal. Some options are low-fat, vegetarian, diabetic, and seafood.

▶ **If you have a layover between flights, use the time to exercise.**

Walk to your gate instead of using moving sidewalks or a bus.

▶ **Bring your own supply of snacks.**

Unless you are flying cross-country or overseas nonstop, you probably won't have a complete meal. And on a plane, even "meals" can be skimpy. You will need snacks! Bring along fresh or dried fruit, whole-grain or graham crackers, string cheese, granola bars, nuts, and other nonperishable snacks.

▶ **Request an aisle seat so you can get up to walk and stretch or go to the restroom.**

Bulkhead seats in the first row of each section offer more leg room.

▶ **If your flight is a long one, drink plenty of fluids before and during the flight.**

Flying can dehydrate you. During long flights, avoid carbonated beverages; they can increase gas.

▶ **Get up and walk around several times during the flight.**

Or, you may want to go to the back of the plane and just stand or stretch for a while. While sitting down, you can do isometric exercises, which can improve circulation.

▶ **Avoid taking heavy carryon luggage unless someone else can carry it for you.**

The weight can increase back pain.

In the Car

▶ **Bring along a small cooler in which you can keep yogurt, cheese, veggies, milk, fruit, and other snacks.**

You can even bring the makings of a sandwich, which can save you money on restaurant food. If you forget a cooler, you can always stop at a grocery along the way and pick up fresh or dried fruit and ready-to-eat raw vegetables.

▶ **Instead of eating regular-size meals when you stop, order appetizers or eat just half a portion.**

Sitting in the car for extended periods of time may induce "boredom eating," yet you won't need as many calories while just sitting. Try to limit snacking to when you are actually hungry.

▶ **Drink plenty of fluids.**

If you are traveling to a higher altitude, your fluid needs will increase. Lack of activity can slow down your digestion and increase constipation. "Pit stops" will allow you to get out and stretch, which can prevent back pain and increase circulation.

▶ **Plan "adventure stops."**

Try to include enough time in your itinerary to make extended stops to see things of interest. Use the stops as your exercise time to walk and stretch.

At Your Destination

▶ **If you are planning to stay at a hotel, try to get a room with a minifridge or kitchenette.**

This will allow you to keep your own snack foods as well as high-fiber cereals for breakfast or snacks.

▶ **Try to make wise food choices when eating out.**

When people eat most meals out, diets tend to be lower in fiber, calcium, vitamin C, and folacin and higher in fat and sodium.[50] (See page 246 for advice on eating out.)

▶ **If you are planning to stay with friends or relatives, bring along a few of the foods you usually eat, such as high-fiber cereal, milk, and extra fresh or dried fruit.**

This way your diet won't be lacking, and you won't have to ask your host to buy special foods for you.

▶ **Make sure you pack nonperishable snacks in your bag for those hectic tourist schedules.**

Good snacks include cheese or peanut-butter crackers, boxes of raisins, wheat crackers, fiber bars, apples, bananas, and individual bags of pretzels. Don't forget the drinks! Juice boxes pack well.

▶ **If you are traveling to a foreign country, talk to your physician before making reservations.**

Vaccinations may be required that you can't take while pregnant. Or, you may need to eat very carefully to avoid bacterial poisoning. You may want to take some nonperishable foods with you to snack on if familiar foods aren't available where you are going, or if food safety may be an issue.

▼

The Positives of Pregnancy

Although most people are familiar with only the negatives of pregnancy, pregnancy also has many positive aspects. For example, some women feel at their best when pregnant. And some women with chronic medical problems go into remission or experience decreased symptoms. By concentrating on the good things that occur during these nine months, life will be much more pleasant. Here are just a few of the good things about being pregnant. Try to think of them often!

- Your hair becomes thick and shiny.
- You radiate a warm, healthy glow.
- People open the door for you.
- Finally, you have a larger bra size!
- You can gain weight without guilt!
- You don't have to tuck in your blouse.
- You now have an excuse for being tired.
- You feel great all over.
- You feel good about taking care of yourself.
- You have a great reason for starting a walking program and for eating right.
- You are the designated driver for the next nine months.

- Your partner brings you meals in bed.
- You're too tired for housework—a good excuse to hire a cleaning service!
- Finally, you have a long vacation to look forward to (maternity leave).
- Your kids learn how to help around the house.
- The love for your yet-to-be-born baby abounds.
- You don't have to worry about forgetting your birth control pill.
- You can wear one-size-fits-all clothes.
- You will become a member of Club Mom.
- You are part of a miracle.
- You have a special new friend living close by.
- This is an experience you'll have only once or a few times in your life. Enjoy it!

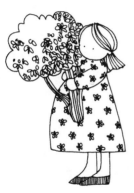

CHAPTER THREE

The First Trimester

What you will find in this chapter:

• How Baby Is Growing
• Weight Gain and Energy Needs
• Protein Needs
• Other Nutrient Needs
• Focus on Fiber
• The Eating Expectantly Eating Plan
• Morning Sickness
• Other First-Trimester Challenges
• Food Planning for the First Trimester

This chapter answers such questions as:

• How much weight should I gain?
• I've read that I should eat 100 grams of protein; how much is that?
• How much protein is in an egg?
• How else can I get protein in my diet if I don't feel like eating meat?
• What can I do about morning sickness?
• How can I avoid constipation?

How Baby Is Growing

During the first three months of pregnancy, good nutrition is vital for your baby's development. Babies born to poorly nourished mothers are more susceptible to birth defects and to infections in early childhood. Read on to learn about the many miraculous events taking place within your body during the first trimester.

At the End of One Week

For the first seven days after the sperm fertilizes the egg, the group of cells, or zygote, is traveling down the fallopian tube toward the uterus. Although the zygote is no larger than the tiniest speck of sand, it carries all the genetic material (DNA) necessary for development. During the first week, the cells are rapidly dividing into what will become organs, skin, hair, bones, and muscle. Even though the DNA and cells "know" the sex of the baby, genital formation has not taken place yet, so we refer to the baby as "it."

The zygote implants in the uterine wall seven to eight days after fertilization; then it is known as an embryo. The mass of cells that includes both the embryo and what will become the placenta is only about the size of a blueberry.

At the End of Four Weeks (One Month)

By this time, you may be confirming your pregnancy and experiencing some of the telltale signs. The embryo is no bigger than a grain of rice, and its heart is beating by the twenty-fifth day. Its digestive system, backbone, and spinal cord are all beginning to form. Tiny limb buds that will become arms and legs are appearing. The next four weeks will be vitally important as development occurs rapidly.

At the End of Eight Weeks (Two Months)

The embryo is now about the size of your big toe, or a little over 1 inch long. All the major organs and systems are formed, yet some are not completely developed. The embryo clearly looks human. Its long arm and leg bones are beginning to form and are visible under its thin skin. The embryo now has a face, and its brain has taken shape. The head makes up almost half of the embryo. The embryo weighs only ¼ ounce!

At the End of Twelve Weeks (Three Months)

From the ninth week on, the unborn baby is called a fetus. The nails are developed, and the fetus can suck its fingers and curl its hands into a fist. The kidneys are beginning to produce urine, and tooth buds for all the baby teeth are appearing. The fetus is only about as long as your middle finger (3 inches) and weighs about 1½ ounces.

Although you may be just starting to buy maternity clothes or adjusting your belt to the next notch, most of your baby's organs and tissues are already formed.

▼

Weight Gain and Energy Needs

Do you believe you have a special license to eat for two because you're pregnant?

Well, your license is being revoked. You do need larger amounts of many nutrients during pregnancy, but you don't need to eat twice the food and calories, especially in the first trimester.

The Subcommittee on Nutritional Status and Weight Gain During Pregnancy of the National Academy of Sciences recommends that you gain about 1 pound (or less) per month during the first trimester. That translates into 135 (or fewer) extra calories per day.[1] Uh oh, there go the visions of sundaes dancing in your head! Later in this chapter we'll talk about how to make your diet a winner without gaining too much weight.

▼

Protein Needs

Protein is essential during pregnancy because your body uses it to build each new cell for your baby. Protein is also needed for the placenta—the lifeline that brings nourishment from you to your baby. Protein helps make new blood cells and muscle tissue that supports your baby. To top it all off, protein is used to make all the hormones that wreak havoc in your body when you're pregnant.

In the first trimester, your protein needs don't increase very much—only about 1⅓ grams extra each day, or the equivalent of ⅙ ounce of meat. The Daily Reference Intake (DRI) for protein throughout pregnancy is 10 grams higher than nonpregnancy needs, or 60 grams per day.[2] The additional protein you need is equal to 1½ ounces of animal protein, 1¼ cups of legumes, 1½ eggs, or 1¼ ounces of cheese.

Several factors influence your body's protein needs. To enable your body to use the protein you eat for building tissues and cells, you must eat enough calories (energy). This is because your body's first priority is supplying energy. If you eat enough protein but not enough calories, your body will use the protein for energy instead of for tissue building and other protein-dependent functions. Let's say you eat 10 ounces of fish and chicken every day. You don't have much of an appetite, so this fills you up and you don't eat much else, making your calorie intake from fats and carbohydrates inadequate. Because your body must use the protein for energy, your body will lack the protein it needs for other important purposes.

Also, you won't have enough glucose (blood sugar) to supply your brain with energy, so your body will start breaking down fat into fragments called ketones. The presence of ketones is a sign that your body can't complete the metabolic process. Large amounts of ketones can be harmful to your body. Avoid the production of ketones by having enough calories and carbohydrates in your diet.

Consuming a certain *quantity* of protein is not the only goal. The *quality* of protein also affects how your body uses it. Protein needs are calculated by determining the need for high biological value, or high-quality, protein. High-quality protein can be turned into body tissues. These proteins include eggs, meat, chicken, milk, and fish. For all the bad press the egg has gotten over the years, it is well respected where protein is

Protein Content of Food Groups		
Food	**Serving Sizes**	**Protein per Serving (grams)**
Legumes	½ cup	7–11
Dairy products	1 cup milk/ 1 ounce cheese	6–8
Meat, poultry, fish	1 ounce	6–8
Bread/cereal	1 slice/1 ounce	2–4
Vegetables	½ cup	2–3
Fruits/juices	1 medium/½ cup	0–1
Fat, oil	Any amount	0

concerned. Egg protein is of the highest quality and is often used as a standard to which other proteins are compared.

If you do not eat animal products, your body will need greater quantities of lower-quality plant proteins to meet protein needs. Vegetarians, don't despair! You can meet your protein needs without eating meat, but you must look carefully at your intake of certain nutrients. (See page 96 for more information on vegetarian protein sources.)

As a rule, Americans eat about twice as much protein as they really need. Pregnant women are no different, eating an average of 75 to 110 grams per day—well above the 60 grams per day recommended by the Food and Nutrition Board. However, some health-care providers and birthing programs recommend up to 100 grams of protein, especially for high-risk pregnancies. A daily diet that contains approximately 100 grams of protein might include four servings of dairy product, 6 ounces of animal protein (or the equivalent), four vegetables, four fruits, and eight servings of starch or bread.

Most women who eat a typical western diet don't have a problem meeting protein needs. In fact, the National Academy of Sciences advises pregnant women not to use specially formulated high-protein supplements, protein powders, or high-protein beverages because some evidence suggests that these products might be harmful.[3]

Why You May Need to Work to Meet Your Protein Needs

You might not be able to meet your protein needs if you:

- don't drink milk or eat dairy products and also don't eat many other protein sources.
- have nausea or vomiting that prevents you from eating much of anything.
- just don't have the desire to eat meat.

If you eat or drink the recommended four servings of dairy products each day, you will be meeting half your protein needs. If you don't, you'll need to increase protein from other sources.

If you just don't feel like eating meat, you are not alone. Most pregnant women have some food aversion; your stomach may turn at the thought of eating what used to be your favorite food.

If your favorite high-protein foods turn your stomach, you can eat more dairy products, which are also good sources of protein, or you can turn to other sources. Many of the women I've talked to could tolerate eggs and cheese even if they couldn't eat meat. You may also tolerate many vegetarian protein sources. See page 67 for a list of protein sources and experiment to find what works for you.

If you can't eat much of anything due to first-trimester morning sickness, eat what you can. (See Chapter Thirteen for first-trimester recipes.) If the condition persists to the point where you are losing weight, alert your health-care provider, who may treat your nausea more aggressively or refer you to a registered dietitian for individual counseling.

▼

Other Nutrient Needs

All vitamins and minerals play specific, essential roles during pregnancy, so be sure to have adequate amounts in your diet for the whole nine months.

Water is one of the most important nutrients in the first trimester—especially if you are suffering from morning sickness. Dehydration can be very serious! Folate is not only important in neural development but is also critical for cell production and division, which occur in leaps and bounds during the first trimester. Manganese is needed for developing the organs used for hearing. Vitamin A is needed for developing tissues. A low intake of zinc early in pregnancy is related to a threefold increase in the risk of very preterm delivery.[4] Phosphorus, calcium, and vitamin D work together to produce strong bones.

Focus on Fiber

Fiber is one of those things most people don't eat enough of, even though every day new studies cite its benefits.

The old saying "An apple a day keeps the doctor away" may well refer to an apple's fiber content. Here's why:

- Fiber-rich whole grains may protect against cancer, especially breast cancer and gastrointestinal cancers.[5]
- Soluble fiber has been shown to reduce cholesterol, thus reducing the risk of heart disease. Trace minerals and antioxidants in whole grains may also help cut heart disease risk.
- Soluble fiber helps control blood glucose, which is particularly beneficial to people with diabetes.[6]
- Fiber fills you up, not out!
- Fiber keeps your bowels moving, which can help prevent constipation and hemorrhoids.

Fiber Tips

Following are a few simple ways to make sure you get enough fiber every day:

▶ **Follow the National Cancer Institute's slogan "Five a Day for Better Health."**

You'll be on your way to having adequate dietary fiber if you eat five fruits and vegetables daily.

Snack Tip

The fig may be the world's most under-appreciated fruit! Not only do figs have the highest amount of dietary fiber of any common fruit, nut, or vegetable, they are also higher in potassium than bananas and are considered a good calcium source. Eat this sweet, healthy treat as a between-meal snack.

Stuffed Figs

Cut a large slice in a fresh or dried fig. Fill it with low-fat or fat-free cream cheese, or purée cottage cheese in a blender until it's the consistency of cream cheese. Add a dash of cinnamon or nutmeg for more flavor.

▶ **Choose whole-wheat bread, crackers, and pasta.**

The American Dietetic Association supports the recommendation of three servings of whole-grain products daily.[7] Look at food labels; "whole grain" or "whole-wheat flour" should be the first ingredient.

▶ **Eat brown rice, bulgur, or quinoa instead of white rice.**

▶ **Start your day with a high-fiber cereal.**

Choose cereals containing at least 5 grams of fiber per serving.

▶ **When baking, replace part of the white flour with wheat bran, whole-wheat flour, or oatmeal.**

Fiber Content of Foods

Food	Serving Sizes	Dietary Fiber (grams*)
Fruits		
Figs	5	9
Apple, fresh with skin	1 medium	4
Blackberries, raw	½ cup	4
Raspberries, fresh	½ cup	4
Dates	5	4
Pear, fresh with skin	1	4
Prunes	5	3
Banana	1 medium	3
Orange, fresh	1	3
Nectarine, fresh	1	2
Raisins	⅓ cup	2
Pineapple, fresh	2 slices	2
Most other fruits contain 1–3 grams of fiber per serving.		
Vegetables		
Artichoke	1 medium	16
Potato with skin	1 medium	5
Green peas	½ cup	4
Spinach, cooked and drained	½ cup	3
Broccoli, cooked and chopped	½ cup	3
Sweet potato, baked in skin	1 medium	3
Rhubarb, cooked	½ cup	3
Corn, canned	½ cup	2
Cereals, Grains, and Legumes		
Black beans	½ cup	8
Baked beans, canned	½ cup	7
Wheat germ or wheat bran, unprocessed	¼ cup	6
Refried pinto beans, canned	½ cup	6
Bulgur or quinoa	½ cup	5
Triscuits	7	4
Corn tortillas	2	3
Nutrigrain waffle	1	2–3
Bran muffin	1	2–3
Popcorn	3½ cups	2–3
Whole-wheat bread	1 slice	2
Brown rice, instant cooked	½ cup	2
Baked Tostitos	1 ounce (20 chips)	2

*Numbers rounded to the nearest whole number.

Sources: Pennington, J. *Bowes and Church's Food Values of Portions Commonly Used.* 17th Edition. Philadelphia: Lippincott Williams and Wilkins, 1998.

▶ **Snack on high-fiber foods such as bran muffins, dried fruit, fresh fruit, vegetables, and whole-grain crackers.**

If your diet is normally low in fiber, increase the fiber in your diet gradually. Adding a lot of fiber to your meals all at once can result in bloating and gas. Also, remember to drink plenty of fluids while eating high-fiber foods. Without enough fluids, high-fiber foods can cause constipation.

If you follow the advice above, you will be sure to get the 20 to 35 grams of fiber currently recommended by the National Cancer Institute.[8] But if you want to be really aware of the specific amounts of fiber found in foods, look at the chart on page 54.

▼

The Eating Expectantly Eating Plan

What's the best way to eat for a healthy pregnancy? The guide below will help you plan your meals and snacks so that you obtain the nutrients you and your baby need. It may be helpful to write down what you eat for a few days and compare it to the Eating Expectantly Eating Plan.

Eating Expectantly Eating Plan

8 or more servings of grains
1 serving is 1 slice any type bread; ½ small bagel, pita bread or English muffin; 1 6-inch tortilla; ½ cup cooked rice or pasta; ½ cup cooked cereal, barley, bulgur, or quinoa; 1 ounce ready-to-eat cereal, 3–4 crackers, or 2 cookies.

Note: 3 or more of your 8 daily grain servings should be whole-grain.

4 or more servings of calcium-rich foods
1 serving is 1 cup any type milk or yogurt, 1½ ounces natural cheese, 2 ounces processed cheese, or 1 cup calcium-fortified orange juice or soymilk.

4 or more servings of fruit
1 serving is 1 medium fresh fruit; ½ grapefruit, mango, or papaya; ½ cup canned or cut fruit; ¼ cup dried fruit; or ¾ cup fruit juice.

4 or more servings of vegetables
1 serving is ½ cup cooked vegetables, 1 cup leafy vegetables, 1 small potato, or ¾ cup tomato or vegetable juice.

Note: Be sure to eat at least one fruit or vegetable that is high in vitamin C and one that is dark green or orange every day.

3 servings of protein foods
1 serving is 2–3 ounces (the size of a deck of cards) cooked lean meat; 2 eggs; ½ cup tuna; ½ cup legumes, tofu, or textured vegetable protein; or 2 tablespoons nuts or nut butter.

Note: Eat a variety of protein foods, including fish at least once a week. Eat an additional ½ protein serving for each cup of milk that you don't drink.

Fats and sweets: Eat sparingly.
Most fat and sugar is hidden in foods, so watch out for fried foods, full-fat dairy foods, sodas, and so on.

Sample Meal Plan

Breakfast

Raisin bran cereal with strawberries

Whole-wheat bagel with light cream
cheese

Milk

Snack

Vegetable juice

Whole-grain crackers

Low-fat string cheese

Lunch

Lean roast beef sandwich on wheat bread

Raw carrots and broccoli with dip

Melon balls

Sugar cookies

Milk

Snack

Popcorn

Dinner

Grilled salmon steak

Grilled corn on the cob

Spinach salad with tomato and mushrooms

Whole-grain roll

Fresh orange

Milk

Snack

Peanut butter and graham crackers

Yogurt with dried fruit

▼

Morning Sickness

A touch of the queasies may be your first
clue that you are pregnant. If you have
morning sickness, you may need to figure
out how to survive the day before you can
even think about eating. Here's some information to help you through this trying time.

The Facts on Morning Sickness

- You are not alone. Morning sickness is
  the most common problem of pregnancy,
  occurring in as many as 90 percent of
  pregnancies. A very small percentage of
  pregnant women have severe nausea
  and vomiting (hyperemesis gravidarum),
  which can lead to weight loss, dehydration, and hospitalization.
- Despite its name, morning sickness can
  (and often does) occur any time of the
  day or night.
- While nausea often subsides by the second trimester, for some women it doesn't.
  According to Miriam Erick, M.S., R.D.,
  author of *No More Morning Sickness* and
  *Take Two Crackers and Call Me in the
  Morning*, the average duration of morning sickness is seventeen-and-a-half
  weeks. Some women have morning sickness throughout their pregnancies.
- Morning sickness may be a sign that
  your hormones are at a healthy level.
  Women with morning sickness have a
  lower risk of miscarriage—unless they
  suffer significant weight loss.

- While no one knows exactly what causes morning sickness, some have theorized that pregnancy hormones—specifically estrogen and human chorionic gonadotrophin (HCG)—are to blame. Heightened sense of smell has also been blamed as a potential cause.

Morning Sickness Survival Tips

If morning sickness is making you miserable, the following tips may help you feel better. The first five tips are summarized from Miriam Erick's *No More Morning Sickness: A Survival Guide for Pregnant Women* (Plume, 1993).

Note: If you experience severe nausea and vomiting, consult your health-care provider. Do not self-treat with medication, vitamins, or herbal supplements without your health-care provider's approval.

1. Track your environment.

Erick recommends keeping score of how you feel throughout the day to determine whether certain environments tend to make you sick. Are you more sensitive to smells? To noise? To light? Are you more likely to feel sick when you are tired or hungry? Do certain food tastes or textures make you feel better?

2. Take the sniff test.

Because a pregnant woman may have a heightened sense of smell, any odor could trigger nausea. It might be an unpleasant odor like your neighbor's cigarette smoke or the body odor of the person next to you on the train, or it might be a smell you normally love, like garlic or your partner's cologne. Try to identify and avoid odors that make you turn green. Alternatively, experiment with smells that make you feel better. (Erick has found the smell of lemon to be helpful for many women.)

3. Change your environment.

If smells bother you, try to get rid of them. This might mean eating only cold foods for a while, eating outside, or having someone else do the cooking. If a coworker's cologne is the problem, ask him or her not to wear it for a while. If the drive to work makes you queasy, try walking, riding public transit, or working at home.

4. Trust your intuition.

Sometimes it's most important just to keep something down—no matter what it is. Ask yourself: "What would make me feel better? Something sweet, salty, crunchy, sour, soft, bland, or wet?" Erick has found that the food that often does the trick is potato chips. I once had a bout of morning sickness on the morning of a TV interview. What sounded good at the moment? Pretzels and a cola. It definitely wasn't the healthiest breakfast—but after eating it, I was able to get on with my day and eat healthier foods.

5. Drink enough fluids.

Dehydration, which can be fatal, is the biggest danger of morning sickness. Women with severe morning sickness are often hospitalized to be rehydrated intravenously. "Fluids are the most necessary nutrients and the hardest to get in," Erick says. Most pregnant women need 10 cups of fluids per day.

Some women find sparkling water appealing, while others get their fluids from fruits with high water content, like watermelon, cantaloupe, and grapes. Popsicles, slushy drinks, ginger ale, and lemonade may also be appealing.

6. Avoid having an empty stomach.

Eat small, frequent meals with snacks in between to keep your stomach from emptying out completely. This might mean eating a little something as often as every thirty minutes. Some women carry a box of crackers with them all day to keep nausea at bay.

7. Eat a substantial bedtime snack.

Eating a bedtime snack with protein, such as half a sandwich and milk or peanut butter and crackers, may keep your blood sugar up during the night and prevent morning sickness.

8. Avoid greasy, spicy, and strong-smelling foods.

Such foods can aggravate nausea as well as heartburn. However, if this kind of food sounds really good to you, it's worth a try!

9. Eat a snack before breakfast.

Leave food beside your bed at night or have your partner bring you a snack in the morning before you get out of bed. (Now there's a fine habit to cultivate!)

10. Eat slowly and drink fluids between (not with) meals.

This strategy may help you keep your food down. Remember that fluids are vital to your health, so be sure to get them one way or another!

11. Eat cold foods or have your partner do the cooking.

The look of raw food or the smell of strong foods cooking may make you feel sick. Use the cooking time to take a walk or do some shopping. You might also want to eat outside when possible to get more fresh air.

12. Think differently.

Some alternative therapies may help morning sickness. Acupressure and Sea-Bands (for motion sickness) have been shown to ease nausea during pregnancy. The use of ginger, hypnosis, and vitamin B_6 has also helped some women. Vitamin B_6 can be toxic in large amounts, so consult your health-care provider before self-treating! Prescription drugs may also be a safe and effective treatment for your morning sickness.[9]

▼

Other First-Trimester Challenges

Frequent Urination

In those first few months, you might feel as though you're wearing a path in the carpet with all your trips to the bathroom. The increased frequency of urination may be an early hint that you're pregnant. Your baby, within the uterus, sits right above your bladder. As your uterus engorges with blood and your baby grows, the pressure on your bladder increases and the space for storing urine decreases.

What You Can Do:

▶ **DON'T decrease your total fluid intake!**

However, if you're getting up several times during the night to urinate, you might want to slightly decrease your intake of fluids during evening hours.

▶ **Sleep on your side.**

Lying on one side may help relieve pressure on your bladder.

▶ **Start doing Kegel exercises now and continue during and after your pregnancy.**

These exercises tone up the muscles that hold in urine. Have you ever sneezed or coughed and felt as though you nearly emptied your bladder? This can happen more frequently during pregnancy and again later in life. The weakened bladder control may be due to poor muscle tone in the area, along with added pressure from baby. Keeping these muscles toned during pregnancy can also help you get back in shape and heal more quickly after you have the baby. Ask your health-care provider or childbirth educator for more information.

Note: If urination is painful, contact your health-care provider.

Fatigue

You may feel as though you could sleep for the rest of your pregnancy. During the first trimester, when your hormones are playing tag and you're it, fatigue is common.

What You Can Do:

▶ **Accept your need for rest and slow down your lifestyle.**

▶ **Eat regular, balanced meals that are high in the essential nutrients.**

If you're not eating enough calories or not getting enough essential nutrients, your diet could be partly to blame for the fatigue. (See page 28 for more information on essential vitamins and minerals.) During the first trimester, your health-care provider will probably check the amount of iron in your blood. Iron-deficiency anemia can cause fatigue and is fairly common in pregnancy due to the greatly increased need for this mineral. Consuming adequate amounts of dietary iron before and during pregnancy can prevent anemia. (See pages 72–73 for good sources of iron.)

▶ **Exercise regularly.**

Even though you may not feel you have the energy to exercise, afterward you'll be glad you did. (See Chapter Ten: Fitting Fitness In.)

Cravings and Aversions

We've all heard stories about the husband who runs to the store in the middle of the night to get his wife a pint of chocolate-fudge ice cream. You may be experiencing something similar. No one is sure what causes cravings. Sometimes, a craving signals a dietary need. (No, we don't have a DRI for chocolate-fudge ice cream yet!) Some women crave nonfood items like clay, starch, dirt, or ice. This particular type of craving, called pica, usually stems from an iron deficiency. Other cravings may be due to—you guessed it—those crazy, mixed-up hormones.

Cravings for sweets can be explained by drops in blood sugar, which can happen easily if you don't eat often enough. In this case, your body needs any carbohydrate food and you may, for example, turn the need into a craving for your favorite high-carbohydrate food, such as ice cream.

Cravings can often be healthy. I'm generally not a grapefruit eater, but when pregnant with my second child, I asked for grapefruit frequently. I also often wanted a stick-to-your-ribs food like a bean burrito or hamburger. This may have been due to the need for more calories or protein.

Aversions to certain foods are just as common as cravings, so don't be surprised if your favorite food now turns you off. Sometimes an aversion (to cigarettes or alcohol, for example) acts to protect your baby. Meat is often unappealing during pregnancy, while eggs, cheese, milk, and beans are often more easy to tolerate. (See Chapter Six for vegetarian eating tips.)

Whatever your particular fancy, rest assured it will probably change during your pregnancy and will be different during your next pregnancy!

What You Can Do:

▶ **To keep cravings in check, make sure to eat regular meals and snacks, including breakfast.**

▶ **If you *must* have something, then have it!**

If the craved food is less than nutritious, try to eat a small amount. Or, try to steer your craving toward a healthier alternative—such as a whole-wheat raisin bagel instead of a doughnut.

Breast Changes

Breast enlargement and sensitivity are common early signs of pregnancy. In the first trimester the fat layer of your breast thickens, and the number of milk glands increases. The veins close to the surface enlarge due to your increased blood flow. Your nipples and areolas (the dark areas around your nipples) will enlarge and probably get darker.

What You Can Do:

▶ **Wear a good supportive bra, preferably one with flexible straps.**

If you plan to breast-feed, a nursing bra is a wise choice.

▶ **If you are large-busted, you might want to sleep in a lightweight bra.**

Teeth and Gum Changes

Hormones and increased blood flow affect many areas of your body, including your gums. They can soften and become more prone to infections.

What You Can Do:

▶ **Eat a balanced diet that contains plenty of vitamin C.**

Good nutrition is the first defense against gum disease.

▶ Don't neglect your teeth and gums during pregnancy.

Continue regular flossing, brushing, and professional cleaning. Have a dental checkup during your pregnancy. However, be sure your dentist knows that you are pregnant before your visit.

Note: If you are planning a pregnancy, visit your dentist first for a checkup and for any dental work that might be needed.

? Questions You May Have

Q: What if I skip meals—is that bad for the baby?

A: Yes, and for you, too! During pregnancy, your baby depends entirely on you for energy. When you don't eat, your baby may not get the energy and nutrients it needs and will then use your nutrient stores, which may leave you depleted. When you skip meals, you often eat much more food later to make up for it, and you may store those extra calories as fat. Try to avoid the feast-or-famine approach by taking the time to eat regular meals and snacks.

Q: I usually eat fast food for lunch every day. How can I eat more nutritiously?

A: I recommend planning ahead and taking the time to shop and cook. The time and

effort will be well spent. Eating typical fast food is costly—both in dollars and to your health. Fast food provides lots of calories, but not many nutrients. To improve on a typical fast-food meal, have fruit with it. Good news: Fast food is improving, and eating nutritiously on the run is getting easier. (See page 325 for "Meals in Minutes," and page 249 for "Choosing Nutritious Fast Foods.")

Q: What if I just can't eat much at all? My "morning" sickness occurs all the time.

A: As noted earlier, extra calories aren't a priority in the first trimester. What is important is keeping your baby's environment safe, having an adequate intake of folic acid, and keeping well hydrated. Eat whatever you can to get through your nausea and make sure to drink plenty of fluids. The baby will draw on your stored nutrients if you aren't able to eat much. However, make your calories count. When you *are* able to eat, eat the most nutritious foods you can, and when your morning sickness has subsided, eat well to restock your body's nutrient stores.

▼

Food Planning for the First Trimester

During the first trimester, cooking and eating can be a big challenge. If you're looking for practical, realistic menus for your situation, browse the list below and refer to Chapter Thirteen for menu details and delicious recipes.

Menus

- Don't Feel Like Eating
- Don't Feel Like Cooking
- Don't Feel Like Eating or Cooking
- Feel Like Staying in Bed, but Can't
- Feel Great
- Blender Breakfasts (or Snacks to Go)
- Snack Ideas
- High-Energy Snack Ideas

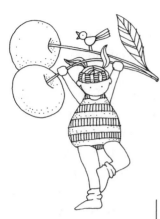

CHAPTER FOUR

The Second Trimester

What you will find in this chapter:

- How Baby Is Growing
- Weight Gain and Energy Needs
- How's Your Diet?
- Protein Needs
- Other Nutrient Needs
- The Power of Soy
- Focus on Calcium
- Focus on Iron
- "Thrive on Five"
- Smart Snacking
- Second-Trimester Challenges
- Food Planning for the Second Trimester

This chapter answers such questions as:

- Doesn't my prenatal vitamin have enough calcium?
- Which foods are high in iron?
- What's a good snack?
- What about chocolate milk?
- Which has more calcium: milk or yogurt?
- When will I feel my baby move?

You've made it through the first trimester–congratulations! The second trimester includes the thirteenth through the twenty-sixth weeks and is usually when pregnant women feel their best. During this time you'll have lots of energy, especially if you're eating right and exercising. You'll mark the halfway point of your pregnancy and you'll feel your baby move!

How Baby Is Growing

The development of all the major organs and systems is either started or complete. From now on, the fetus will start to gain more weight. Your body is producing more blood in order to nourish your baby, so you need to be drinking plenty of fluids, preferably 10 cups per day of water, milk, juice, or soup. Anything with caffeine can cause you to lose your needed fluids.

At the End of Sixteen Weeks (Four Months)

Your baby is quite active, even though you might not feel it yet. Making facial expressions, swallowing, rotating feet, kicking, sleeping, waking, and even listening to you are all part of your baby's daily routine. Downy hair called lanugo is developing on the head. The fetus is now 6 to 7 inches long and weighs 6 to 7 ounces, the weight of a large apple.

At the End of Twenty Weeks (Five Months)

A growth spurt has occurred within the last month. The fetus now measures between 8 and 12 inches and weighs about 1 pound. Lanugo now covers the whole body, and the hair on the head is getting thicker. Eyebrows and eyelashes are developing. You are beginning to sense your baby's movements as its muscles develop and it becomes stronger at turning and rolling.

At the End of Twenty-Four Weeks (Six Months)

Baby is now between 11 and 14 inches long and weighs between 1½ and 1¾ pounds. The fetus looks like a wrinkled old man. Its skin is covered in vernix, a thick waxy coating that protects its skin while in the amniotic fluid. Baby opens and closes its eyes and can hear and respond to external noise and music. Its distinct fingerprints and footprints are formed. (Even identical twins have different fingerprints.) The alveoli in the lungs are just beginning to develop. If the baby were born at this time, it would need extremely specialized care.

Weight Gain and Energy Needs

During the last two trimesters of your pregnancy, your body needs about 300 more calories per day than it needed before you were pregnant. Eating at this rate will result in a 25-to-35-pound weight gain—considered optimal for a healthy baby. However, many things will affect your energy needs, including prepregnant weight, activity level, and current weight. Some women are less active during the last half of pregnancy; others remain active and burn even more calories due to their increasing weight.

From now on, you should try to gain about 1 pound per week.[1] Remember that the extra calories and protein you are eating work toward creating a healthy environment for your baby to live in until birth. The extra nutrients are required for increased blood volume, placental growth, increased fat storage, increased breast tissue, and production of amniotic fluid. In addition, nutrients provide the building materials for your growing fetus.

In the next few weeks—usually between sixteen and twenty weeks gestation—you should feel a fluttering in your uterus; this is your baby moving! It's a very exciting feeling and also a reminder that during these special months you must take good care of yourself by eating right, exercising moderately, and trying to improve other lifestyle habits.

Now is a good time to take inventory of your diet and health habits. Complete the survey below to find out how your diet compares with the dietary needs of a mother-to-be.

How's Your Diet?

First write down in the spaces that follow everything you've eaten during the last day (or on a typical day). Then refer to the Eating Expectantly Eating Plan on page 55 to tally the number of servings of each food type you've eaten. Compare your totals for the day with those recommended.

Breakfast

_____

_____

_____

Snack

_____

_____

Lunch

_____

_____

_____

Snack

_____

_____

Dinner

_____

_____

_____

Snack

_____

_____

_____

How Did You Do?

Your diet should contain at least:

8 or more servings of grains
Best choices: whole grains, whole-wheat bread and cereal, sweet potatoes, winter squash, potatoes, dried beans, peas, corn, wheat crackers, and popcorn.
Note: Don't forget that three servings should be whole grains.

4 or more servings of fruits
Best choices: papaya, mango, melon, berries, apricots, peaches, grapefruit, orange, and kiwi.

4 or more servings of vegetables
Best choices: broccoli, cauliflower, carrots, spinach, cabbage, leaf and romaine lettuce, greens, sweet peppers, and tomatoes.

Note: Don't forget to eat at least one vitamin-C-rich and one vitamin-A-rich fruit or vegetable every day!

4 or more servings of calcium-rich foods
Best choices: skim and low-fat milk and yogurt, fat-free and low-fat cheeses, and tofu made with calcium.

3 servings of protein foods
Best choices: fish and shellfish, dried beans and legumes, tofu, poultry, lean beef, lamb, and pork. Be sure to eat a variety, and include fish at least once a week!

Fats and sweets: Eat sparingly.
Best choices: avocado, nuts, nut oils, seeds (especially flaxseed), canola and olive oil or products made with these oils.
Note: Remember that baked goods, fried foods, whole-milk products, and desserts

have many hidden fats. Fat has twice as many calories as carbohydrate or protein.

8 to 10 cups of fluid

You should be drinking to thirst, or at least 8 cups of fluid per day, most of it from water.

Visit www.healthyfoodzone.com for more eating tips.

Protein Needs

Protein is very important during the second trimester for the growing tissue of the fetus and placenta, your increasing blood volume, and your growing breast and uterine tissues.

All protein is not equal. Proteins are composed of amino acids, and for proteins to be used most efficiently, all the essential amino acids must be present in certain amounts and proportions. The term *complete protein* describes protein that contains all the essential amino acids (those your body can't produce) in the amounts needed to build proteins. *Incomplete proteins* lack one or more amino acids or contain small amounts of amino acids. This distinction is important for people who don't eat animal protein. In the past, nutritionists believed that we needed to combine incomplete proteins during the same meal. Now we know that eating a variety of different proteins throughout the day is adequate.[2]

Foods that contain complete protein include beef, poultry, fish, milk, eggs, and cheese. Foods considered incomplete-protein sources include beans, rice, grains, peanut butter, nuts, pasta, soy products, and some vegetables. (Fruit contains very small amounts of protein.) Various protein sources supply different nutrients, so eat a variety of foods, both those that contain complete protein and those that contain incomplete protein. (See the chart on page 67 to learn the protein content of many common foods.) Even if you are not vegetarian, I encourage you to eat nonanimal protein sources, especially soy. Consider eating one or two meatless meals per week.

If you aren't much of a meat eater, eat smaller amounts of the higher-protein meats or eat more vegetable protein sources. (See Chapter Six: Vegetarian Eating for more information.)

Other Nutrient Needs

Iron is important during the second trimester because the fetus starts to store iron for the future and you continue to need more iron for increased blood volume. Your body needs potassium for nerve impulse transmission. If you vomited a lot during the first trimester, your body may be depleted of potassium. Vitamin C is necessary to produce collagen, a binding substance used in muscle, blood vessels, and nerves. Chromium is a trace mineral used in the regulation of blood sugar, and inadequate intake may contribute to gestational diabetes, which often occurs during the second trimester.

Protein Content of Common Foods

The Dietary Reference Intake (DRI)* for pregnancy is 60 grams; for breastfeeding, 65 grams.

Food	Serving Sizes	Protein (grams†)
Complete Protein Foods		
Turkey, light meat	3 ounces	26
Chicken breast	3 ounces	26
Beef, chuck arm roast	3 ounces	25
Pork, center loin	3 ounces	25
Canned tuna, drained	3 ounces	22
Flounder	3 ounces	21
Beef, ground, extra lean	3 ounces	21
Shrimp	3 ounces	18
Scallops	3 ounces	16
Ham	3 ounces	16
Cottage cheese	½ cup	15
Eggs	2 large	12
Yogurt	1 cup	9–11
Milk, any type	1 cup	8
Cheddar cheese	1 ounce	7
Beef frankfurter, any type	1	6
American cheese, Kraft	1 ounce	5
Quinoa (a high-quality grain)	½ cup	4
Incomplete Protein Foods		
Tofu, firm	½ cup	20
Split-pea soup with ham	1 cup	20
Lentils, cooked	1 cup	18
Miso or tempeh (soy products)	½ cup	16
Garden Chef Hamburger Style Gardenburger	1	14
Green peas	1 cup	9
Peanut butter	2 tablespoons	8
Egg noodles	1 cup	8
Soymilk	1 cup	7
Nuts	1 ounce	6–7
Bulgur, cooked	1 cup	6
Brown rice, cooked	1 cup	5
White rice, cooked	1 cup	4
Whole-wheat bread	1 slice	3

*Formerly known as RDA

†Numbers are rounded to the nearest whole number.

Sources: Pennington, J. *Bowes and Church's Food Values of Portions Commonly Used,* 17th edition. Philadelphia: Lippincott Williams and Wilkins, 1998.

U.S. Department of Agriculture. USDA Nutrient Database for Standard Reference, Release 13, 1999.

Food and Nutrition Board. *Recommended Dietary Allowances.* Revised 1989. Washington, D.C.: National Academy Press, 1998.

The Power of Soy

Soy may just be the health food of the century. Several components of soy—protein, fiber, and phytochemicals (plant substances that are biologically active)—appear to have various benefits:

- Regular consumption of soy foods is linked to reduced risk of breast and rectal cancer.
- Soy protein seems to significantly lower serum cholesterol, low-density-lipoprotein (LDL) cholesterol, and triglycerides.[3] Soy-protein-based diets also significantly lowered cholesterol in children who had hereditary high cholesterol.[4] If high cholesterol runs in your family, eating soy regularly could help keep your cholesterol under control.
- Isoflavones, phytoestrogens found in soy foods, may affect how much calcium is lost from bones—an important consideration for those who have osteoporosis risk factors like family history of osteoporosis and fair skin.[5]

So how do you get soy into your diet? First, leave all preconceived ideas about tofu behind. Tofu is a bit like plain yogurt; it doesn't have much taste on its own. However, tofu will pick up any flavor you decide to give it. Textured vegetable protein (TVP) is dehydrated tofu and is a good substitute for hamburger in sloppy joes, chilies, and soups. Be creative and try some soy in your diet! (See Chapter Six:

Vegetarian Eating and Chapter Fifteen: Menus and Recipes for the Third Trimester for more ideas.)

Focus on Calcium

Calcium is a vital mineral for your baby's bone development. Unfortunately, it's a mineral that adults often delete from their diets when they cut down on dairy products. Although the DRI is 1,000 milligrams,[6] a National Institute of Health Consensus Conference on calcium intake recommended an intake range of 1,200 to 1,500 milligrams per day; 4 to 5 cups of milk contain this amount. Milk and dairy products also provide such important nutrients as protein, magnesium, vitamin D, and riboflavin. If you don't use dairy products, you should consume calcium-fortified products like juices and high-calcium vegetables—and you'll have to eat a lot of them! You should try to get your calcium from food before considering supplements.

Twelve Ways to Sneak Calcium into Your Diet

If you don't like milk, the following foods contain good sources of calcium yet don't taste like milk. If you think creatively, you can sneak calcium into your diet in dozens of ways. Here are just a few ways to increase the calcium in your diet:

1. Make creamy soups (homemade or canned) with milk or evaporated milk.

2. Use evaporated milk, which has twice the calcium, when preparing food like mashed potatoes, pudding, and cream sauces.

3. Eat dairy desserts such as pudding, frozen yogurt, milk shakes, and Berry Mousse Parfait (page 319).

4. Add reduced-fat or fat-free cheese to your mashed potatoes, vegetables, pasta, sandwiches, and sauces. Instead of meat, use low-fat cheese or tofu made with calcium in your lasagna or Spinach-Stuffed Shells (page 362).

5. Eat more corn tortillas! A meal of two bean tostadas contains almost 400 milligrams of calcium.

6. Add molasses to homemade quick breads, cookies, and pancakes (or add it to your mix). Sesame seeds and tahini (sesame-seed paste) are also high in calcium and can be added to snack bars, cakes, vegetables, and dips. (See Favorite Snack Cake, page 367, and Quick and Healthier Pancakes, page 298.)

7. Add nonfat milk powder to prepared soups, prepared muffin and pancake mixes, milk shakes, and cream sauces.

8. Use plain yogurt as a base for salad dressing or veggie dip, or use fruit-flavored yogurt as a sauce for fruit salad or as a dip for fresh fruit.

9. Eat fish with small bones. Salmon Pâté (page 267) contains both salmon and fat-free cream cheese. (Make sure to leave the skin off the salmon.)

10. Prepare Broccoli Quiche (page 350) or egg custard, both of which contain milk. Eat more vegetables that are good sources of calcium.

11. Instead of buying regular orange juice, buy Minute Maid Premium calcium-enriched orange juice. It contains 300 milligrams of calcium in 8 ounces.

12. Use silken tofu as a base for dips, puddings, and salad dressings; use firm tofu as a meat substitute in lasagna and "meatloaf." (See Tofu Loaf, page 363.) Check the label to make sure the tofu has calcium added.

? Questions You May Have

Q: I can't tolerate milk! What can I do?

A: Many African Americans, Asians, Native Americans, and Hispanics have lactose intolerance, meaning they have trouble absorbing and digesting lactose, or milk sugar. The result is uncomfortable gas, stomachaches, and in some cases, diarrhea.

If you have lactose intolerance, don't give up on dairy products! Research shows that as pregnancy progresses, especially in the third trimester, women who are lactose intolerant can break down much more lactose. This may be a compensatory effect, since the body needs large amounts of calcium in the third trimester.[7]

Lactase, the enzyme that is lacking in lactose-intolerant people, can be purchased in drops (to put into milk) or in pills (to take directly before drinking milk). Lactase is sold over the counter in pharmacies under such names as Lactaid, Lactrace, and Dairy Ease. You can also purchase Lactaid milk, which is 2-percent milk with reduced lactose content.

Some lactose-intolerant people can tolerate milk with food, especially with food that contains fiber, such as milk over raisin bran at breakfast.[8] Cocoa may stimulate the body to produce more lactase, thereby increasing the tolerance of chocolate milk or hot cocoa.[9]

I've found that some women tolerate whole milk better than skim or low-fat milk. This may be because the fat slows digestion of the milk and thus improves lactose digestion. For those who can use the extra calories and energy, chocolate milk is an option for increasing calcium in the diet. Other low-lactose dairy options are yogurt, buttermilk, sweet acidophilus milk, and cheese.

If none of these solutions works for you, the last resort is to take a calcium supplement.

Calcium Content of Animal-Based Foods and Beverages

The DRI* for pregnancy and breastfeeding is 1,000 milligrams.

Food	Serving Sizes[†]	Calcium (milligrams)
Carnation Instant Breakfast, any flavor	1 serving with 1 cup 1% milk	500
McDonald's milk shake	1 small	350
Yogurt, fruit-flavored, with nonfat dry milk	1 cup	314
Alba dairy shake mix	1 cup	300
Low-fat milk (1% fat)	1 cup	300
Lactaid milk	1 cup	300
Wendy's Frosty dairy dessert	small	300
Whole milk (3.5% fat)	1 cup	291
Cheese pizza, thin crust	2 slices	290
Buttermilk, cultured	1 cup	285
Chocolate milk (2% fat)	1 cup	284
Swiss cheese	1 ounce	272
Cheddar cheese	1 ounce	204
Salmon, canned with bones	3 ounces	203
Cottage cheese (2% fat)	1 cup	155
Taco Bell Gordita Supreme, steak	1	150
American cheese	1 ounce	150
Taco Bell taco	2 small	140
Kraft macaroni and cheese	1 cup	100
McDonald's reduced-fat ice cream	1 cone	100

*Formerly known as RDA

[†]1 cup = 8 ounces

Sources: Pennington, J. *Bowes and Church's Food Values of Portions Commonly Used*, 17th edition. Philadelphia: Lippincott Williams and Wilkins, 1998.

U.S. Department of Agriculture. USDA Nutrient Database for Standard Reference, Release 13, 1999.

Manufacturers' labels.

Food and Nutrition Board. *Dietary Reference Intakes*, 1999.

Note: See page 250 for fast foods highest in calcium.

(See page 38 for more about calcium supplements.)

Q: What about drinking chocolate milk?

A: Until recently, it was thought that the calcium in chocolate milk was absorbed poorly because of oxalate, another element in the milk. However, now we know that the amount of calcium in chocolate milk is similar to that found in regular milk (284 milligrams in 8 ounces) and also that the amount of calcium absorbed from chocolate milk is similar to that absorbed from whole milk, yogurt, and cheese.[10]

Another concern about drinking chocolate milk has been its caffeine content. You'll be happy to know that 8 ounces of chocolate milk contains only 5 milligrams of caffeine—or about the amount found in 5 ounces of decaffeinated coffee. If you prefer chocolate milk to white milk and can afford the calories (179 calories for 8 ounces

Calcium Content of Vegetarian Foods and Beverages

The DRI* for pregnancy and breastfeeding is 1,000 milligrams.

Food[†]	Serving Sizes[‡]	Calcium (milligrams)
Agar (a product made from algae), dried	3½ ounces	625
Collard greens	1 cup	358
Rhubarb, frozen, cooked	1 cup	348
Blackstrap molasses	2 tablespoons	344
Orange juice, calcium-fortified	1 cup	300
White Wave soymilk, chocolate or vanilla	1 cup	300
Spinach, frozen, boiled[§]	1 cup	278
Firm tofu made with calcium sulfate (a processing agent)	4 ounces	200+ (varies)
Turnip greens, fresh, boiled	1 cup	198
Kale, frozen, cooked	1 cup	180
Okra	1 cup	177
Sesame seeds	2 tablespoons	176
Kombu (a sea vegetable), raw	3½ ounces	168
Mustard greens, frozen, boiled	1 cup	152
Wakame (a sea vegetable), raw	3½ ounces	150
Tortillas, corn	2	90
Nori (a product made from algae), raw	3½ ounces	58

*Formerly known as RDA

†Foods are cooked unless otherwise noted.

‡1 cup = 8 ounces

§Spinach contains oxalates, which can significantly cut down on calcium absorption.

Sources: Pennington, J. Bowes and Church's Food Values of Portions Commonly Used, 17th edition. Philadelphia: Lippincott Williams and Wilkins, 1998.

U.S. Department of Agriculture. USDA Nutrient Database for Standard Reference, Release 13, 1999.

Manufacturer's labels.

Food and Nutrition Board. Dietary Reference Intakes, 1999.

of 2-percent chocolate milk compared to 120 calories for 8 ounces of plain 2-percent milk), then drink and enjoy!

Q: Doesn't my prenatal vitamin have enough calcium?

A: No, even though the pill is big. If it did contain all the calcium needed, you *really* wouldn't be able to swallow it! Most prenatal vitamins contain only a small percentage of the DRI for calcium. You must obtain the majority of calcium you need from your diet.

▼

Focus on Iron

Sometime between the twenty-fourth and twenty-eighth week, your health-care provider will probably test your blood again for iron-deficiency anemia, a somewhat common problem during pregnancy. Because your blood volume increases up to 50 percent, you need twice as much iron as you needed before you were pregnant.

Iron Content of Animal-Based Foods

The DRI* for pregnancy is 30 milligrams; for breastfeeding, 15 milligrams.

Food[†]	Serving Sizes	Iron (milligrams)[‡]
Clams	3 ounces	24
Oysters, Pacific (also a great source of zinc)	3 ounces	8
Mussels	3 ounces	6
Chili with meat[§]	1 cup	2–5
Roast beef sandwich	1	4
Stuffed green pepper with beef and crumbs[§]	1	4
Spaghetti and meatballs with tomato sauce[§]	1 cup	4
Shrimp	3 ounces	3
Egg McMuffin	1	3
Green pepper steak[§]	10 ounces	3
Beef and vegetable stew[§]	1 cup	3
Cheeseburger, Burger King	1	3
Lasagna with meat sauce	1 cup	2–3
Bass, freshwater	3 ounces	2
Chicken breast	3 ounces	1

*Formerly known as RDA
[†]Foods are cooked, as applicable, unless otherwise noted.
[‡]Numbers are rounded to the nearest whole number.
[§]Also contains a significant amount of vitamin C, which helps absorption of iron.

Sources: Pennington, J. *Bowes and Church's Food Values of Portions Commonly Used*, 17th edition. Philadelphia: Lippincott Williams and Wilkins, 1998.

Food and Nutrition Board. *Recommended Dietary Allowances*. Revised 1989. Washington, D.C.: National Academy Press, 1998.

Knowing a few things about iron will help you prevent anemia and improve your iron status if you are anemic.

Iron is best absorbed from animal sources such as beef, eggs, and so on. If you are not a big meat eater, combine a small amount of animal protein with vegetable protein. This helps you absorb more iron from vegetable foods. For example, mix a small amount of ham with your pinto beans, or chop a hard-boiled egg into your cooked spinach or spinach salad.

You can also increase the amount of iron your body absorbs from food by eating a vitamin C food along with it. For example, have an orange, some melon, or berries for dessert after a meal, or have raw or cooked tomatoes, tomato juice, broccoli, cabbage, greens, cauliflower, or bell pepper as your veggie. Or, drink citrus juice, vegetable or tomato juice, or vitamin-C-fortified apple juice with your meal.

Factors that inhibit iron absorption are:

Iron Content of Vegetarian Foods

The DRI* for pregnancy is 30 milligrams; for breastfeeding, 15 milligrams.

Food[†]	Serving Sizes	Iron (milligrams)[‡]
Quinoa (a grain)	1 cup	16
Tofu, firm	½ cup	13
Soybeans	1 cup	9
Blackstrap molasses	2 tablespoons	7
Black or navy beans, canned	1 cup	5
Pinto beans, canned	1 cup	4
Chickpeas (garbanzo beans), canned	1 cup	3
Prune juice	8 ounces	3
Spinach[§]	1 cup	3
Potato[§]	1 medium	3
Peas, frozen, boiled	1 cup	3
Soy yogurt, plain	1 cup	3
Figs, dried	5 medium	2
Bulgur	1 cup	2
Raisins	⅔ cup	2
Pumpkin, canned	½ cup	2
Green beans or broccoli[§]	1 cup	1
Tomato or vegetable juice[§]	8 ounces	1

*Formerly known as RDA

[†]Foods are cooked, as applicable, unless otherwise noted.

[‡]Numbers are rounded to the nearest whole number.

[§]Also contains a significant amount of vitamin C, which helps absorption of iron.

Sources: Pennington, J. *Bowes and Church's Food Values of Portions Commonly Used*, 17th edition. Philadelphia: Lippincott Williams and Wilkins, 1998.

Food and Nutrition Board. *Recommended Dietary Allowances*. Revised 1989. Washington, D.C.: National Academy Press. 1998.

- Coffee
- Tea
- Calcium supplements
- Antacids
- Dairy products
- Soy protein
- Wheat bran
- Fiber

Factors that aid iron absorption are:

- Vitamin C. Vitamin C foods include tomato, greens, cabbage, citrus, peppers, pineapple, mango, and papaya.
- Cooking with an iron skillet. The iron content of about 3 ounces of spaghetti sauce increases from 3 milligrams to 87 milligrams of iron when cooked in an unenameled iron skillet.[11]

▼

"Thrive on Five"

The National Cancer Institute uses the slogans "Thrive on Five" and "Five a Day for Better Health" to encourage Americans to eat more fruits and vegetables. Why? Fruits and vegetables are great sources of vitamins, minerals, and fiber. All plant foods also contain phytochemicals, biologically active substances that are widely believed to have many beneficial effects on health, such as prevention of cancer and heart disease.

The great thing about filling up on fruits and vegetables is that when you do so, you are less likely to eat chips, cookies, and other less-nutrient-dense foods. Try to eat a variety of fruits and vegetables from day to day.

Do you think that five fruits and vegetables per day sounds like a lot of food? Here are a few easy tips for adding fruits and vegetables to your meals:

Breakfast

▶ **Add mashed banana, dried fruit, or applesauce to pancake batter.**

Top pancakes and waffles with strawberries or other fresh fruit.

▶ **Whip up a fruit shake. (See pages 282–287 for recipes.)**

▶ **Add dried fruit, peaches, strawberries, blueberries, bananas, or other fresh fruit to your cereal.**

▶ **Eat a fruit or drink some juice before you have anything else.**

▶ **If you eat omelets, add tomatoes, mushrooms, and red or green peppers.**

Lunch

▶ **Add apple, raisins, pineapple, mango, or mandarin orange slices to your chicken, tuna, or tossed salad.**

▶ **Have a salad or raw veggies before your meal.**

Use darker greens, such as romaine or leaf lettuce or spinach, for your salads.

▶ **Drink vegetable or tomato juice before or with your meal.**

▶ **Add leaf lettuce, thinly sliced cucumber, finely shredded cabbage,** or spinach and tomatoes to your sandwiches.

▶ Stuff leftover veggies or salad in a pita pocket with cheese.

▶ To save time, buy ready-to-eat salads, carrots, broccoli, and so on. Talk about fast food!

Dinner

▶ Do a stir-fry for dinner. You can even buy the vegetables cleaned, chopped, and ready to go!

▶ Zip up your spaghetti sauce with bell pepper, zucchini, carrots, or eggplant.

Shred or chop these vegetables finely and they will cook quickly. If you have picky children at home, you can purée the cooked vegetables. Your kids will never know the veggies are there!

▶ Use puréed roasted red pepper or another vegetable as the base for a sauce. (See page 364 for recipe.)

▶ Start dinner with a vegetable-based soup, such as minestrone or gazpacho. (See page 300 for recipe.)

▶ Make a fruit salsa to accompany your grilled chicken or seafood. (See page 352 for recipe.)

▶ Make an appetizer of oven-fried zucchini sticks or eggplant slices. (See page 274 for recipe.)

Dessert

▶ A mixed fresh fruit salad makes a great finish.

▶ Top angel food or pound cake with fresh or canned fruit.

▶ Make a fruit shake with frozen strawberries, raspberries, and milk. (See page 287 for recipe.)

▶ Try a fruit sorbet.

▶ Have a frozen yogurt layered with fruit.

▶ Munch on a frozen banana or frozen grapes.

▶ Top off a grilled dinner with grilled fruit kebabs.

▶ Dip strawberries in a yogurt dip or chocolate sauce. (Everyone needs an occasional splurge!)

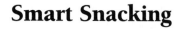

Smart Snacking

When I ask my clients if they snack, they usually look embarrassed. You would think *snack* is a four-letter word. Most people think of snacking as eating foods they shouldn't or cheating. Actually, snacking can be healthy, and it's a must during pregnancy. Snacking helps you get all the nutrients you need when you can't eat much at a meal. It also gives you more energy during those times when baby seems to be sapping it all.

What Are the Best Snacks?

The best snacks are those that offer the most nutrition per calorie. Fruits and vegetables are tops; they offer lots of nutrition, virtually no fat, and few calories. Their fiber and fluid content are additional benefits.

The Center for Science in the Public Interest, publisher of *Nutrition Action Healthletter,* recently published a list of the healthiest fruits, based on their nutrient and fiber content. Here are the top fifteen: papaya, cantaloupe, strawberries, oranges, tangerines, kiwis, mangos, apricots, persimmons, watermelon, raspberries, red or pink grapefruit, blackberries, dried apricots, and white grapefruit.[12] Don't despair if your favorite fruit isn't on this list; just try to include the above fruits more often to get the most nutrition.

The second category on our list of good snacks is other high-carbohydrate foods. These also provide energy, little fat, and contain fiber. Of course, they also taste good! Third on our list are dairy and protein food combinations. Try to eat a variety of snacks during the day. Here are some ideas to get you started:

Healthy Snacks

Fruits and Vegetables
- Dried or fresh fruit (Since dried fruits are concentrated, they are a great source of vitamins, minerals, and fiber. You can also keep them in your purse or desk drawer.)
- Raw vegetables (You can buy them ready to eat and keep them in your refrigerator.)

At Last, Low-Fat Chips

As I write this, I'm snacking on tortilla chips that aren't fried—and they taste great! Guiltless Gourmet Inc. did what was thought to be impossible: They made tortilla chips, as well as black bean and pinto bean dips, salsas, and queso dips, without added fat! One ounce of chips also provides 80 milligrams of calcium. Other baked chips are also available: Baked Tostitos, Baked Lay's, and many other brands. It is better to eat naturally low-fat chips than those made with Olestra (a fat substitute) while you are pregnant.

- Leftover vegetables (Heat them up for a healthy snack.)
- Fruit or vegetable juice, fruit juice mixed with club soda, or a fruit smoothie

High-Carbohydrate Foods
- Health Valley Granola Bars (I like these because they are sweetened with fruit and are high in fiber.)
- Dehydrated bean soup in a cup
- Raisin bran or other high-fiber cereal
- Rice or popcorn cakes (For a sweet tooth, Quaker Caramel Corn Popcorn Cakes are my favorite!)
- Popcorn (Choose the one with the least fat, or pop your own.)
- Rye or wheat crackers
- Graham crackers
- Fig Newtons

• Guiltless Gourmet No Oil Tortilla Chips, Baked Tostitos, or other baked chips with salsa

Dairy Foods

• Milk
• Yogurt
• Low-fat cheese
• Dip made with cottage cheese or fat-free cream cheese
• Milk shake made with fresh fruit (See pages 282–287 for yogurt shakes.)

High-Protein Snacks

Add protein foods for a big appetite. Eating a snack that contains protein before you go to bed at night can prevent low blood sugar in the morning.

• Peanut butter on crackers or with banana or apple
• Whole-grain cereal with milk
• Cheese and apple
• Tortilla rolled up with ham and cheese or with refried beans and cheese
• Yogurt with grape nuts or granola
• Cottage cheese and fruit
• Fat-free cheese on celery, carrots, and broccoli
• Tortilla chips and fat-free refried beans

See page 261 for lots more snack ideas!

▼

Second-Trimester Challenges

Vaginal Discharge

Increased discharge is considered normal during pregnancy. It is usually whitish and is the result of an increased supply of blood and glucose to the vaginal walls and increased production of mucus by the endo-cervical glands. The acid level of your mucus changes during pregnancy, making you more susceptible to vaginal infections. If you have severe itching, irritation, or a foul odor, contact your health-care provider.

What You Can Do:

▶ **Continue to bathe daily.**

▶ **Wear cotton underwear.**

▶ **Avoid feminine deodorants, powders, and bubble baths.**

Constipation

Progesterone, a pregnancy hormone, slows down the movement of food in your intestine, causing more water and nutrients to be absorbed, and constipation is often the result. The pressure of the growing baby on your intestines and rectum can also cause this problem. An iron supplement can further worsen it.

What You Can Do:

▶ **Drink plenty of fluids—at least 8 to 10 glasses daily, mostly from water.**

▶ **Eat high-fiber foods. Eating at least five fruits and vegetables per day will keep constipation away! (See page 53, "Focus on Fiber.")**

▶ **Exercise regularly.**

▶ **Avoid foods that cause constipation. Some people are constipated when they eat certain foods, such as cheese or bananas.**

▶ **Avoid caffeine, since it can cause a loss of even more fluid, which can make the stools hard.**

Hemorrhoids

Hemorrhoids are swollen or enlarged veins in the rectum. Hormones once again play a role in this problem, as does straining during a bowel movement. As the baby grows, greater pressure from the uterus displaces intestines, which can lead to constipation and then hemorrhoids.

What You Can Do:

▶ **Prevent constipation.**

▶ **Discuss hemorrhoids with your health-care provider.**

Your health-care provider may advise a stool softener or high-fiber laxative such as Metamucil. If you do take a stool softener, keep in mind that it can take as long as three

days to work. Don't take more than one type of stool softener at the same time.

▶ **DON'T take over-the-counter laxatives, stool softeners, or hemorrhoid treatments without your health-care provider's approval.**

▶ **Taking warm baths and sitting on soft pillows can relieve the pressure.**

▶ **Avoid heavy lifting, pushing, and standing for long periods of time.**

Stress

We all live with stress. If you don't manage your stress, it can lead to chronic medical problems such as ulcers and heart disease. Pregnancy offers its own special stresses. Just wondering whether you are doing all the right things for your baby is a stress. You may be debating whether to work after you have the baby or preparing another child for your new arrival. You may be trying to figure out how you'll pay for the delivery or all those baby things you'll need to buy. And pregnancy hormones can bring mood swings, causing you to cope less effectively with stress.

According to the March of Dimes, some studies show that extreme stress can play a role in low birth weight.

What You Can Do:

▶ **Set realistic goals.**

You probably can't physically do what you did before pregnancy. You must put yourself first; take more time for rest, exercise, and planning and preparing healthy meals. Pare down your busy schedule if necessary.

▶ **Use relaxation techniques such as biofeedback and meditation.**

Many audio- and videotapes with relaxing music and scenery are available, and these can help you take a mental vacation. A daily walk can also relieve stress and help you put things in perspective.

▶ **Try to find support in your partner, friends, and coworkers or on the internet.**

Other new moms or moms-to-be will be especially empathetic. Remember that your partner will also be feeling stress and will probably need support, too. Below are some internet pregnancy resources that you may find helpful:

www.babysoon.com
www.pregnancyguideonline.com
www.pregnancycalendar.com
www.fitpregnancy.com
www.epregnancy.com

Food Planning for the Second Trimester

Most women feel their best during the second trimester. Your appetite may be robust, and you may feel like spending more time in the kitchen. The menus listed below and detailed in Chapter Fourteen are a bit heavier than those I've recommended for the first trimester, and some of the recipes require more preparation.

Menus

• A Month of Breakfast Ideas
• Menus for a Hungry Appetite
• I Could Cook All Day
• Company's Coming!

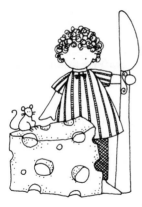

CHAPTER FIVE

The Third Trimester

The third trimester is an important time for many reasons. It's the homestretch of your pregnancy, a time when you will be completing preparations for your baby's arrival. Likewise, your baby will be growing rapidly to prepare for its birth into the world.

How Baby Is Growing

Your baby is now rapidly filling your uterus. With less elbow room, the baby will be turning flips less often. You might, however, feel rhythmic movements. These are hiccups!

At the End of Twenty-Eight Weeks (Seven Months)

A baby born at this time is considered able to live outside the uterus, though its lungs are still not mature. Your baby did a lot of growing in the last month and should weigh between 2½ and 3 pounds. It is 14 to 17 inches long. Baby is now storing calcium, and its bones are hardening. Many babies now find they fit better upside down and start to position themselves for birth. Your health-care provider can determine if your baby is positioned head down.

At the End of Thirty-Two Weeks (Eight Months)

All your baby needs to do now is develop lung surfactant (which enables the lungs to inflate and deflate properly) and store some fat. Baby is beginning to store minerals such as iron, calcium, and phosphorus. The kicks are strong and vigorous, and many women can feel a heel, fist, or elbow through their abdomen. Your baby now weighs between 4½ and 5 pounds and is between 16½ and 18 inches long.

What you will find in this chapter:
- *How Baby Is Growing*
- *Weight Gain and Energy Needs*
- *Other Nutrient Needs*
- *Focus on Vitamin B₆ and Zinc*
- *What about Sugar?*
- *Tips for Keeping Your Energy Up*
- *Third-Trimester Challenges*
- *Food Planning for the Third Trimester*

This chapter answers such questions as:
- *What if I have gained too much weight?*
- *I feel so tired; what can I do?*
- *What can I do for heartburn?*
- *I can't sleep; any advice?*
- *I have backaches and swollen ankles. Help!*

At the End of Thirty-Six Weeks (Nine Months)

Baby is now making great strides in growth and is gaining close to ½ pound per week. The bones in the head are soft and ready for delivery. Lanugo and vernix are disappearing. Fat deposits under the skin help fill out the body and eliminate the wrinkling of the skin. Baby will settle lower into your pelvis and may seem to slow its activity. However, you should still feel your baby move at least ten times in a twelve-hour period. If you don't, contact your health-care provider.

At the End of Forty Weeks (Ten Months)

Your baby is not considered full-term until thirty-eight weeks. At this time, the baby has a well established sleeping pattern and individual styles of responses. The baby will continue to gain weight until the time of delivery. These last few weeks can be tiring as you wait for the arrival of your new little one.

▼

Weight Gain and Energy Needs

During the last trimester you will probably gain a large proportion of your total pregnancy weight. Just when you think you cannot gain another pound or expand your belly another inch, you do! Remember that as you prepare for the baby's arrival, you still need to eat well and make wise food choices.

You should continue to gain about a pound a week during this time. Remember that if you are overweight or underweight, your weight gain should be adjusted accordingly. If you find that you have exceeded your goal weight already, discuss this with your health-care provider. He or she will still want you to continue gaining weight, but perhaps at a slower rate. Never try to lose weight while pregnant, no matter how much weight you have gained. Your baby needs you to eat adequately so that it can grow and develop enough to survive on its own in our world.

In the third trimester many women find that their get-up-and-go got up and went. Regular exercise (even a simple walk around the block) will improve your endurance and keep you from feeling like a couch potato. If you find that you are much less active now, you may not need the entire 300 extra calories I recommended earlier for the second and third trimesters. However, you still need all the added nutrients, so if you do cut down on food intake, you must make your food choices with even more care.

On the other hand, you may find that with your baby's arrival just around the corner, you have renewed energy! You may need to increase your calories. (See page 263 for high-energy snack ideas.)

As your due date gets closer, you might consider getting more of your calories from complex carbohydrates. Competitive athletes often load up on carbohydrates before a big event. Labor and delivery constitute such an event! Building up your store of carbohydrate may give you a bit more energy for labor.

Weighing In

Are you one of those weight-conscious women who weigh themselves daily? Don't! Although being aware of your weight is a good idea, during the third trimester you are more prone to water retention and fluctuations in weight gain. So when you panic, thinking you've gained a pound in two days, the weight gain may simply be a result of water retention. Develop a healthy attitude about weight by weighing yourself just once a week at the same time of day under the same conditions. This will give you a truer idea of how your weight gain is progressing.

Note: If you do find that you have gained 2 or more pounds in two days; notice extreme swelling in your hands, face, or feet; or have headaches or vision trouble, notify your health-care provider. This may be a sign of preeclampsia. (See page 128 for more information.)

▼

Other Nutrient Needs

Your need for vitamins and minerals during the third trimester remains essentially the same as during the second trimester. Calcium is important during the third trimester for the laying down of calcium in the baby's bones. Brain development during the third trimester makes zinc a key nutrient. Zinc is critical throughout pregnancy, and a deficiency is related to premature delivery and many other problems. Vitamin B_6, essential for the use of protein, is necessary for the building of tissues, including brain and muscle tissue. B_6 is needed in proportion to the protein in your diet; the more protein you eat, the more B_6 you need. Also important for brain development are omega-3 fatty acids, primarily found in cold-water fish such as salmon and tuna. Try to eat fish at least once or twice a week.

Keep in mind that certain water-soluble vitamins such as thiamin, riboflavin, and niacin are required in amounts relative to your calorie intake. Thus, if you increase your calories, make sure your diet contains foods rich in these vitamins. Women who follow strict vegetarian diets (no animal protein) should take a vitamin B_{12} supplement of 2.6 micrograms per day.[1]

Research data shows that pregnant women's diets do not meet the Dietary Reference Intakes (DRIs) for vitamin B_6, vitamin D, vitamin E, folate, iron, zinc, calcium, and magnesium.[2] How does your diet stack up? Answer "yes" or "no" to the following questions.

1. I eat a variety of foods daily.
2. I eat an orange or dark green vegetable daily.
3. I eat a citrus fruit or another fruit or vegetable high in vitamin C daily.
4. I eat two to three servings of protein food daily.
5. I eat a variety of protein sources, including plant proteins.
6. I eat three servings of whole grains almost every day.
7. I eat six fruits and vegetables on most days.

8. I eat four servings of dairy products or high-calcium food daily.
9. I am gaining about 1 pound per week.
10. I avoid caffeine, alcohol, and drugs.

If you answered "yes" to seven or more questions, you're doing pretty well. Fewer than that? Well, you know what you need to work on.

▼

Focus on Vitamin B₆ and Zinc

Vitamin B_6 is necessary for many reactions in the body, namely building protein from amino acids and forming hemoglobin and neurotransmitters in the brain. Women usually don't have enough B_6 in their diets. Most recently, however, vitamin B_6 has made the news with the discovery that adequate amounts of B_6 help decrease blood levels of homocysteine, an amino acid that increases the risk of heart disease.

The more protein in your diet, the more B_6 you need. (Luckily, high-protein foods are good sources of vitamin B_6.) Also, women who take birth control pills seem to need more of the vitamin. If you have recently been taking birth control pills, try to have extra B_6 in your diet. Remember that vitamin B_6 is water-soluble and can be destroyed by cooking and processing.

Zinc performs many functions during pregnancy; it is necessary for conception, for every phase of growth, and for the immune system. Zinc even helps to ensure that your

Good Sources of B₆		

The DRI* for pregnancy is 1.9 milligrams; for breastfeeding, 2.0 milligrams.

Food	Serving Sizes†	B₆ (milligrams)
Animal Sources		
Chicken, light meat	3 ounces	.51
Pork loin	3 ounces	.34
Ham	3 ounces	.34
Halibut	3 ounces	.34
Tuna, light	3 ounces	.29
Vegetable Sources		
Chickpeas, canned	1 cup	1.14
Sweet potato, mashed	1 cup	.80
Potato, baked with skin	1 medium	.70
Banana	1 medium	.66
Prune juice	1 cup	.56
Bran flakes	⅔ cup (1 ounce)	.50
Soybeans	1 cup	.40
Lentils	1 cup	.35
Brown rice, medium	1 cup	.29
Wheat germ, toasted	¼ cup	.28
Pinto beans	1 cup	.275
Dates, dried	10	.16

*Formerly known as RDA

†Values represent cooked foods, as applicable.

Sources: Pennington, J. *Bowes and Church's Food Values of Portions Commonly Used*, 17th edition. Philadelphia: Lippincott Williams Wilkins, 1998.

Food and Nutrition Board. *Dietary Reference Intakes*, 1999.

baby is not premature. Low zinc intake has been related to neural tube defects and other birth defects. Unfortunately, zinc is a mineral that nonpregnant women often don't get enough of. High-fiber diets can interfere

Good Sources of Zinc

The DRI* for pregnancy is 15 milligrams; for breastfeeding, 19 milligrams.

Food	Serving Sizes†	Zinc, (milligrams)
Animal Sources		
Oysters, fried	3 ounces	74
Chuck arm pot roast	3 ounces	7.4
Crab, Alaskan	3 ounces	6.5
Prime rib	3 ounces	6.0
Veal roast, sirloin	3 ounces	4.0
Lamb chop, lean	3 ounces	2.8
Lobster	3 ounces	2.5
Pork roast, rump	3 ounces	2.4
Clams	3 ounces	2.3
Shrimp	3 ounces	1.3
Vegetable Sources		
Wheat germ, toasted	¼ cup	4.8
Chickpeas, canned	1 cup	2.5
Green peas, frozen	1 cup	1.5
Bran flakes	1 ounce	1.5
Bran muffin	1 medium	1.5
Spinach	1 cup	1.4

*Formerly known as RDA

†Values represent cooked foods, as applicable.

Sources: Pennington, J. *Bowes and Church's Food Values of Portions Commonly Used*, 17th edition. Philadelphia: Lippincott Williams and Wilkins, 1998.

Food and Nutrition Board. *Recommended Dietary Allowances*. Revised 1989. Washington, D.C.: National Academy Press, 1998.

with absorption of zinc. Beef and shellfish are generally rich in zinc; vegetarian women need to eat plenty of zinc-rich legumes and whole grains.

▼

What about Sugar?

Sugar has gotten a lot of bad press over the years. Many myths are still circulating about sugar. Here are the facts:

- Sugar doesn't cause diabetes, though it does cause the body to produce more insulin in order to use the sugar. This happens with any carbohydrate food, but the effect is more pronounced with simple sugars.

- Sugar doesn't appear to cause hyperactivity. A review of twenty-three studies showed that sugar had no effects on either behavior or cognitive performance. In fact, sugar has been shown to have a calming effect on newborns in pain.[3] The increased activity of children who have consumed sugar may often be caused by the accompanying caffeine, as in a cola. Another explanation may be that the settings in which children usually eat a lot of sugar, such as birthday parties and Halloween outings, promote increased activity. However, individual reactions to any food are possible.

- Sugar does cause tooth decay, as do many other carbohydrate foods.

- Americans have increased their calorie intake in recent years, and most of the extra calories come from added sugars. It is estimated that nearly one-quarter of our daily calories come from added sugar—mainly from soft drinks. Since high-sugar foods are often low-nutrient foods, they can have a negative impact on the overall diet. *Dietary Guidelines for Americans 2000* recommends choosing foods and beverages that limit sugar intake.[4]

▼

Tips for Keeping Your Energy Up

You may have heard that the third trimester (especially the last month) is a real challenge. You feel as though you can't possibly get bigger. Getting out of your chair or bed (especially if you have a waterbed) is sometimes tough, and your energy level may need a boost. On the other hand, many women feel great and enjoy sudden bursts of energy (often called the nesting syndrome) when they want to get everything done. The following tips will help you feel your best during the last months of pregnancy.

▶ **Put up your feet from time to time.**

Some swelling in the feet and legs is considered normal during the last few months. Keep in mind that the extra 20 to 30 pounds you are now carrying are putting a lot of pressure on your legs, knees, and feet. Wear flat, supportive shoes; support hose may also be a good idea.

▶ **Take catnaps at lunch if you can,** *after* **you've eaten.**

I remember taking several naps on my boss's couch during lunch when I was pregnant.

Baby Pick-Me-Up: A High-Energy Drink
(2 servings)

1 frozen or ½ cup canned peach or nectarine (Freeze for 45 minutes or more.)

½ banana

½ cup frozen strawberries

1 cup low-fat vanilla yogurt or 1 cup milk plus sweetener to taste

2 tablespoons nonfat dry milk

Combine all ingredients in blender. Makes approximately 2 cups. If you don't have frozen fruit, adding ice to desired consistency will increase the volume.

Nutrient analysis per serving:

274 calories

8 grams protein

6 grams fiber

2 grams fat

Percentage of DRI* for pregnancy:

46% vitamin C

23% vitamin B$_{12}$ and calcium

29% potassium

* Formerly known as RDA

▶ **Let the housework go!**

It's good practice for the first few months with baby. Start putting your feelings first and the housework second. Do only what has to be done (laundry, for example) or enlist the help of your partner or children.

▶ **Don't forget those in-between snacks– they help boost your energy.**

Keep a snack stash in your drawer: peanut-butter crackers, raisins, dried figs, prunes, apricots, graham crackers, and granola bars.

▶ **Keep up with your exercise program.**

Exercise is probably the last thing you want to do when you feel tired, but it really will help in the long run. I don't like to swim very much, but when I attended a water exercise class for pregnant women, I loved it. You feel weightless in the water–and that is a nice feeling! After a long workday, being in the water can be very refreshing.

▼

Third-Trimester Challenges

Backache

As pregnancy progresses and the uterus enlarges, spine curvature increases. Also, hormones cause the pelvic joints to loosen. You may notice that the way you walk is a bit different than before you were pregnant. This may be due to loosening of joints and an adjustment in posture to compensate for carrying a big load out front.

What You Can Do:

▶ **Practice good body mechanics and posture.**

▶ **Avoid bending over and lifting heavy objects (including children, if possible).**

Bend at the knees and keep your back straight.

▶ **Wear low-heeled shoes.**

▶ **Learn to do pelvic tilts; they will relieve pressure on your back and stretch and tone your muscles.**

Ask your health-care provider or childbirth educator for instructions, or see page 195.

▶ **Bend your knees slightly when standing in place.**

Edema (Swelling)

Many women experience ankle swelling in the last trimester because blood and fluid circulation (between the heart and the lower extremities) becomes more and more difficult. Let your health-care provider know if you have swelling in your hands or face; this could be a sign of preeclampsia.

What You Can Do:

▶ **Elevate your legs to the level of your hips as often as possible.**

▶ **Avoid standing for long periods of time.**

▶ **If you must sit for long periods, try to stand up, stretch, and move around a bit to improve circulation.**

▶ **Avoid anything that will restrict circulation: stockings with tight bands, tight slips or pants, tight knee-highs, and so on.**

▶ **Don't restrict fluid intake!**

Heartburn

As the baby grows, it compresses your stomach, leaving minimal space for food. The hormones that slow down your digestion also relax the sphincter muscle that keeps food in your stomach. These changes cause stomach acid to back up into your esophagus, causing a burning sensation that feels as though it's around your heart.

What You Can Do:

▶ **Eat small, frequent meals.**

▶ **Stay away from gassy, spicy, and greasy foods.**

▶ **Don't overeat.**

▶ **Stand or walk around after eating, instead of lying down immediately after a meal.**

▶ **Keep your head slightly elevated when you're in bed.**

▶ **Cut down on caffeine; it causes heartburn for some women.**

▶ **Wear comfortable clothes.**

▶ **Talk with your doctor before using antacids; some contain sodium bicarbonate, which may interfere with absorption of some nutrients.**

Sleepless Nights

As your body gets larger, you may find that getting comfortable in bed is quite a chore. The baby kicking, heartburn, and anxiety about the arrival of the new person in your life can add to sleeplessness.

What You Can Do:

▶ **Try a bedtime ritual: warm bath, decaffeinated mint tea or warm milk, and soft jazz or easy-listening music.**

▶ **Support yourself with pillows.**

One new mom says, "Our bed was a virtual oasis of pillows! I used two behind me to support my back, one between my knees to relieve back pressure, and one for my head."

▶ **Practice the relaxation and breathing techniques that you learned in childbirth class.**

▶ **Continue regular exercise; it has a calming effect and can help with insomnia.**

Another new mom shares, "My husband and I enjoyed a leisurely walk every evening after dinner. It gave us quiet time to talk and helped me sleep better at night. Of course we always had other things we could do, such as cleaning the house or paying bills, but we made our walk together a priority."

Food Planning for the Third Trimester

The main problems with eating during the last months of pregnancy are:

1. You get full quickly.

2. Fatigue may prevent you from wanting to cook.

3. Heartburn may restrict the variety or amount of food you eat.

4. You may be so busy getting ready for the baby that you neglect your own nutrition needs.

5. You may be trying to cut food expenses to accommodate costly necessities for your baby.

The third-trimester menus in this book are designed with the above in mind. Look over the list that follows and refer to Chapter Fifteen for details.

Now is a good time to prepare some foods to freeze for those first few days or weeks with your new baby.

Menus

• Using Leftovers with Flair
• Meals in Minutes
• Feel Full Menus
• Best Bite Snacks
• Vegetarian Budget Menus

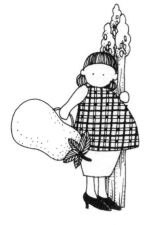

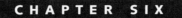

CHAPTER SIX

Vegetarian Eating

What you will find in this chapter:

- *Vegetarians: The Healthy Minority*
- *The Pregnant Vegetarian*
- *Nutrients of Special Concern*
- *The Eating Expectantly Vegetarian Eating Plan*
- *Vegetarian Shopping List*
- *Vegetarian Food Planning*
- *Eating Out Vegetarian-Style*
- *Vegetarian Convenience-Food Choices*
- *Eating after Delivery*

This chapter answers such questions as:

- *How can I get enough calcium in my diet if I'm vegetarian?*
- *I'm diabetic; how do vegetarian foods fit into my diet?*
- *How can I get vitamin B_{12} in my diet if it is only found in animal foods?*
- *Must I buy special vegetarian foods to have a good diet?*

Vegetarian eating is on the rise as more people realize the benefits of eating plant proteins. (See Chapter Four for more on soy protein.) Even if you just "lean" toward vegetarian eating, you can receive many of the same health benefits.

Most people eat some vegetarian foods without even thinking about it. The teen who picks up a bean burrito is doing it, the parent who makes pasta with marinara sauce and cheese is doing it, and of course the vegan who eats no animal products is doing it, too. People eat vegetarian for a variety of reasons: because eating vegetarian is healthy, because they're concerned about the environment or animal rights, or simply because vegetarian food is tasty and cheap.

The Food Guide Pyramid depicts a healthy eating pattern for everyone. What many people don't realize is that a vegetarian

Food Guide Pyramid
Suggested Daily Servings

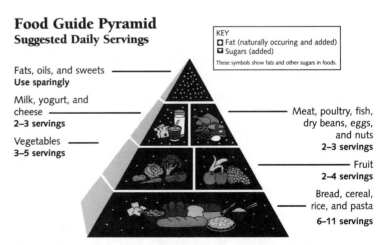

KEY
☐ Fat (naturally occuring and added)
☑ Sugars (added)
These symbols show fats and other sugars in foods.

Fats, oils, and sweets — **Use sparingly**

Milk, yogurt, and cheese — **2–3 servings**

Vegetables — **3–5 servings**

Meat, poultry, fish, dry beans, eggs, and nuts — **2–3 servings**

Fruit — **2–4 servings**

Bread, cereal, rice, and pasta — **6–11 servings**

Source: U.S. Department of Agriculture/U.S. Department of Health and Human Services.

diet (based on grains, fruits, and vegetables, with smaller amounts of protein, dairy, fat, and sugar) exemplifies this eating pattern.

▼

Vegetarians: The Healthy Minority

Many people would like to have the health records that vegetarians have. Vegetarians have lower body mass index (BMI), lower cholesterol, and lower risk of heart disease than meat eaters have. They may also have lower risk of constipation, diverticular disease (an intestinal condition), gallstones, and appendicitis.[1] It appears that vegetarians are also less likely to have adult-onset diabetes, cancer, and high blood pressure.[2] Research shows that a low-fat vegetarian diet along with stress management and exercise can actually reverse coronary heart disease.[3] Vegetarians are generally closer to their ideal body weights than are nonvegetarians. Some studies show that vegetarians have lower rates of osteoporosis, cancer, kidney stones, gallstones, and diverticular disease.

Good genes? Not necessarily. Most vegetarian diets are low in saturated fat and thus can prevent high cholesterol levels and heart disease. Vegetarians eat many fruits and vegetables; this increases their intake of healthy phytochemicals and fiber, both of which are thought to be cancer fighters. Lacto-ovo vegetarians have adequate calcium in their diet, which may be protective against colon cancer. Vegetarians may also have beneficial lifestyle habits that contribute to good health, such as regular exercise and abstinence from tobacco and alcohol. Maintaining ideal body weight can reduce the risk of heart disease, high blood pressure, and diabetes.

The position of the American Dietetic Association states, "Appropriately planned vegetarian diets are healthful, are nutritionally adequate, and provide health benefits in the prevention and treatment of certain diseases."[4] The key word here is *planned*. Even a vegetarian diet can be unhealthy if it contains too much fat and sugar or if it doesn't include a variety of foods, especially protein sources. If you are currently a vegetarian, your diet is probably on its way to meeting the dietary guidelines. If you are contemplating becoming vegetarian, you can become part of the healthy minority, too!

▼

The Pregnant Vegetarian

Some pregnant women turn to vegetarian foods when they find they can't tolerate meat. Sometimes eggs, cheese, or black beans go down a lot easier than a steak. Of course, many women are practicing vegetarians before they become pregnant. Vegetarianism has several levels:

Vegan

This person is the "true" vegetarian. A vegan eats no animal products whatsoever and should be sure to consume reliable sources of vitamin B_{12}, which is found only in animal products or fortified foods. The vegan's need for calcium is actually less than that of meat eaters who consume larger amounts of protein. However, the vegan may have to make an effort to consume enough vegetable sources of calcium. Like meat-eating pregnant women, vegan women may also have difficulty getting enough iron. Vegan women living in northern latitudes and those who get very little exposure to the sun in winter may have a problem producing enough vitamin D, which is made in the skin after exposure to sunlight and is also found in dairy products.

Lacto-Ovo Vegetarian

This person eats no red meat, poultry, or fish, but does eat dairy products and eggs. Lacto-ovo vegetarians have little trouble meeting nutrient needs for iron, calcium, vitamin B_{12}, or vitamin D.

No-Red-Meat "Vegetarian"

This person is someone who avoids red meat but does eat dairy products, fish, and/or poultry. Although people who eat no red meat may call themselves vegetarians, vegetarian organizations do not regard them as such. No-red-meat "vegetarians" generally have no problem meeting nutrient needs, except perhaps iron, which is found in lesser amounts in white meats.

Comparison of Vegan and Nonvegetarian Diets of Women Ages Twenty to Forty		
Expressed in percentages of the Dietary Reference Intakes (DRIs)*		
Nutrient	**Vegans**	**Nonvegetarians**
Calcium	72	119
Folic acid	231	49
Iron	118	102
Magnesium	141	108
Vitamin B_6	117	101
Vitamin C	310	193
Vitamin A	336	205
Vitamin B_{12}	25	189
Zinc	71	92
*Previously known as RDA		

Nutrients of Special Concern

How does pregnancy affect vegetarians? Most pregnant vegetarians can expect to meet or exceed their nutritional needs. In fact, a study that compared the diets of health-conscious vegetarian women and nonvegetarian women showed that vegetarian nonpregnant women ate more of most nutrients than meat eaters ate, except for vitamin B_{12}, calcium, and zinc.[5] (See the chart above.) This is a cause for concern since B_{12}, calcium, and zinc are very important during pregnancy.

Vegetarians should pay particular attention to a handful of nutrients: vitamin B_{12}, iron, calcium, and vitamin D. Since vitamin B_6 and zinc are nutrients lacking in all women's diets, we'll address them, too.

Vitamin B$_{12}$

Since vitamin B$_{12}$ is found only in animal products and fortified foods such as commercial breakfast cereals, you should make sure that you have a source of vitamin B$_{12}$ in your diet while you are pregnant and breast-feeding. Because product formulations often change, be sure to check labels.

According to Suzanne Havala, M.S., R.D., Nutrition Adviser to the Vegetarian Resource Group, "Some vegetarian specialty foods thought by many to be good sources of vitamin B$_{12}$, such as tempeh and spirulina, are in fact not reliable sources. Food labels listing the vitamin B$_{12}$ content of these foods include forms of the vitamin that are not active for humans and may compete for absorption with cyanocobalamin, the form we use."

If your diet contains neither animal products nor foods fortified with vitamin B$_{12}$, you probably need a vitamin supplement. Ask your health-care provider.

Vitamin-B$_{12}$-Fortified Cereals

Each of these cereals provides 100% of the Daily Value for vitamin B$_{12}$. However, since product formulations often change, read the labels to make sure these products still contain added vitamin B$_{12}$.

Kellogg's Special K Plus

Kellogg's Product 19

General Mills Multi-Grain Cheerios Plus

Kellogg's Smart Start

Note: Many other cereals contain 25% of the Daily Value for B$_{12}$.

Source: Manufacturers' labels

Iron

Even though intakes for iron are about the same for vegetarians and nonvegetarians, the type of iron that vegetarians eat may not be absorbed as well as the iron in meat. Vitamin C consumed with nonheme iron (the form of iron found in plant foods) helps increase the absorption of the mineral. Vegetarian diets are usually high in vitamin C.

Although anemia is no more common among vegetarians than meat eaters, anemia can occur in any pregnant woman due to the high iron requirement during pregnancy.[6] Thus, a supplement of 30 milligrams of ferrous iron is recommended for all pregnant women. (See page 73 for vegetarian sources of iron.)

Calcium

Calcium isn't usually a challenge for vegetarians unless they are vegan, are lactose intolerant, or just aren't milk drinkers. Since vegetarians generally eat less protein, this may affect how much calcium is lost in their urine. However, since calcium needs have not been established for vegans, it is best to follow the Dietary Reference Intake (DRI) for calcium, which is 1,000 milligrams.[7] If you are lactose intolerant, see page 71 for information on nondairy foods high in calcium. If you don't like milk by itself, but do eat other dairy products, see page 68 for tips on sneaking calcium into your diet.

Some sea vegetables are good sources of calcium and other minerals. If you eat sea vegetables regularly, be aware that if they come from polluted waters, they could contain heavy metal pollutants. You should make sure your seaweed comes from a controlled source, such as a sea vegetable farm in the United States.

Oxalates and phytates, substances found in leafy green vegetables and whole grains, can affect absorption of calcium. The high oxalate content of vegetables like spinach, Swiss chard, rhubarb, and beet greens make the calcium in these vegetables largely unabsorbable. High-fiber foods also high in phytates—especially wheat bran—can decrease the absorption of calcium from milk. But overall, the absorption of calcium from vegetables and legumes is equal to or better than absorption of calcium from milk.[8]

If you are concerned about your calcium intake, talk to a registered dietitian about increasing the calcium in your diet or ask your health-care provider about a supplement.

Vitamin D

The need for supplemental vitamin D is rare because the body can usually produce all that it needs from exposure to sunlight. Few foods are naturally high in vitamin D; milk, soymilk, and some cereals are fortified with it. If you are strictly vegan and you either live in a northern latitude or have very limited sun exposure, you may need a supplement of not more than 100 percent of the DRI.

Exposing the hands, arms, and face for five to fifteen minutes per day is believed to provide enough vitamin D from sunshine. People who use sunscreen, have dark skin, or live at northern latitudes or in cloudy or smoggy areas may need increased exposure

or may need to get their vitamin D from fortified foods or a supplement.[9] It has been recently proposed that for vegans who get no sun exposure, the current DRI may not be adequate. Ask your health-care provider for more information.[10]

Vitamin B_6

All women seem to have a problem getting enough vitamin B_6. Your body needs this vitamin in proportion to your protein intake, so if your diet is especially high in protein foods, you may need even more B_6. (See page 84 for a list of vegetarian sources of B_6.)

Zinc

Zinc is a very important nutrient for a developing fetus. It is widespread in such foods as legumes, shellfish, whole grains, and cheese. Many people don't have enough zinc in their diet.

One study that evaluated the diets of vegans and lacto-ovo vegetarians found that neither group met the DRI for zinc. The mean intake for vegan women was only 13 percent of the DRI, while lacto-ovo vegetarian women's average intake was 71 percent of the DRI. The women's food choices in this study were mostly low-zinc foods such as fruits, salads, and vegetables.[11]

Factors that may affect absorption of zinc include fiber, phytates, and some minerals. To obtain an adequate amount of zinc, vegetarians—especially vegans—must make careful food choices. Consult the list on page 85 to see how much zinc your diet supplies.

Essential Fat

Vegetarian diets don't contain docosahexanenoic and eicosapenaenoic acid (DHA and EPA), omega-3 essential fats that are necessary for fetal brain and eye development. Vegetarians generally do have a source of alpha-linolenic acid—a fatty acid that is converted to DHA and EPA. However, vegetarians also have a much higher intake of linoleic acid—another essential fat that can decrease the conversion of alpha-linolenic acid into DHA and EPA. Therefore, it is recommended that the ratio of intake of alpha-linolenic to linoleic acid be between five to one and ten to one. Sources of alpha-linolenic acid include linseed oil, flaxseed, walnuts, canola oil, walnut oil, and soybean oil. It is also helpful to substitute monounsaturated fats such as canola oil and olive oil for oils that are high in linoleic acids, such as safflower, sunflower, corn, and cottonseed oils.[12]

Protein

Protein is important during pregnancy, and although vegetarians have just a little less protein in their diets than nonvegetarians have, their intake still exceeds the DRI. The list of foods below will give you an idea of foods that can supply you with the 10 extra grams of protein needed daily during your pregnancy. Keep in mind that eating a variety of protein foods throughout the day is important so that your body can utilize the protein for building tissue.

Vegetarian Foods That Contain 10 Grams of Protein:

Black beans (or any legume), ¾ cup
Brown rice, 2 cups
Cashews, ½ cup
Peas, 1¼ cup
Peanut butter, 2¼ tablespoons
Quinoa, 1 cup
Soy yogurt, 1 cup
Tofu (firm), 2 ounces
Veggie burger, ⅔ to 1 patty

▼

The Eating Expectantly Vegetarian Eating Plan

This diet covers both vegan and lacto-ovo vegetarians and is meant as a guideline only. Eating a variety of high-nutrient foods without following a structured diet will provide the nutrition you need.

8 or more servings of grains
1 serving is 1 slice any type bread; ½ small bagel, pita, or English muffin; 1 6-inch tortilla; ½ cup cooked rice or pasta; ½ cup cooked cereal, barley, bulgar or quinoa; 1 ounce (¾–1 cup) ready-to-eat cereal; 3–4 crackers; or 2 cookies.

Note: 3 or more of your daily grain servings should be whole-grain.

4 or more servings of milk or milk substitute
1 serving is 1 cup any type milk, soymilk (calcium-fortified), or yogurt; 1½ ounces natural cheese; or 2 ounces processed cheese.

4 or more servings of fruit

1 serving is 1 medium fresh fruit; ½ grape-fruit, mango, or papaya; ½ cup canned or chopped fruit; ¼ cup dried fruit; or ¾ cup fruit juice.

4 or more servings of vegetables

1 serving is ½ cup cooked vegetables, 1 cup leafy vegetables, 1 small potato, or ¾ cup tomato or vegetable juice.

Note: Be sure to eat at least one fruit or vegetable that is high in vitamin C and one that is dark green or orange every day.

3 or more servings of legumes, nuts, and meat substitutes

1 serving is ½ cup legumes, tofu, tempeh, or textured vegetable protein; 2 eggs; 2 table-spoons nuts, seeds, or nut butter; or 1 veggie burger patty.

Note: Eat ½ more serving for each cup of milk or milk substitute that you don't drink.

Fats and sweets: Eat sparingly.

While most vegetarians need to limit fats and sweets, some may need to increase them to supplement their calorie intake.

Sample Vegan Menu

This menu contains about 2,400 calories and exceeds the DRIs for all major nutrients except vitamin D. (It contains 0 percent of the DRI for vitamin D.) Vitamin D can be produced in the skin with adequate exposure to sunshine.

Breakfast

  1 cup oatmeal with 1½ tablespoons molasses and 2 tablespoons raisins

  1 piece whole-wheat bread with 1 table-spoon peanut butter

  1 cup soymilk

Snack

  1 cup Minute Maid Premium calcium-enriched orange juice

Lunch

  1 cup navy bean soup with 1 piece whole-wheat bread

  Broccoli and tofu stir-fry with 1 cup tofu, ½ cup broccoli, and 1 cup brown rice

  1 cup soymilk

Snack

  1 apple

Dinner

  Salad with 1 cup romaine lettuce, ½ tomato, ¼ avocado, and vinaigrette dressing with 2 teaspoons canola oil

  Stuffed bell pepper with ½ cup bulgur, 1 cup black beans, and ½ tomato

  ½ cup corn

  1 cup soymilk

Snack

  Shake with 1 cup soymilk and ¾ cup frozen strawberries

Sample Lacto-Ovo Vegetarian Menu

This menu, which contains eggs and dairy products, contains approximately 2,400 calories and exceeds all of the DRIs for pregnancy.

Breakfast

1½ cups Bran Chex with 2 tablespoons
raisins and ½ banana

1 cup skim milk

1 piece toast with 2 teaspoons peanut
butter

Snack

1 ounce string cheese

1 apple

1 ounce baked tortilla chips

Lunch

1½ cups split-pea soup

1 cup spinach salad with ½ tomato, mushrooms, ¼ avocado, 1 ounce grated
reduced-fat Cheddar cheese, croutons,
and vinaigrette dressing with 2 teaspoons canola oil

1 piece whole-wheat bread

1 orange

8 ounces low-fat yogurt

Snack

1 cup milk

2 cups popcorn

Celery sticks

Dinner

1 cup Black Bean and Corn Salad (page
270)

1 serving Broccoli Quiche (page 350)

Whole-wheat roll with 1 teaspoon
reduced-fat butter or margarine

1 cup skim milk

Snack

Strawberry Shake (page 287)

Complementary Proteins: An Old Myth

A myth about complementary proteins
has been passed down for years. Even
recently, vegetarians have been advised
to eat the traditional legume with grain,
grain with dairy, or nut with grain to
have a "complete protein." Current
thinking is that as long as a vegetarian
eats a variety of foods with enough
calories, he or she will have enough of
all the amino acids. According to the
position of the American Dietetic
Association on vegetarian diets, "Plant
sources of protein alone can provide
adequate amounts of essential amino
acids if a variety of plant foods are consumed and energy needs are met.
Research suggests that complementary
proteins do not need to be consumed at
the same time."[13]

Vegetarian Shopping List

Now that you are pregnant, you are probably much more aware of what you buy at
the store. This handy shopping list can be
reproduced and used weekly. (See page
201 for more information about shopping
and label reading.)

Produce

Vegetables: asparagus, artichokes, broccoli, Brussels sprouts, beets, cabbage, carrots, cauliflower, celery, corn, eggplant, garlic, green beans, lettuce (romaine, leaf, Boston), mushrooms, onions (white, red), peppers (green, red, yellow), potato (sweet, white, new), rhubarb, rutabaga, spinach, summer squash, Swiss chard, tomatoes, turnips, winter squash, zucchini

Fruit: apples, avocados, bananas, blueberries, canteloupe, cherries, grapes, grapefruit, honeydew melon, lemons, oranges, pears, peaches, plums, pineapple, raspberries, strawberries, watermelon

Other: _____

_____

Note: Fruits and vegetables that aren't in season should be bought frozen.

Dry/Bulk Foods

Grains/flour/etc.: barley, bulgur, nutritional yeast, oats, quinoa, wheat germ, wheat pastry flour, whole-wheat flour

Rice: basmati, brown, instant, long- and short-grain, wild

Dried fruit: apricots, dates, prunes, raisins

Nuts and seeds: almonds, cashews, peanuts, sesame seeds, walnuts

Breads: rye, whole-wheat, bagels, English muffins, pitas, tortillas (corn, flour)

Pasta: whole-grain, regular

Snack foods: rice cakes, crackers, popcorn cakes, pretzels, graham crackers, granola bars, cookies

Mixes: falafel, hummus, refried beans, burgers

Other: _____

_____

Canned Goods/Jar Goods/Packaged Items

Beans: adzuki, black, kidney, navy, pinto, refried, chickpeas (garbanzo beans)

Nonfat evaporated milk

Fruit: peaches, pears, pineapple

Spreads/dips: chutney, fruit spread, peanut butter, tahini spread

Soups

Tomatoes: paste, sauce, spaghetti sauce, whole

Vegetarian specialty foods: veggie burger mix, sea vegetables, miso

Other: _____

_____

Refrigerated Foods

Cheese: American, low-fat Cheddar, low-fat cottage cheese, mozzarella, soy, Swiss

Tofu

Milk: low-fat, skim, soy

Yogurt: dairy, soy

Eggs

Fresh pasta

Biscuits

Spreads: butter, margarine

Other: _____

_____

Oils/Condiments

Flavored vinegar

Low-fat salad dressings

Low-sodium soy sauce, tamari sauce, mayonnaise, mustard

Oils: olive, canola, walnut

Spices: _____

_____

Sweeteners: honey, molasses, sugar (brown, white)

Frozen Foods

Frozen meals _____

_____

Fruits _____

_____

Meat substitutes _____

_____

Pancakes, waffles _____

_____

Sorbet, tofutti, frozen yogurt, sherbet

_____

Vegetables _____

_____

Veggie burgers, hot dogs _____

_____

Seitan

Tempeh

Wraps, burritos

Drinks

Juices: frozen, bottled (vegetable, fruit)

Sparkling water

Decaffeinated coffee, tea, Cafix

Other: _____

_____

Nonfood Items

Paper goods

Soaps

Toiletries

Other: _____

_____

▼

Vegetarian Food Planning

In Chapter Fifteen, you will find two weeks of budget menus modified to fit pregnancy needs.

▼

Eating Out Vegetarian-Style

As more people eat meatless, restaurants are adding vegetarian and vegan options to their menus. Some restaurants are very accommodating and will put together vegetarian meals that aren't even on the menu. Below are some healthy vegetarian entrées you're likely to find at various kinds of sit-down restaurants. Not all meatless entrées are vegan, so if you are concerned about animal-derived ingredients, you should consult the restaurant manager.

Vegetarian Entrées at Restaurants

Asian/Chinese

Any tofu (also called bean curd) dish
Egg foo yung
Noodle dish with vegetables and/or tofu

Bistro

Veggie burger
Vegetable platter
Spinach-and-artichoke dip
Veggie wrap
Stuffed potato

Continental

Quiche
Ratatouille
Vegetable risotto
Bean soup

Indian

Vegetable curry dish
Lentils
Spinach paneer

Italian

Cheese- or vegetable-stuffed ravioli or
   manicotti
Stuffed eggplant
Pasta primavera
Pasta e fagioli (pasta-and-bean soup)
Cheese or veggie pizza
Vegetarian lasagna

Mexican

Bean burrito
Huevos rancheros
Cheese or green chili enchilada
Bean Tostadas

Middle Eastern

Falafel (ground chickpea fritters often
   served in pita bread)
Hummus (chickpea dip)
Tabouli (bulgur salad)
Baba ghanouj (eggplant dip)
Ful medames (fava bean and chickpea dish)

Steak House

Vegetable or bean soup
Salad bar
Baked potato bar
Steamed vegetables

Thai

Vegetarian basil rolls
Vegetable boat
Tofu mussaman curry

Vegetarian Fast Food

In the United States, only a handful of fast-food restaurants offer vegetarian options besides ordering a sandwich or burger without the meat. Veggie burgers are common in restaurants on the West Coast, but they still are not on menus at the big burger chains—at least in the United States. (Burger King does have a veggie burger in its Irish, British, and European restaurants.) Progress may be made if many people contact the corporate offices of these chains to request more vegetarian choices.

Here are a few options: Taco Bell, Taco John's, and other Mexican fast-food restaurants offer several dishes based on refried beans and cheese. Subway has sandwiches containing lots of veggies, with or without cheese. Some Subway locations even have veggie burgers or soy "turkey" subs. At fried chicken restaurants, you can choose from a wide variety of vegetables like baked beans, corn on the cob, mashed potatoes, and green beans. Wendy's has a stuffed baked potato, which is a staple in many restaurants. Salad bars are also a good option, as are hearty bean soups and vegetarian chilis.

For more information on vegetarian options in restaurants or about ingredients in restaurant foods, contact the Vegetarian Resource Group (VRG). This nonprofit organization publishes a booklet called *Vegetarian Journal's Guide to Fast Food*. It also publishes *Vegetarian Journal* and many other resources, including vegetarian dining guides for major cities in the United States and abroad. Visit VRG's website at www.vrg.org or call the organization at 410-366-VEGE.

▼

Vegetarian Convenience-Food Choices

Going meatless is getting popular, and vegetarian foods are now widely available at grocery stores. The fat in some products is still surprisingly high, though, so be sure to read labels if fat is a concern for you. On the next page is a table that lists the nutrient information for some products currently available at large natural foods stores. The nutrient contents given are per serving as listed on labels.

Following are just some of the frozen entrées, either vegetarian (containing cheese or milk) or vegan, found in most grocery stores. To make a complete meal, add milk or yogurt, vegetable, fruit, and in some cases beans or another protein source.

Budget Gourmet Macaroni and Cheese with Cheddar and Parmesan

Budget Gourmet Three-Cheese Lasagna

Healthy Choice Manicotti with Three Cheeses

Healthy Choice Pasta Shells Marinara

Lean Cuisine Angel Hair Pasta

Lean Cuisine Cheese Ravioli

Lean Cuisine Fettuccini Primavera

Lean Cuisine Macaroni and Cheese with Broccoli

Michelina's Spaghetti Marinara

Weight Watchers Kung Pao Noodles and Vegetables

Weight Watchers Parisian-Style White Beans with Vegetables

Weight Watchers Pasta and Spinach Romano

Weight Watchers Paella Rice and Vegetables

Weight Watchers Peking-Style Rice and Vegetables

Weight Watchers Pilaf Florentine

Weight Watchers Risotto with Cheese and Mushrooms

Weight Watchers Santa Fe-Style Rice and Beans

Here are some ideas for convenience foods you can buy at the grocery store to form the foundation of a vegetarian meal.

Bird's Eye Meal Starter Oriental Stir Fry

Bird's Eye Meal Starter Primavera

Bird's Eye Meal Starter Teriyaki Stir Fry

Green Giant Create-A-Meal Garlic Herb

Nutrient Information for Some Products Currently Available at Large Natural Foods Stores					
Food	Calories	Protein*	Carbohydrate*	Fat*	Fiber*
Amy's Shepherd's Pie	160	5	27	4	5
Amy's Black Bean Ranchero Breakfast Burrito	230	9	38	5	5
Amy's Tomato-and-Spinach Pizza (3 slices)	300	12	38	12	2
Boca Burger	97	13	9	1	4
Cascadian Farm Indian Vegetarian Meal (3½ cups)	340	12	62	5	9
Cascadian Farm Szechuan Vegetarian Meal (3½ cups)	340	14	56	9	8
Cedarlane Veggie Wrap Vegetarian Pizza	220	17	32	3	2
Garden Chef Garden Burger	140	8	21	2.5	5
Lightlife Smart Deli Meatless Franks	80	16	4	0	1
Morningstar Farms Chik Patties	150	9	15	6	0
Natural Touch Garden Vege Pattie	110	10	8	2.5	3
Natural Touch Vegetarian Dinner Entrée	220	19	2	15	2
Soy Boy Ravioli	180	10	31	3	0
White Wave Baked Tofu, Thai Style (1 piece)	120	13	3	6	1
White Wave Mushroom-and-Gravy Stroganoff	90	11	10	0	3
White Wave Tempeh	150	10	10	6	6
Yves Veggie Pepperoni Slices (4)	90	17	5	0	1

*In grams

Source: Manufacturers' labels.

Green Giant Create-A-Meal Szechuan Stir Fry

Green Giant Harvest Burgers

Healthy Choice Split Pea, Garden Vegetable, or Country Vegetable Soup

Health Valley Vegetarian Chili

Morningstar Farms Veggie Burgers

Progresso Lentil or Black Bean Soup

Rosarita or Kuner's Vegetarian Refried Beans

▼ Eating after Delivery

Your doctor orders the diet that you receive in the hospital. Make sure your doctor understands that you want vegetarian meals and specify which type. Many hospitals have options for vegetarians, but they usually aren't vegan.

In addition, a dietary technician or registered dietitian may visit you to see if you have specific likes or dislikes or if you are having any problems eating. Make your preferences known, and try to select your own menu if possible. Be polite but persistent!

See page 175 for more information about eating after delivery. You can also read *Hospital Survival Guide* by Suzanne Havala, M.S., R.D., and *Vegetarian Journal Reports,* by Vegetarian Resource Group, 1990.

Eating after Surgery

If you have a cesarean section, you may not eat solid food for a day or so, depending on the type of anesthesia you receive. The progression from "nothing by mouth" to "regular diet" usually starts with clear liquids, such as clear juices, broth, gelatin, coffee, tea, and soda. As your tolerance increases, your diet will progress to a full liquid diet, which includes such foods as thinned hot cereals, cream soups, and dairy products.

You should be able to omit the nonvegetarian foods and eat double portions of the other foods. Again, make sure that your doctor leaves instructions for you to have vegetarian meals once you can eat solid food.

❓ Questions You May Have

Q: I just found out I have gestational diabetes. How can I fit vegetarian foods into my meal plan?

A: Actually, a vegetarian diet fits very well into a diabetic diet. Depending on your blood sugar, your dietitian may want you to eat less carbohydrate and more fat. To do this you could increase your intake of nuts, avocado, peanut butter, and cheese. Visiting with a registered dietitian can help in planning a vegetarian diet to meet your specific needs. On the next page you will find a table of some typical vegetarian foods with their diabetic exchanges.

Q: Is a vegetarian diet lower in fat than a diet containing meat?

A: Generally, yes, but not always. For example, lacto-ovo vegetarians may eat a lot of cheese, eggs, and low-fat or regular dairy products, which raise the fat content of the diet. A diet that is not well planned can have as much fat (including saturated fat) as the typical American diet.

A vegan diet can also be high in fat, although most of the fat would be unsaturated (unless you regularly use coconut products and palm or palm kernel oil). For example, nuts, tahini, avocado, and nut butters, staples for some vegetarians, are very high in fat. Other hidden fats can find their way into the diet through such goodies as tofu ice cream and carob.

The important feature for any type of diet is that high-fat foods—especially those high in saturated fat—be eaten in moderation.

Q: I'm worried about being able to eat vegetarian while I'm in the hospital. Any advice?

A: If you preregister at your hospital, you might be able to request a vegetarian diet then. When you go to the hospital in labor, you will probably be allowed to eat only ice chips or perhaps clear liquid, such as apple juice. This is because if you need anesthesia, your stomach should be empty. During this time, you might want to remind your doctor that when you *can* eat, you would

like a vegetarian diet. You might even want to write down your request before you go to the hospital.

After you have your baby, you will probably be allowed to eat a "real meal." Your meal may depend on what's left in the kitchen, which in turn depends on what time your baby is born. Babies seem to love arriving at off hours, and that may mean slim pickings for a very hungry new mom! A simple meal would be a cheese sandwich, fruit, and juice. For vegans, the selection may be very limited after hours. You may want to bring some nonperishable snacks from home for after delivery.

Exchanges for Special Vegetarian Foods		
Food	**Serving Sizes**	**Exchanges**
Beans, dried, cooked	½ cup	1 starch + 1 very lean meat
Brewer's yeast	3 tablespoons	1 starch
Bulgur, cooked	½ cup	1 starch
Carob flour	⅛ cup	1 starch
Kefir (a dairy drink)	1 cup	1 milk + 1 fat
Loma Linda Veggie Links	1 ounce	1 high-fat meat
Morningstar Farms Grillers	1 ounce	1 high-fat meat
Miso (a bean and grain paste)	3 tablespoons	1 vegetable
Seaweed, cooked	½ cup	1 vegetable
Soy flour	¼ cup	1 lean meat + ½ bread
Soy grits, raw	⅛ cup	1 lean meat
Soymilk	1 cup	1 milk + 1 fat
Tahini	1 teaspoon	1 fat
Tempeh	4 ounces	1 starch + 2 lean meats
Tofu, soft	½ cup	1 medium-fat meat
Tofu, firm	½ cup	2 medium-fat meats
Wheat germ	3 tablespoons	1 starch

Source: Modified from *Vegetarian Journal Reports*, Vegetarian Resource Group.

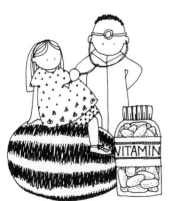

CHAPTER SEVEN

Special Care for High-Risk Pregnancies

What you will find in this chapter:

- *Expect the Unexpected*
- *Dealing with Your Emotions*
- *Preexisting Diabetes*
- *Gestational Diabetes*
- *The Diabetic Eating and Exercise Plan*
- *High Blood Pressure*
- *Multiple Births*
- *Coping with Bed Rest*
- *Older Moms*
- *Teen Pregnancy*

This chapter answers such questions as:

- *What kind of diet should I follow if I have gestational diabetes?*
- *Should I cut my salt intake if I have high blood pressure during pregnancy?*
- *How can I prepare and eat healthy meals if I'm on bed rest?*
- *Are artificial sweeteners safe?*
- *How much weight should I gain if I'm expecting twins?*
- *How many calories should I eat if I'm seventeen?*
- *Should I eat differently if I'm over thirty-five?*
- *What are some healthy snacks for a diabetic diet?*

Expect the Unexpected

The unknown can be awfully scary—especially when you're pregnant. To equip you for the unexpected, this chapter tells you how some special conditions may affect you and your baby and what you can do to deal with them. There are other complications associated with pregnancy, but this chapter will discuss only those that can affect or can be affected by your diet. Being informed is the key to taking charge of your health and having the healthiest pregnancy possible.

Dealing with Your Emotions

When you discover that you have a high-risk pregnancy, you will probably find yourself on an emotional roller coaster. You may experience guilt, fear, anger, denial, depression, or loneliness. Emotions are sometimes helpful in getting you through rough times, but emotions can be unhealthy if they prevent you from taking care of yourself.

For example, guilt and fear may motivate you to change your lifestyle to protect your baby, and denial may give you time to get used to the idea of a high-risk condition. However, depression and loneliness may alienate you from people who can help you. Identifying your feelings can help you adjust and seek support from others. If any of your emotions hinder you from dealing with your situation or significantly affect your sleeping or eating patterns, speak with your physician.

When I was put on bed rest for eleven weeks with my second

child, I had many of the emotions mentioned earlier. At one point I got so upset that I was ready to walk out the front door and away from my problems. Of course that wasn't possible, but it did give me an emotional release. (And looking back, the idea of walking away from my own belly is pretty funny!) What helped me the most was the support I received from others and reading about the experiences of women on bed rest.

Whatever happens, and whatever you have to do to carry out your pregnancy, it will be worth it when you see your healthy baby!

You Are Not Alone

One of the hardest aspects of a high-risk pregnancy is feeling like you are the only person with your problem. You're not alone; many women have faced or are facing the same challenges.

Sidelines National Support Network is a network of local support groups for women and families experiencing high-risk pregnancies. You can request phone or e-mail support and be matched up with one of five thousand women who have gone through a similar high-risk pregnancy. Many states have local chapters of Sidelines. You can contact them by visiting www.sidelines.org, or writing to P.O. Box 1808, Laguna Beach, CA 92652, or calling 949-497-2265.

The Confinement Line will find a woman to act as your support line while you are on bed rest. Write to The Confinement Line Childbirth Education Association, P.O. Box 1609, Springfield, VA 22151 or call 703-941-7183.

The American Diabetes Association is the best resource for information on all types of diabetes. On this organization's website you can find a multitude of resources, including several consumer and professional magazines. Visit www.diabetes.org or call 800-DIABETES (800-342-2383).

▼

Preexisting Diabetes

If you were diabetic before pregnancy, you probably already know the importance of managing your diabetes. Before conception and during pregnancy are critical times to control your blood sugar. Before you attempt to become pregnant, consult your physician, who will want you to be in tight control and will want to monitor you closely.

The Importance of Tight Control

High blood sugar in the first six to ten weeks of gestation is related to birth defects. Consequently, babies of women who have diabetes are at a higher risk for birth defects. However, moms who maintain acceptable blood sugar control are at no more risk for having babies with birth defects than the general population.[1]

The American Diabetes Association suggests that *before* conception, diabetic moms-to-be keep fasting (overnight fast) and just-before-meals blood sugars between 70 and 100 milligrams, one-hour-after-meals blood sugars less than 140 milligrams, and two-hours-after-meals blood sugars under 120 milligrams. Be sure to work out your individual goals with your health-care provider.[2]

The Health-Care Team

Before we go further, we should talk about a group of people who are very important to the health of your baby: the health-care team. You will need some specialized professionals to help in your care. If you are not already working with these health professionals, you can find them by calling a local medical society, asking your family physician, or calling a local chapter of the American Dietetic Association or the American Diabetes Association.

A diabetologist, endocrinologist, or physician who specializes in the care of people with diabetes is someone you should talk to before you become pregnant to make sure you are in good control of your diabetes.

A perinatologist is an obstetrician who specializes in high-risk pregnancies or who has experience working with pregnant women with diabetes. Some women consult a perinatologist before they get pregnant if they have had previous problems in pregnancy.

An endocrinologist is a physician who specializes in caring for people with diabetes and who treats other conditions that involve hormones. If you aren't already under an endocrinologist's care, your obstetrician may refer you to one to help manage your diabetes during pregnancy.

A certified diabetes educator (C.D.E.) will probably be a registered nurse, but dietitians and physicians can also hold this title. A C.D.E. is someone who has many hours of experience working with people who have diabetes and who has also passed a certification exam. This will probably be the person with whom you work closely for day-to-day management of your diabetes.

A registered dietitian (R.D.) is someone who will develop an individual eating plan for you. An individual plan is important because it is designed with your specific activity level, work schedule, lifestyle, and favorite foods in mind. The dietitian usually works closely with the C.D.E. Your dietitian can also work with you after you have your baby to help with diet for breastfeeding and weight loss.

A pediatrician or neonatologist is someone who provides medical care for your newborn baby. Since babies of diabetics sometimes have health problems, a neonatologist (who specializes in newborns up to six weeks old) might be needed.

You are the most important member of your health-care team. You are responsible for the day-to-day management of your diabetes, including contacting other members of the team to let them know how you are doing or when you need help.

What to Expect

If you are taking insulin, you will probably have to adjust your doses with the help of your health-care team. Some pregnant women need to adjust their insulin dosages as often as every five days because of increased need.[3] If your diabetes was controlled with diet or oral medications (type II or noninsulin-dependent) before pregnancy, there is a good chance you will be put on insulin during pregnancy. However, after you have your baby, you will likely return to your prior mode of treatment, especially if you return to your ideal body weight and exercise regularly.

Some women take injections before every meal to keep their sugar under control. Others use a pump. Be prepared to take more shots if needed. Taking more shots will probably mean checking your blood sugar more often.

Possible Effects on Mom

Women with preexisting diabetes have a higher risk of preterm birth, C-section, and hypertension. Their risk of preeclampsia is also higher, and the risk increases with the severity of diabetes.[4]

What to Watch For:

Some common conditions of pregnancy can be a real challenge for women with diabetes. And some common conditions for women with diabetes are more challenging during pregnancy.

Insulin resistance: As pregnancy progresses, especially around the twenty-fourth to twenty-eighth weeks, a hormone produced by the placenta resists insulin. Therefore, the body needs much more insulin. Diabetic moms-to-be may need twice the insulin they usually take.

Sign of Insulin Resistance
increased blood sugar

Ketoacidosis: Ketones are byproducts of fat breakdown and are a sign that glucose is not available and the body is breaking down fat stores for energy. As ketones increase in the bloodstream (usually as a result of high blood sugar from not having an adequate dose of insulin), the pH level of the blood changes and ketoacidosis occurs. Because of changing insulin needs and energy requirements during pregnancy, ketoacidosis can occur more quickly and if not treated, can lead to coma.

Signs of Ketoacidosis
If you have any of these signs, seek medical attention fast! Some symptoms are similar to signs of hyperglycemia, but are much more intense.

excessive urination
excessive thirst
fruity, acetone, or alcohol breath
listlessness, total lack of energy
nausea
abdominal pain
vomiting
labored breathing

Hypoglycemia (low blood sugar): Low blood sugar can occur because of increased activity, inadequate meals or snacks, excessive exercise, fetal energy demands, too much time between meals, or too much insulin. Always have glucose tablets or glucose gel with you, or keep in your purse a food that is a quick source of energy, such as chewable candy, fruit juice, or nondiet soda. Be sure to have a more substantial snack, such as a half sandwich or cheese and crackers, about a half-hour later. Add milk for an even more substantial snack.

If you have low blood sugar more than once a week, report it to your health-care provider. If you can pinpoint the cause of your low blood sugar, try to remedy it with the guidance of your health-care team. Preventing low blood sugar is often just a matter of eating before exercise, eating a bigger meal, or adding a snack. You may, however, need a different insulin schedule. Many people are surprised to find that they have been giving their injections incorrectly, even though they may have been doing it for years. This could also affect your blood sugar.

Signs of Hypoglycemia

These signs may develop very quickly.

  nervousness
  shakiness
  dizziness
  perspiration
  cold, clammy skin
  hunger
  headache
  disorientation, difficulty paying attention
  irritability, sudden mood changes
  pale skin

Hyperglycemia (high blood sugar):

Hyperglycemia is elevated blood sugar. It can be caused by changes in how your insulin is being used (see insulin resistance); by being less active, by being under mental or physical stress (such as illness); by eating more food or different types of foods than usual; or by a combination of any of these factors. Elevated blood sugar can cause your baby to grow larger and fatter than normal (macrosomia), which may lead to a difficult delivery.

Signs of Hyperglycemia

These signs occur gradually.

  blurred vision
  dry, itchy skin
  frequent urination
  increased thirst
  headache
  fatigue

Infections: Even minor infections can increase blood sugar and change insulin requirements. This can cause a breakdown of fat and lead to ketoacidosis (see definition on page 110). If you have the symptoms of ketoacidosis, seek medical attention immediately!

Sick-Day Rules

If you are sick with a virus or infection, your blood sugar will increase, even though you may not be eating much. The following rules are important to remember:

▶ **Contact a member of your health-care team.**

This is the first sick-day rule during pregnancy, especially if you are vomiting or have diarrhea.

▶ **Continue to take your insulin.**

Talk to your physician to see if you should take the same dose. You may actually need more.

▶ **Check blood sugar more frequently.**

Your doctor or diabetes educator will let you know how often. This will prevent any potential problems of high blood sugar and ketoacidosis. Your doctor may also want you to check your urine for ketones more frequently.

▶ **Prevent dehydration.**

Do this by drinking at least half a cup of fluid each hour. If you can't keep much food down and you are taking insulin, you must have carbohydrate in liquid form; this will give your body energy and will prevent dehydration. Examples of liquids (as well as some easy-to-digest solid foods) that contain 10 to 15 grams of carbohydrate are:

Fruit Juice or Sweetened Drinks
⅓ to ½ cup apple juice
½ cup orange juice
⅓ to ½ cup soda or fruit punch (not diet)
¼ to ⅓ cup lemonade

Solid Foods Easy to Digest
4 saltine crackers
¼ cup sherbet
½ Popsicle
¼ cup regular Jell-O
10 ounces chicken-noodle soup
10 ounces chicken-and-rice soup
8 ounces cream-of-mushroom soup
   (prepared with water)

▶ **If you can eat solids, drink plenty of calorie-free drinks to avoid dehydration.**

Good examples are water, broth, decaffeinated tea, sugar-free and caffeine-free soda, sugar-free fruit drinks, or Popsicles.

▶ **Replenish lost sodium or potassium.**

If you are losing a lot of fluid through vomiting or diarrhea, you will need to replenish your body with these important minerals. Here are good sources:

Sodium: Broth, canned soups, salted crackers, and Gatorade. (Choose regular or sugar-free depending on your ability to eat other solids.)

Potassium: Orange juice, melon, papaya, banana, orange-pineapple-banana juice, pineapple juice, tomato juice, vegetable juice, and dried fruits.

How Diabetes May Affect Your Baby

Blood sugar crosses the placenta from you to your baby. High blood sugar causes the baby to produce more insulin. Large amounts of sugar and insulin can cause serious risks, including a greater chance of stillbirth. However, stillbirth is not common.

Birth defects occur more often in babies of mothers who are diabetic. Fortunately, pre-pregnancy planning, early prenatal care, and keeping blood sugar in a narrow range can dramatically decrease that risk. If possible, seek medical counseling before you consider pregnancy.

Women with diabetes are prone to having bigger babies (macrosomia). High levels of blood glucose in mom, especially during late pregnancy, are thought to be responsible. After thirteen weeks gestation, your baby can start producing its own insulin in response to high blood glucose levels. Insulin acts as a growth hormone, causing baby to deposit excess fat, and the increased size may make a C-section necessary.

Babies of women with diabetes sometimes

have hypoglycemia (low blood sugar) immediately after delivery and must take glucose or sugar water. They are also prone to having higher bilirubin levels, or jaundice, which is easily treated with special lights in the hospital. Babies of diabetic moms may have a higher chance of respiratory distress syndrome.[5]

Children of diabetic mothers are at increased risk of obesity and impaired glucose tolerance by the time of puberty. Breastfeeding is encouraged because it decreases the risk of obesity and in some populations decreases the risk of diabetes.[6]

If your diabetes is advanced and you have some blood vessel damage, you may have restricted blood flow to the placenta, so your baby may have problems growing and may be small for gestational age.

What You Can Do

To Keep Your Diabetes under Good Control during Pregnancy:

▶ See your doctor before you become pregnant.

The American Diabetes Association recommends a prepregnancy care program, which involves evaluation by your health-care team to improve your chances of becoming pregnant as well as the outcome of your pregnancy.[7]

▶ Eat more high-fiber foods and whole grains.

Soluble fiber helps keep blood sugar under control by slowing digestion. Foods high in soluble fiber include oatmeal, peas and other legumes, barley, fruits, and vegetables. The antioxidants and insoluble fiber found in whole grains have additional benefits, such as preventing constipation.

▶ Monitor your blood sugar.

Your physician will give you the blood sugar range within which you should stay. The blood sugar range during pregnancy is much stricter than when you are not pregnant. Remember that blood glucose values reflect what has happened in the last one to three hours.

▶ Eat regular meals and snacks.

You will want to eat balanced meals at regular intervals. Most pregnant women need 2,000 to 2,400 calories per day, divided between carbohydrate (40 to 50 percent), fat (30 to 40 percent), and protein (20 to 25 percent).[8] Your calories should be divided among three meals and three snacks, with a space of two to three hours between meals and snacks. You may be instructed to use carbohydrate counting alone or in addition to exchanges. It is best to avoid combining milk and fruit alone for a snack. Including protein in snacks is recommended. Especially important is the bedtime snack, which should contain carbohydrate, fat, and protein. Eating a snack before bedtime (especially one that contains protein) can prevent hypoglycemia in the middle of the night. Some women even need a snack in the middle of the night (such as a glass of milk) to keep their blood sugar up.

▶ **Exercise.**

You should ask your physician about specific guidelines for frequency and duration of exercise and when NOT to exercise (such as when blood sugar is too low or too high). Regular exercise can decrease your need for insulin and can also make you feel more energetic. When you exercise, always take glucose gel or tablets, fruit juice, or hard candy with you, and eat a snack or meal before you begin. Never exercise when you know your blood sugar is low or when ketones are present. Also, don't give your insulin injection in an area that you will use immediately in exercise. For example, don't give it in the leg if you will take a brisk walk immediately afterward. (See page 188 for other tips on exercising.)

Labor and Delivery

Many doctors will induce labor for pregnant women who are diabetic. With all the high-tech equipment available, your physician can tell just when the baby is developed enough to enter our world. About one-half of all women with diabetes need cesarean delivery because their babies are too big to fit through the birth canal or because of other complications.[9]

During the first twenty-four to forty-eight postpartum hours, your insulin requirements can drop dramatically. You may need to watch for signs of hypoglycemia. Within a week after delivery, your insulin needs should return to prepregnant levels.

How to Cope

▶ **Keep stress low.**

Remember that stress can also raise blood sugar. Learn techniques to handle your stress, such as relaxation, visualization, and advance planning. Again, seek cooperation from others to help reduce your stress.

▶ **Remember that the extra hassle and discomfort you experience now will only last nine months.**

When you have your healthy baby, it will all be worth it.

▶ **Seek out a diabetes support group, preferably one for pregnant women.**

Research shows that women who have more social support can follow their dietary and self-monitoring regimens better.[10]

▶ **You and your family need to be committed to your pregnancy and to the unborn child.**

Everyone should learn how insulin works, the importance of dietary management, and what to do in case of hypo- or hyperglycemia. You'll also need your family's emotional support and understanding.

"It was really tough to put myself first," says Cindy, a woman who has been diabetic for fifteen years. "When I was pregnant with my second child, I felt guilty when I had to stop whatever I was doing to get myself something to eat because of low blood sugar. But I learned that I had to put myself first for the sake of my baby."

▶ **Learn to recognize the early warning signs of hypoglycemia, hyperglycemia, and ketoacidosis so you can take action.**

▶ **Always be prepared to handle a low blood sugar reaction.**
See page 110 on how to treat hypoglycemia.

▼

Gestational Diabetes

About 4 percent of all pregnant women will have diabetes of pregnancy, or gestational diabetes mellitus (GDM).[11] Diabetes mellitus is a disorder that prevents the body from using a simple sugar called glucose. GDM is a type of diabetes that occurs only during pregnancy and usually disappears after delivery.

Glucose is a simple sugar that is the final product of carbohydrate digestion. Carbohydrate is found in all starchy foods, such as bread, potatoes, and corn, and also in milk, fruits, and vegetables. Forms of simple carbohydrate that enter the bloodstream more quickly are found in candy, jam, syrup, honey, and table sugar. Your body can also make glucose from protein and stored carbohydrates. Every cell in the body uses glucose for energy.

Insulin is the hormone produced by the pancreas that allows glucose to enter your body's cells. A trace mineral called chromium is necessary for insulin to work. Supplementation studies have shown that chromium improves glucose tolerance in women with gestational diabetes and

people with type II diabetes. While chromium supplementation is not recommended, it couldn't hurt to eat more foods high in chromium: brewers yeast, American cheese, whole grains, apples with skin, spinach, oysters, carrots, and chicken breast.[12]

During pregnancy, women need two to three times more insulin. This is due to increased body weight and increased levels of hormones that work against insulin. These hormones peak during the twenty-fourth to twenty-eighth weeks. When the body cannot produce the insulin it needs, high blood sugar and diabetes are the result.

Effects on Mom

Many women have no symptoms of GDM. Some of the symptoms are also the typical signs of pregnancy, such as fatigue and frequent urination, so it may be hard to tell them apart. Some women have the symptoms of high blood sugar or low blood sugar listed on page 111.

Women with GDM have increased risk of high blood pressure, preeclampsia (a hypertensive disorder of pregnancy), and urinary tract infections. Symptoms of urinary tract infections include burning during urination and frequent urination.[13]

Effects on Baby

The most common problem is macrosomia, delivering a large baby, which may make for a difficult delivery, trauma to the baby during delivery, and/or increased need for a C-section.

Less common problems sometimes seen

in babies of mothers with GDM include premature delivery, hypoglycemia (low blood sugar) at birth, increased bilirubin in the blood (jaundice), and respiratory distress syndrome.[14]

One study showed that intensified management of blood glucose resulted in similar rates of macrosomia, C-section, stillbirth, and respiratory complications in children of diabetic and nondiabetic women.[15]

Children of women with gestational diabetes are at increased risk of obesity and impaired glucose tolerance by the time of puberty. Breastfeeding is encouraged because it decreases the risk of obesity and in some populations decreases the risk of diabetes. You should inform your child's health-care provider that you had GDM so he or she can recommend preventive measures.[16]

Who Is at Risk?

For Gestational Diabetes

Risk factors for gestational diabetes include overweight, family history of diabetes, and adverse pregnancy outcomes such as stillbirth, miscarriage, and congenital malformations. Risk also increases with age and with each subsequent pregnancy.[17]

For Type II Diabetes

Unlike type I diabetes, which generally begins during childhood and requires insulin treatment from then on, type II diabetes is usually diagnosed during adulthood and does not as a rule require insulin injections.

It is estimated that half of all people with diabetes in the United States haven't even been diagnosed. Your chances of becoming diabetic are greater if you:[18]

- have a close blood relative who is diabetic.
- were diagnosed with GDM in a previous pregnancy.
- are more than 20 percent over your ideal body weight.
- have had a baby that weighed 9 pounds or more at birth.
- are African-American, Native-American, Hispanic-Latino, Asian-American, or a Pacific Islander.
- are over forty-five years old.
- have been previously diagnosed with impaired glucose tolerance or impaired fasting glucose.
- have high blood pressure.
- have high-density lipoprotein (HDL) cholesterol less than 35.
- have a triglyceride level over 250.

Are You at Risk?

Take a test that shows your level of risk at www.diabetes.org/ada/risktest.asp.

Testing for Diabetes

When you are between the twenty-fourth and twenty-eighth weeks of pregnancy, your health-care provider will ask you to take a glucose challenge test that looks for sugar in the blood. This test is done without special preparation, such as fasting or eating certain foods. First, you will be asked to drink a very sweet drink called glucose (it tastes like cola syrup before the carbonated water is added). One hour later your blood will be drawn, and the amount of sugar (or glucose) in your blood will be tested. If your blood sugar is over 140 milligrams, this is considered a positive, or abnormal, test. You may be asked to:

- see a registered dietitian for meal-planning guidance

OR

- take a glucose tolerance test, which is similar to the glucose screening test but lasts three hours. You will need to follow a special high-carbohydrate diet for three days prior to the test. Your health-care provider will give you specific instructions. After drinking the glucose, a health professional will draw your blood every hour for three hours.[19]

If your physician diagnoses you with GDM, you may be referred to a specialist, such as an endocrinologist or a perinatologist, who probably works with a staff of diabetes educators. However, your physician may decide to treat the diabetes aspect of your pregnancy by working closely with an R.D., who will give you a diabetic meal plan, and a C.D.E., who will teach you about monitoring your blood sugar. (If you aren't referred to an R.D., you should request a referral!)

Keys to Controlling Gestational Diabetes

▶ Eat balanced meals at regular intervals.

See a registered dietitian to make a personal meal plan.

▶ Keep your activity level up.

Talk to your doctor about recommending a daily exercise program; most physicians approve of walking or swimming.

Note: DON'T exercise if your blood sugar is elevated or if ketones are present in your urine; contact your physician. (See Chapter Eleven: Fitting Fitness In for more information on exercise during pregnancy.)

▶ Divide the food you eat daily into three meals and two to three snacks.

The bedtime snack is especially important. It should include some starch, protein, and fat.

▶ Keep a handle on weight gain by making wise food choices.

Choose foods that are low in saturated fat.

▶ Avoid emotional eating, such as eating when you are sad, angry, or stressed-out.

▶ Eat more whole-grain foods and legumes.

Avoid concentrated sweets such as cookies, candy, pie, sugar, honey, and chocolate. Also, limit or avoid fruit juices, even unsweetened ones. They contain concentrated amounts of fruit sugar, which can raise your blood sugar.

▶ Expect to monitor your blood sugar; your diabetes educator will teach you how to do this.

Your blood sugar level will show you how your diet is affecting the amount of glucose in your blood and will be used to adjust your diet and exercise regimen.

At first, your health-care provider will ask you to test your blood sugar as often as four to five times per day for the first week. This could include testing in the middle of the night, when blood sugar sometimes drops. When your blood sugar is under good control, you will probably test less often.

▶ **Keep your diet high in fiber.**

Fiber helps stabilize blood sugar. So stay away from foods made with white flour as much as possible. Try to eat raw (instead of cooked) fruits and vegetables. Eat high-fiber cereal with milk as a snack. (See page 53, "Focus on Fiber.")

▶ **Smile!**

You have a unique opportunity to improve your family's diet! Try to make the changes permanent.

▼

The Diabetic Eating and Exercise Plan

Many people think that going on a diabetic diet means they must give up all their favorite foods. This is just not true!

The diabetic eating plan is simply a way of eating that includes balanced amounts of carbohydrate, fat, and protein in each meal. All foods are allowed except simple sugars like table sugar, honey, jam, and syrup and foods that contain a lot of sugar like cakes, pies, cookies, and candy. However, foods with small amounts of sugar are allowed in moderation. For example, graham crackers, animal crackers, and angel food cake are allowed in moderation when your blood sugar is under good control.

The goal in managing your diabetes is to keep your blood sugar within a certain range. General guidelines are listed on page 108 under "Preexisting Diabetes." However, your doctor or diabetes educator may have individual recommendations for you. You can control your blood sugar by not eating too many carbohydrates at one time and balancing your meals with protein and fat. The protein and fat slow digestion and cause a slow, gradual rise in blood sugar, instead of a fast rise that would occur if you ate a carbohydrate food by itself.

Carbohydrate is found in starchy foods like bread, crackers, cookies, rice, potatoes, corn, milk, yogurt, dried beans, fruit, and fruit juice. Carbohydrate is also found in smaller amounts in nonstarchy vegetables like green beans, carrots, and squash. The Sweet Success Program in California recommends staying away from fruit juices and processed and refined starch products such as instant potatoes, instant noodles, instant hot cereals, cold processed cereals, canned soups, and packaged stuffing. It also recommends avoiding sugar-containing sauces such as teriyaki and barbecue. On the other hand, it encourages eating whole-grain breads, noninstant oatmeal, legumes, and lentils because of their small effect on blood glucose.[20] Of course, any food containing concentrated sugars also provides concentrated sources of carbohydrates and should be avoided.

Your meal plan will be arranged with your current eating pattern, individual lifestyle, and activity level in mind. The calories, carbohydrate, protein, and fat that you need in a day will be calculated and then divided between your meals and snacks. Snacks are important because they allow you to eat smaller meals and prevent your blood sugar from dropping too low. (See page 121 for snack ideas.) Follow-up visits with a dietitian are important because assessing the energy needs and eating patterns of a person is difficult in just one visit. Your meal plan may need adjusting as your activity level increases or decreases.

Your Meal Plan

A common meal pattern is one that contains three meals and three snacks comprising 40 to 45 percent carbohydrate, 20 to 25 percent protein, and 30 to 40 percent fat. Hormones sometimes cause higher blood sugar in the morning. For this reason, a low-carbohydrate breakfast (for example, two eggs and one to two pieces of toast) containing 15 to 30 grams of carbohydrate is recommended. Fruit, fruit juice, and milk should be avoided in the morning because of their high simple sugar content. However, fruit and milk are encouraged the rest of the day.

Bev Spears, R.D., of The Diabetes Center of New Mexico starts her GDM patients with just one serving of a starchy food (such as one piece of toast) at breakfast. If the blood sugar testing shows that the amount is well tolerated, the carbohydrate is increased. The preliminary diet excludes milk and juice, because many diabetic women are sensitive to the simple carbohydrates found in these drinks. Milk may be added back into the diet as tolerated.[21] Generally, fruit juices (even ones with no added sugar) should be avoided, since they can increase blood sugar at any time. Vegetable juice and tomato juice are okay.

Your diet will probably be based on the Exchange Lists for Meal Planning and/or the carbohydrate counting method (both from the American Diabetes Association and the American Dietetic Association). Your diabetes educator will determine which method of meal planning is best for you.

Carbohydrate counting is a relatively new method of meal planning in the United States, but it has been the primary approach in the United Kingdom for years. Its focus is balancing the amount of carbohydrates eaten at meals and snacks.

The exchange method of meal planning uses a combination of foods from six food groups: starch, fat, milk, meat, fruit, and vegetable. Each food serving within a group has approximately the same number of calories and other nutrients, so the foods within a group can be exchanged for each other. For example, one serving of starch has 80 calories and 15 grams of carbohydrate. You won't have to worry about those numbers, but do get to know the serving sizes. See page 120 for an abridged exchange list. Your dietitian will give you a complete list of exchanges from the American Diabetes Association.

The following meal plan has about 2,200 calories and is an example of a meal plan that your dietitian might develop for you.

Your calorie needs will vary depending on your size, ideal body weight, and activity level. An individualized diet developed just for you is very important. The sample below is an example only and is not intended to replace individual counseling by a diabetes educator.

Breakfast

1 medium-fat meat = 1 egg

2 starches = 1 piece whole-wheat toast, ½ cup old-fashioned oatmeal

2 fats = 2 teaspoons tub margarine

1 milk = 8 ounces sugar-free or ¾ cup plain yogurt

Snack

1 starch = ¾ ounce whole-grain crackers

1 fruit = 1 small apple

1 medium-fat meat = 1 ounce string cheese

1 skim/very-low-fat milk = 1 cup sugar-free low-fat fruit yogurt

Exchange List	
1 starch =	1 piece bread; 1 tortilla; 6 crackers; ½ cup pasta, bulgur, corn, potatoes, or hot cereal; ⅓ cup rice; ½ cup beans, peas, or lentils (also counts as 1 very lean meat); or ¾ cup flaked cereal
1 fat =	1 teaspoon margarine, oil, mayonnaise, or butter; 1 tablespoon diet margarine (30 to 50% oil) or low-fat mayonnaise; 1 tablespoon salad dressing or 2 tablespoons low-fat dressing; ⅛ avocado; 20 small peanuts; 8 large olives; 2 tablespoons sour cream; or 1 slice bacon
1 milk =	*Skim/very-low-fat:* 1 cup skim milk; ½ or 1%-fat milk or buttermilk; 1 cup nonfat or low-fat sugar-free yogurt; or ¾ cup plain nonfat yogurt
	Low-fat: 1 cup 2%-fat milk or ¾ cup plain low-fat yogurt
	Whole: 1 cup whole milk or 1 cup kefir
1 meat/meat substitute =	1 ounce unless specified
	Very lean: fish; shellfish; chicken or turkey breast; fat-free cheese; sandwich meats with 1 gram or less fat per ounce; ¼ cup nonfat or low-fat cottage cheese; or ½ cup cooked dried beans, peas, or lentils (also counts as 1 starch)
	Lean: round, sirloin, or flank steak; pork tenderloin; ham; veal; leg of lamb; dark meat of chicken (no skin); cheese and lunch meats with 3 grams fat or less per ounce
	Medium fat: most other beef; mozzarella cheese; cheese with less than 5 grams fat per ounce; 1 egg; dark-meat chicken with skin; salmon; tuna in oil (drained); ground turkey; or ½ cup tofu
	High fat: spareribs, sausage, regular cheese, hot dogs, or sandwich meats with 8 grams fat or less per ounce
1 fruit =	1 medium fresh; ½ banana; 12 cherries; 15 grapes; or ½ cup canned, unsweetened
1 vegetable =	½ cup cooked vegetables; ½ cup vegetable juice; or 1 cup raw vegetables

Source: *Exchange Lists for Meal Planning,* The American Diabetes Association and The American Dietetic Association, 1995.

Lunch

3 starches = 2 slices whole-wheat bread, 1 ounce pretzels

2 very lean meats = 2 ounces tuna packed in water

1 fat = 1 tablespoon reduced-fat mayonnaise

2 vegetables = 1 sliced tomato, raw veggies, romaine lettuce

1 skim/very-low-fat milk = 1 cup 1% milk

Snack

1 starch + 1 very lean meat = ½ cup low-fat refried pinto beans

1 starch = ¾ ounce baked corn tortilla chips

1 fruit = 1 orange

Dinner

3 lean meats = 3 ounces grilled tenderloin steak

2 vegetables = ½ cup each broccoli and carrots

2 starches = 1 small baked potato, 1 whole-wheat roll

2 fats = 1 teaspoon tub margarine or butter, 2 tablespoons sour cream

1 skim/very-low-fat milk = 1 cup 1% milk

1 fruit = ½ frozen banana

Bedtime Snack

1 starch = ½ whole-wheat bagel

1 very lean meat = 2 tablespoons peanut butter

1 fruit = 1¼ cups berries

After You Start a Diabetic Diet

Don't be alarmed if you have a small weight loss after you start a diet to control your blood sugar. This is fairly common, especially if you are now eating fewer carbohydrate foods than you did previously. Just remember that weight loss should be temporary, lasting no more than about five days. If the weight loss continues, talk to your doctor or dietitian.

You may be asked to self-monitor your blood glucose to find out how much sugar is in your blood. Some physicians randomly test blood sugar during office visits.

Blood sugar monitoring involves pricking your finger and letting a drop of blood fall on a test strip. The test strip is placed in a tiny machine that reads the blood glucose level and displays it on a panel. Your blood sugar and ketone testing records are good tools to see if you are eating enough food. Go over these records with your health-care team.

If you find that your blood sugars are consistently low at certain times of the day, try to figure out why. Some possibilities are:

- You didn't eat enough food at the previous meal or snack.
- You need to add a snack two hours or so before your sugar is low.
- You're not eating the right kind of snack. (Read on for good snack ideas.)
- You are more active or are exercising close to this time and need more food.

Healthy Snacks

A diabetic snack should contain some carbohydrate, fat, and protein. You may be able to have a carbohydrate snack alone, as long as it is not juice. Your lifestyle, activity level, and weight gain will dictate the type of snacks you need. Again, your individual snack needs should be discussed with your dietitian, diabetes educator, or physician.

Balanced Snacks

Each snack equals one starch or one fruit, one meat, and one fat exchange. To add a milk exchange, add 1 cup milk or 1 cup plain or sugar-free yogurt.

- 1 ounce Swiss cheese and 6 rye crackers
- 2 tablespoons peanut butter and 2 popcorn cakes
- 1 piece whole-wheat bread and 1 ounce light cream cheese
- 1 small bran muffin and ¼ cup cottage cheese
- 1 pear and 1 ounce string cheese
- ½ ham sandwich on rye bread with 1 teaspoon mayonnaise
- 1 apple with Caramel Dip (see recipe on page 335)
- ⅓ cup refried beans with 1 ounce cheese
- 9 Wheat Thins and 1 ounce turkey
- 2 tablespoons peanut butter and ½ small banana
- Raw veggies, 1 ounce cheese dip, and 6 crackers

Starchy Snacks

Each snack is equal to one serving of starch.
- ½ whole-wheat pita bread
- 6 rye crackers
- 2 to 3 cups light popcorn
- 2 rice cakes
- 5 Triscuits or other whole-wheat crackers
- ½ cup tabouli (bulgur salad)
- ½ cup black beans
- 1 ounce baked tortilla chips

"Free" Snacks

These foods have very few calories, so they can be eaten as desired when you don't have any exchanges left in your meal plan. Do not eat these snacks alone before exercise, because they will not affect your blood sugar.

- Raw vegetables with 2 tablespoons fat-free dressing
- Sugar-free Jell-O or sugar-free Popsicles (if your doctor allows artificial sweeteners)
- Vegetable broth
- Lettuce and raw greens
- Cucumbers
- Celery

Exercise: A Shot in the Arm

Imagine something that makes you feel more energetic and relaxed, makes your body muscular instead of flabby, allows you to eat more without gaining too much weight, and reduces your long-term risk of heart disease. This something also helps you avoid taking insulin or reduces your dose. Would you go out and buy it by the bucketful? Exercise is this wonderful something, and it is strongly recommended for women who have diabetes.

Health-care providers generally recommend that you exercise twenty to thirty minutes daily, and at least three times per week; some suggest a daily walk or water exercise. However, you should talk to your health-care provider to see what specific guidelines he or she has for you. Regular exercise improves the efficiency of your body's insulin, which can help control blood sugar levels so that you don't have to take insulin.

A study done at the Sansum Medical Research Foundation in Santa Barbara found that regular exercise normalized fasting and postprandial (after-meal) glucose levels, which prevented the need for insulin. The women worked out on arm ergometers (stationary bicycles that use the arms to pedal) three times per week for six weeks.[22] Lois Jovanovic-Peterson, M.D., writes in her book *Managing Your Gestational Diabetes,* "If your doctor tells you to restrict physical activity due to premature labor, you may still be able to do upper-arm exercises—such as lifting 2-pound weights while sitting in a chair." You can do this while watching the news or your favorite soap! You can do such exercises on a daily basis, split between two ten-to-twenty-minute sessions.[23]

We would all like to exercise regularly, but may have trouble finding time for exercise in our busy schedules. The solution is to *make* exercise a priority and *make* time for it regularly. (See Chapter Ten: Fitting Fitness In for tips on "exercising without exercising." Also found in Chapter Ten are exercise guidelines for pregnancy.)

If you start exercising when your blood sugar level is normal, you could have low blood sugar when you finish. Here are some tips for avoiding low blood sugar during exercise:[24]

- If you know your blood sugar is low, delay exercise until after you have had a meal or snack.
- If your blood sugar is within normal range, eat one serving of fruit before a thirty-minute activity.
- If your blood sugar is within normal range, eat one serving of starch and one

serving of fruit before an activity that lasts an hour or more.
- If your activity is more strenuous, you may need to increase the amount of food for your snack.
- If your activity (such as a hike) is longer than two hours, eat before you go and also bring snacks to eat along the way.
- Always carry hard candy or glucose tablets with you in case you have low blood sugar or an insulin reaction. Packaged peanut-butter or cheese crackers are also good to keep in your purse.

The Scoop on Sweeteners

There are three types of sweeteners: nutritive sweeteners, which contain calories; sugar alcohols, which contain fewer calories; and nonnutritive sweeteners (also called artificial sweeteners), which contain virtually no calories. The different types of sweeteners and their use during pregnancy (and as they relate to diabetes) are described below.

For more information about sweeteners, visit the International Food Information Council at www.ificinfo.health.org, the American Dietetic Association at www.eatright.org, or the Center for Science in the Public Interest at www.nutritionaction.org.

Sucrose and Other Sugars

If you have diabetes while pregnant, you should avoid foods with concentrated sugars—even if you could use sugars in your diabetic meal plan before you were pregnant. You can find the different types of sugars on food labels by looking for these words: *sugar (brown, confectioner's, invert, raw, cane, crystallized cane, turbinado), honey, corn syrup, dextrin, fruit juice concentrate, maple syrup, corn sweetener, malt,* and *molasses.* Less-processed sugars like honey, molasses, and brown sugar have the same calories as processed sugars and can have the same effect on your blood sugar. Small amounts of sugar are common in many foods. That's okay; simply choose foods with the least amount of sugar. Keep in mind that 4 grams of sugar is equivalent to 1 teaspoon.

Sugar Alcohols (Polyols)

You may have seen the ingredients sorbitol, mannitol, and xylitol on food labels. These are sugar alcohols, types of sugar that are not completely absorbed in the intestines. Sugar alcohols therefore have fewer calories than sugar and do not raise blood sugar the way regular sugars do. Sorbitol and mannitol, often found in diet candies, can cause diarrhea if eaten in large amounts. Isomalt, lactitol, maltitol, hydrogenated starch hydrolysates (HSH), and erythritol are other sugar alcohols that you will be seeing more of in the future. Check with your dietitian about fitting foods with sugar alcohols into your eating plan.[25]

Artificial Sweeteners

If you are avoiding sugary foods and drinks, you may still want an occasional something sweet. Should you eat products sweetened with artificial (nonnutritive) sweeteners? Saccharin (found in Sweet 'n Low), aspartame (found in NutraSweet), acesulfame K (found in Sweet One and Sunette), and sucralose (found in Splenda) have all been approved for use during pregnancy, but there are some caveats.

Many physicians would prefer that their patients limit or avoid artificial sweeteners. Moderation is usually a good rule to follow when it comes to food. A moderate intake of artificial sweeteners would be one to two servings per day. Consult with your health-care provider for individualized recommendations.

Saccharin

Saccharin has been shown to cause bladder cancer in rats and remains somewhat controversial. Because saccharin can cross the placenta and remain in fetal tissues for a while, it has been suggested that women consider careful use of saccharin during pregnancy.[26]

Aspartame

Aspartame is a widely used sweetener in the United States. Almost 80 percent of the world's supply of the sweetener is used here. Although aspartame is popular, some people have reported reactions such as dizziness and headaches after ingesting it. People with a metabolic disorder called phenylketonuria (PKU) should avoid it.

How much aspartame is too much? The Acceptable Daily Intake (ADI) set by the Food and Drug Administration (FDA) is 22.7 milligrams of aspartame per pound of body weight (or 50 milligrams per kilogram of body weight). A 12-ounce diet soda contains approximately 225 milligrams; an 8-ounce yogurt or 4-ounce gelatin dessert contains about 100 milligrams; ½ cup of frozen yogurt contains about 47 milligrams; and a packet of aspartame sweetener contains 37 milligrams. To exceed the ADI, a 150-pound woman would have to drink more than fifteen diet sodas in a day!

Most people keep within the ADI for aspartame without even trying. If you have a sweet tooth, though, you should keep an eye on how much aspartame you use. You may find yourself eating a lot of foods sweetened with aspartame.[27] Also, be aware that sometimes aspartame and saccharin are found together in a product. Be sure to read food labels carefully.

Acesulfame K

The safety of consuming acesulfame K during pregnancy was determined by rat studies. Several well-respected scientists have said that the carcinogenicity testing was flawed. Given this possibility and the fact that acesulfame K can cross the placenta, it is best to avoid acesulfame K while you are pregnant.[28] Keep in mind that acesulfame K and sucralose are sometimes mixed in a product, so read food labels carefully.

Sucralose

Sucralose was approved in the United States in 1998 and has been used by millions of people around the world since 1991. It's the only nonnutritive sweetener made from sugar. Sucralose has been approved for use in beverages, baked goods, desserts, syrups, jams, chewing gum, and more. It was determined not to pose any carcinogenic, reproductive, or neurological risks to humans on the basis of one hundred studies conducted over twenty years. According to the Center

for Science in the Public Interest (CSPI), a consumer watchdog group, sucralose is safer than saccharin and doesn't raise the concerns that aspartame and acesulfame K do.[29]

The ADI for sucralose is 11 milligrams per pound of body weight (5 milligrams per kilogram of body weight). A tabletop packet of sucralose sweetener contains 12 milligrams.

Sweeteners Awaiting FDA Approval

Alitame is currently awaiting FDA approval pending more research. Alitame is approved for use in food and beverages in Australia, New Zealand, Mexico, and the People's Republic of China.

Stevia, which is much sweeter than sugar without the calories, is made from the stevia shrub and has been used for years in South America and Japan. Although it is sold in the United States as a dietary supplement, it has not been approved as a food sweetener by the United States, Canada, or the European Union. European animal tests have indicated fertility and reproductive problems and have deemed stevia unacceptable as a sweetener. It is best to avoid using stevia until it is approved as a sweetener in the United States.[30]

Diet Foods

It's not just sugar and calories that diet products may be lacking; some are also missing vitamins and minerals, which are so important for you and your baby. One mineral that diet sodas do have is phosphorus, which can be a problem in large amounts. It is thought that a high proportion of phosphorus to calcium in the diet causes leg cramps during pregnancy.

If you choose to use artificially sweetened products, moderation is the key. What's moderation? Most professionals consider one to two servings per day moderate—a serving being one diet soda (caffeine-free) or one serving of diet gelatin, pudding, or hot cocoa.

For more information on sweeteners, contact the International Food and Information Council for brochures about artificial sweeteners, additives, and food safety. Write to 1100 Connecticut Avenue NW, Suite 430, Washington, DC 20036 or call 202-296-6540. You can also call NutraSweet Consumer Affairs at 800-321-7254.

? Questions You May Have

Q: Will I have to take insulin?

A: If your blood sugar can't be controlled by diet and exercise, you will probably take insulin in the form of a self-administered shot. You may take one or several insulin shots daily. Even if you don't take insulin, you will probably be asked to monitor your blood sugar.

Blood glucose monitoring is a great way to see how you are doing with your diet. You may be following your meal plan closely, yet seeing high blood sugars. This is because some foods affect your blood glucose quite differently, even though they are similar in carbohydrate value and calories. Also, some women can tolerate carbohydrates better than other women.

Q: What else can affect my blood glucose?

A: Many other factors can affect your blood glucose or blood sugar level:

- The combination of protein, fat, carbohydrate, and fiber you eat at a meal.
- How much fiber is in your diet. Fiber slows down digestion, causing slower release of glucose into the bloodstream.
- Your activity level. Exercise uses up extra glucose and causes insulin to work more efficiently, thus keeping your blood sugar down and reducing the likelihood that you will have to take insulin.
- Your overall health. Infection and illness can increase blood sugar levels. (See page 111 for "Sick-Day Rules.")
- Your stress level. Emotional stress can also increase your blood sugar level.

Q: Can hypoglycemia harm my baby?

A: One animal study indicates hypoglycemia in mom does cause hypoglycemia in baby, and that baby will produce glucose from other sources, such as fat, to meet its energy needs. Recurrent bouts of hypoglycemia could cause poor growth in baby.[31]

If you take insulin, some doctors recommend having a glucagon kit available for severe hypoglycemic reactions. (Glucagon is a hormone that increases blood sugar.) Make sure that relatives, friends, and coworkers know what to do for you if you start having the symptoms of hypoglycemia, including knowing how to use the glucagon kit. Also, be sure to wear a necklace or bracelet that identifies you as diabetic.

Q: What about hyperglycemia?

A: Hyperglycemia is more likely to adversely affect your baby. High blood sugar can cause the baby to have increased body fat, which could cause delivery problems. High blood sugar can also increase your baby's risk of being overweight and having impaired glucose tolerance when he or she is older. It has been suggested that if a baby has hypoglycemia at birth caused by the mother's hyperglycemia, it could cause long-term neurological dysfunction.[32]

Q: I have gestational diabetes. Will I still have diabetes after my baby is born?

A: Most women's blood sugar levels go back to normal shortly after delivery. Only a small number of women continue to have glucose intolerance.

However, over half of the women who have gestational diabetes will be diagnosed with type II (adult-onset) diabetes ten to fifteen years after their children are born. Women who have GDM with one pregnancy are very likely to have it with other pregnancies, too. The American Diabetes Association recommends having your blood glucose tested six weeks after delivery, and if normal at least every three years thereafter.[33] Can you avoid postpregnancy diabetes? Very possibly, if you maintain your ideal body weight and exercise regularly. Eating a balanced diet is also beneficial.

Q: What about my next pregnancy?

A: Women with GDM have a very high chance of having GDM with subsequent pregnancies. Losing excess weight between pregnancies, exercising regularly, and eating well can cut your risk.

Q: What if I get sick and can't eat?

A: If you get ill and don't feel like eating or can't keep food down, you should first contact your health-care provider. Women are usually instructed to continue taking insulin (if applicable) because illness can raise blood sugar levels. You must also continue drinking fluids, so that you don't become dehydrated. (See page 111 for "Sick Day Rules.")

Q: Will my baby be diabetic?

A: Not at birth. However, having diabetes (either preexisting or gestational) does increase your child's risk of being overweight and of having impaired glucose tolerance, which are risk factors for diabetes. Breastfeeding is the first line of defense, since it can decrease the risk of obesity. Your family should also practice a healthy lifestyle, including regular activity, a healthy diet with plenty of high-fiber foods, and close-to-ideal weight.

Q: The week before I had my blood sugar checked, I was eating a lot of candy and soda. Is that what caused my diabetes?

A: No. However, you may have craved sweets because of the diabetes. When your blood sugar is high, but you don't have enough insulin to use the glucose, your body sends out the signal that you need energy.

Sugar does not cause diabetes. However, excess simple sugar and starches in the diet cause the pancreas to secrete more insulin; and if your body cannot produce the amount of insulin needed, the result is high blood sugar.

▼

High Blood Pressure

Sarah was surprised when she went to her doctor's office and found that her blood pressure was elevated. She felt fine! No one in her family had high blood pressure (hypertension), and she had never had a problem with it either. Sarah's condition, called pregnancy-induced hypertension (PIH), is diagnosed in 10 to 20 percent of women pregnant for the first time.

Sarah was asked to take time to rest. Because she was a salesperson at a local department store, resting was virtually impossible while she was at work. However, she did try to put her feet up for a few minutes when she could and rested a lot in the evenings.

After closely monitoring Sarah's blood pressure for several weeks, Sarah's doctor decided she should be on strict bed rest to prevent her blood pressure from getting worse. She took a temporary disability leave, which allowed her to keep receiving some income. After two months on bed rest, Sarah delivered a healthy, blue-eyed boy who weighed 7 pounds.

For Sarah, following the doctor's orders paid off! Keeping her doctor's appointments and staying in bed kept her blood pressure from going up any more and improved her circulation. The improved circulation allowed adequate blood flow and nutrients to her baby so he could grow adequately.

Had Sarah not taken such good care of herself, the PIH might have escalated into more serious conditions called preeclampsia and eclampsia. PIH, preeclampsia, and eclampsia are all hypertensive disorders of pregnancy. Each is a stage of the same disease. These disorders are also known as the toxemias of pregnancy, or simply toxemia. Because the term *toxemia* has been used to describe the hypertensive disorders of pregnancy in the past, some people may still use the term.

The following list of definitions will help you understand high blood pressure during pregnancy:[34]

Pregnancy-Induced Hypertension (PIH) or Transient Hypertension refers to high blood pressure caused by pregnancy. PIH may also be called gestational hypertension. Women with PIH usually have no symptoms, and their blood pressure generally goes back to normal after delivery. They are at risk for developing PIH again in subsequent pregnancies and may also develop chronic hypertension later in life.

Preeclampsia refers to several complications, including high blood pressure, protein in the urine, and edema (excessive fluid retention). Kidney and liver damage can occur if untreated.

Eclampsia is a potentially fatal condition in which the mother can go into convulsions or a coma.

Chronic Hypertension is high blood pressure that existed before pregnancy, or that is diagnosed before the twentieth week of pregnancy.

If preeclampsia were superimposed upon chronic hypertension, the woman would have high blood pressure and the pre-eclampsia symptoms (protein in the urine and edema).

What Happens to Blood Pressure during Pregnancy

Blood pressure usually drops during the first half of pregnancy and then rises to normal levels. Women with mild hypertension may also experience that drop and may have normal blood pressure until midpregnancy. Not until the third trimester does blood pressure increase to the point where some type of treatment (such as bed rest or medication) may be necessary. Once blood pressure increases, it may not drop back to normal levels until after delivery.

Though the causes of PIH are not fully understood, poor nutritional status is one risk factor. PIH appears to occur at a higher rate among women with poor nutritional intake and no prenatal care.

Your overall food intake, including adequate calories, protein, and certain minerals, appears to be important in preventing high blood pressure. If you don't have enough energy or calories from carbohydrate or fat in your diet, your body will use dietary or tissue protein for energy. This can reduce protein available for tissue growth and can also limit the protein used in fluid balance.

Underweight women who fail to gain weight properly have a higher risk of developing PIH.

You are more likely to develop hypertension during pregnancy if you fall into one or more of these categories:[35]

- You are pregnant for the first time.
- You are expecting multiple fetuses.
- You are diabetic.
- You have kidney disease.
- You were overweight before your pregnancy.
- Your mother had preeclampsia.

The information below applies both to women with PIH and to those with chronic hypertension.

Risk to Mom

The biggest danger of high blood pressure during pregnancy is preeclampsia. Restricted activity and bed rest are two treatments to control your blood pressure and ensure that adequate blood and nutrients circulate to your baby.

Risks to Baby

Even if you have no symptoms, high blood pressure can reduce blood flow—and thus oxygen and nutrient flow—to your baby. Your baby may not grow properly and may have intrauterine growth retardation (IUGR). Your physician will probably monitor your baby's heart rate and growth with ultrasound tests. Women with hypertension are also more likely to have a miscarriage or stillbirth. If your blood pressure cannot be controlled, your baby may be delivered prematurely.

What You Can Do

If You Have Chronic High Blood Pressure before Pregnancy:

▶ **See your physician before you become pregnant.**

Establish good blood pressure control and a base-line reading of your blood pressure.

▶ **Lose weight and start a regular exercise program before pregnancy.**

Both can help reduce your blood pressure.

▶ **When you become pregnant, see your physician as soon as possible to start your prenatal care.**

Be sure to keep your appointments with your health-care provider so that you and your baby can be monitored.

If You Are Diagnosed with High Blood Pressure during Pregnancy:

▶ **Get plenty of rest–at least eight hours of sleep per night.**

Also, try to lie down a few hours during the day on your left side to increase blood flow to your baby. When sitting, elevate your legs above your hips to improve circulation.

▶ **Monitor your blood pressure.**

You may go to your doctor's office for a blood pressure check or you may check it at home. Keeping track of your blood pressure will give you and your physician a better idea of your average blood pressure over time.

▶ **Be aware of your sodium intake.**

Because your need for sodium increases during pregnancy, restricting sodium in your diet is not necessary. However, women who are salt-sensitive before pregnancy and follow a sodium-restricted diet may want to continue to watch their sodium during pregnancy. Ask your physician about your specific sodium needs. Foods with excess sodium include pickles; regular canned soups; smoked and cured meats such as bacon, sausage, and ham; and many frozen and ready-to-eat foods. Sodium information can be found on nutrition labels.

▶ **Eat plenty of calcium-rich foods.**

Research has shown that calcium plays a role in reducing blood pressure and may also reduce the risk of preeclampsia and premature birth.[36] Though the evidence isn't conclusive enough to recommend supplementary calcium over the Dietary Reference Intake (DRI), getting plenty of calcium through your diet can only help! Try to have at least four servings of calcium-rich foods every day. If you are lactose intolerant or allergic to milk, a calcium supplement from your physician may be warranted. If you simply don't like dairy products, see page 68 for tips on sneaking calcium into your diet.

▶ **Eat balanced, healthy meals.**

Follow the Eating Expectantly Eating Plan! (See page 55.)

▶ **Watch your activity level.**

Because you will need to restrict your activity or may be on bed rest, you'll need super-speedy meals. (See page 325 for "Meals in Minutes" and page 140 for eating tips for women on bed rest.)

▶ **Avoid caffeine, alcohol, and cigarettes; these substances can increase blood pressure.**

▶ **Keep your stress level low.**

Cut down on commitments and chores. If you're a type A person, learn to slow down! One study has shown that women in high-stress jobs during the first twenty weeks of pregnancy were more likely to have preeclampsia than women in low-stress jobs.[37]

▶ **Continue drinking plenty of fluids, even if you are retaining fluid.**

▶ **Avoid prolonged vigorous exercise, including lifting.**

This is especially important for women with children at home. Instead of picking up your children, squat to their level. Don't bend over with straight knees! Your physician will give you more specific exercise guidelines.

What Can You Expect?

If you have high blood pressure during pregnancy, you may be asked to restrict your activity, be on bed rest, or be hospitalized. Rest has been shown to reduce premature labor, lower blood pressure, and help the body get rid of excess water.[38]

Even if you aren't given special instructions for rest, you should set aside time every day to be off your feet. Making rest a priority on your own may prevent imposed restrictions and medications from your doctor. (See page 140 for "Coping With Bed Rest" if bed rest or hospitalization becomes necessary.)

Elevated blood pressure and preeclampsia may warrant an early delivery of your baby, preferably induced vaginal delivery. However, in cases where a speedy delivery is necessary, a C-section may be done.

In some cases, even bed rest or restricted activity may not adequately control blood pressure. If this happens to you, you may need to be hospitalized, put on medication, or deliver prematurely. For women who have chronic high blood pressure before pregnancy, hospitalization is not uncommon.

Rest during Pregnancy

Tell the typical woman to rest, and she'll say, "Oh, okay," and take a fifteen-minute catnap then go back to her very busy lifestyle. Most people don't realize how vital rest is for pregnant women with high blood pressure.

Kathy said her doctor told her to rest, and she did lay down for a rest "every so often." She didn't realize exactly what the doctor meant. Eventually she was put on strict bed rest. When she went into labor, her blood pressure became very elevated and she had to have an emergency C-section. She wished that someone had explained what "rest" really meant!

If you're told to rest, this is what you should do:

▶ **Rest one to two hours off your feet in both the morning and the afternoon every day. Ask your doctor for specifics.**

▶ **With your supervisor, arrange a rest period at work or a reduced work schedule.**

▶ **Enlist older children to help with household duties. You may also need some extra help with child care.**

▶ **Avoid stressful situations that could further increase your blood pressure.**

? Questions You May Have

Q: How will I know if I am developing preeclampsia?

A: These are specific signs and symptoms of preeclampsia:

• Swelling of hands, face, feet, and legs. Some water retention during the last months of pregnancy is normal. However, if the swelling moves to the upper part of your body, it may be a sign of preeclampsia.

• Sudden increased weight gain. If weight gain is not explained by increased food or fluid intake and occurs over a short period of time, this may also be a symptom. If you gain several pounds over a few days or in less than a week, check with your physician.

• Persistent, violent headache. If you have a severe headache that just won't go away, contact your physician immediately. This may be a warning sign of a convulsion.

• Visual difficulty. Blurred vision or partial-to-complete blindness are signs of preeclampsia. Again, seek medical attention immediately.

• Stomach pain. This can also be a sign of preeclampsia.[39]

Q: Will I still have high blood pressure after delivery?

A: Probably not immediately after delivery, unless you have chronic hypertension. Women who have pregnancy-induced hypertension are very likely to have high blood pressure later in life. You might reduce your risk of hypertension by going back to your ideal body weight after pregnancy, exercising regularly, and eating a nutritious diet containing adequate high-calcium foods. (See page 179 for more information on losing weight after delivery.)

Women with preeclampsia have about the same risk of developing hypertension later in life as those who never had the disease.[40]

Q: What about my next pregnancy?

A: If you have PIH, you have about an 80-percent chance of developing it again in later pregnancies. If you have preeclampsia along with chronic hypertension, your risk of having the same problem with other pregnancies can be as high as 70 percent.[41]

On the bright side: If you do have the

same problem with your next pregnancy, you will be a pro at handling it! You will know how to truly rest, how to monitor your blood pressure, and what to expect during your pregnancy.

For more information on coping with chronic disease during pregnancy, I recommend an excellent book titled *Intensive Caring* by Diane Hales and Timothy Johnson, M.D., Crown Books.

▼

Multiple Births

One way to have an instant family is to deliver twins, triplets, or more! In the United States and other countries that have increased the use of fertility treatments, carrying multiple fetuses is much more common than it used to be. In 1996, one in thirty-eight U.S. births produced twins, and in 1997 that rate rose to one in thirty-three. In 1996, 1 in 795 U.S. births produced triplets. Between 1995 and 1996, quadruplet births rose 53 percent, and pregnancies with five or more fetuses rose 42 percent.[42] The likelihood of having a multiple birth rises with age; a woman who is between thirty-five and forty is three times more likely to have fraternal twins than a woman who is twenty to twenty-five years old.

What Can You Expect?

Before we discuss the potential problems of carrying multiple fetuses, we need to make an important point: You have more control over your pregnancy and the health of your babies than you may think. Some of the small daily choices you make—like eating the right foods, resting when your body tells you to, and following the advice of your health-care provider—can significantly affect your babies' well-being.

Multifetal pregnancies are considered high-risk, and here's why: Newborn multiples tend to be preterm, low-birth-weight, and small for their gestational age. Multiple deliveries accounted for 3 percent of U.S. births in 1997, but 21 percent of all babies that were low-birth-weight.[43] Birth defects, respiratory distress syndrome, cerebral palsy, and other complications are more common among multiples. During a multifetal pregnancy, a woman is more likely to have preeclampsia, iron-deficiency anemia, hyperemesis gravidarum (persistent, excessive nausea and vomiting), placenta previa (abnormal placement of placenta), and kidney problems.[44] Many women carrying multiple fetuses are given tocolytic agents (medication to stop labor) and put on bed rest.

Does this mean that you will have the problems above? No. You may have some—or you may be lucky and have minimal problems. Many women at the University of Michigan Multiples Clinic have beaten the odds. Two-thirds of the moms at this clinic deliver at thirty-six weeks or later—compared with only two-fifths nationwide. Triplets born in this clinic's program weigh 35 percent more than the national average birth weight for triplets. Two-thirds of the clinic's newborns weigh more than 5½ pounds, and one-fourth of the clinic's

More Statistics on Multiples	
Twins	Average gestation is 37 weeks. Average birth weight is between 5 pounds and 5 pounds, 11 ounces. 50% of twins are preterm, and 50% are low-birth-weight.
Triplets	Average gestation is 33 to 34 weeks. Average birth weight is 3.9 pounds. 75% of triplets are preterm, and 90% are low-birth-weight. Average hospital stay is 29 days.
Quadruplets	Average gestation is 30 weeks. Average birth weight is 3 pounds, 12 ounces.

Sources: Brown, J. "Nutrition and Multifetal Pregnancy." Journal of the American Dietetic Association, 100, 3, March 2000. Luke, B. and T. Eberlein. *Expecting Twins, Triplets or Quads*. New York: HarperCollins, 1999.

newborns weigh more than 6½ pounds. That's double the average birth weight of multiples.

What do all these numbers mean? It bears repeating: Careful attention to your health while you're pregnant can significantly affect your babies' well-being.

What Factors Affect the Birth Weights of Multiples?

- Your prepregnancy weight and height (Shorter and lighter mothers are more prone to having smaller babies.)
- How much weight you gain
- The pattern of your weight gain (Weight gain in early pregnancy is important.)
- How long your pregnancy lasts (gestation)
- Your diet (Quality counts!)
- Whether the babies are identical or fraternal (Identical fetuses–produced from one egg that splits–generally weigh less.)
- Number of fetuses (The more there are, the less they will usually weigh.)
- Sex (Girls tend to be lighter.)

The Most Important Factor: Weight Gain

As with single-fetus pregnancies, the amount of weight gained during a multifetal pregnancy is directly related to the babies' birth weight. And because multiples tend to be delivered early and tend to be smaller, weight gain during multifetal pregnancy is even more important.

The Subcommittee on Nutritional Status and Weight Gain during Pregnancy has concluded that a weight gain of 35 to 45 pounds produces the healthiest twins.[45] A study done in Washington state found a weight gain of about 44 pounds was associated with optimum outcome of pregnancies lasting at least thirty-seven weeks and babies weighing over 5.5 pounds.[46] The chart on page 135 outlines weight gain suggested by Dr. Barbara Luke at the University of Michigan Multiples Clinic.

The pattern of your weight gain also affects your risk of preterm delivery and low birth weight. That is: Gaining weight consistently throughout pregnancy is related to a healthier outcome. And early weight gain has a great effect on birth weight, as was found in a large study of twins.[47]

Recommended Weight Gain Pattern for Multifetal Pregnancy					
Type of Pregnancy	Weekly Goal before 24 Weeks (pounds)	Goal by 24 Weeks (pounds)	Weekly Goal after 24 Weeks (pounds)	Total Goal (pounds)	Average Gestation (weeks)
Twins	1	24	2	40–50	36
Triplets	1.5	36	2.5	50–60	32
Quadruplets	2	50	3	65–80	30

Source: Luke, Barbara, and Tamara Eberlein. *When You're Expecting Twins, Triplets, or Quads*. New York: HarperCollins, 1999.

Another twin study revealed that underweight women who gain at least 1.13 pounds per week during the first twenty weeks of pregnancy and 1.92 pounds after twenty weeks of pregnancy were more likely to have twins that weighed at least 5.5 pounds. Normal-weight women who gained 1.5 pounds per week after twenty weeks were more likely to have babies that weighed at least 5.5 pounds.[48]

The suggested pattern of weight gain above will help you make short-term, intermediate, and long-term weight gain goals. You and your health-care provider will probably work out an individual plan for you. Remember to keep your eye on the prize: healthy babies!

Your Diet

Very little research has been done regarding exact nutrient needs of women pregnant with multiples. Calorie needs increase immensely, and the need for some vitamins and minerals increases, too—though no one is sure how much. One thing we do know is that nourishing fetuses takes a lot of good food. Following are some guidelines modified from the University of Michigan Multiples Clinic. Keep in mind that your health-care provider or dietitian may want to develop a more individualized plan for you.

The Need for Specific Nutrients

Calcium

Magnesium sulfate is a common tocolytic agent for multiple pregnancies. Although it is very effective in preventing preterm labor, it alters calcium metabolism, causing large amounts of calcium to be lost in the urine.[49] For one women pregnant with triplets, a postpartum fracture was thought to be due to osteoporosis after bed rest and therapy with magnesium sulfate.[50] Because of magnesium sulfate's effect on calcium metabolism, additional calcium (dietary or supplemental) may be necessary for women on magnesium sulfate therapy.

Iron

Iron is needed in even greater amounts for multifetal pregnancies because of the increase in blood volume. Iron is best absorbed from animal sources. See page 33 for iron-rich and zinc-rich foods. Liver is

Eating for Multiples								
Type of Pregnancy	Total Calories	Dairy (servings)*	Meat, Fish, Poultry (servings)†	Eggs (servings)‡	Vegetables (servings)§	Fruits (servings)‖	Grains (servings)#	Fats (servings)**
Twins	3,500	8	10	2	4	7	10	6
Triplets	4,000	10	10	2	5	8	12	7
Quads	4,500	12	12	2	6	8	12	8

*Serving size: 1 cup milk or ice cream, 1 ounce hard cheese.

†Serving size: 1 ounce. Concentrate on beef and pork, since these are highest in iron.

‡Serving size: 1 egg.

§Serving size: ½ cup cooked or 1 cup raw.

‖Serving size: 1 medium fresh fruit, ½ cup raw, 1 cup berries, ¼ cup dried fruit, ¾ cup juice.

#Serving size: 1 slice bread, 1 ounce (¾ cup) cereal, ½ cup pasta or rice.

**Serving size: 1 teaspoon oil, margarine, or butter; 1 tablespoon salad dressing or mayonnaise.

Source: Modified from *When You're Expecting Twins, Triplets, or Quads* by Dr. Barbara Luke and Tamara Eberlein. New York: HarperCollins, 1999.

the best source of iron and is recommended in the University of Michigan program. However, liver contains large amounts of vitamin A, which can cause birth defects in early pregnancy, which is why you will not find it in any of the food lists in this book.

Vitamin D

Vitamin D appears to be used in larger amounts during multifetal pregnancies. Vitamin D is made in the skin with exposure to sunlight. Since a woman may not get any exposure to the sun during the last half of a multifetal pregnancy, she needs to get adequate vitamin D from fortified foods (milk and some breakfast cereals) or a supplement.[51]

Essential Fatty Acids

Essential fats (discussed in detail in Chapter Two), are important for development of the nervous system (including the brain) and retina. This development occurs at the end of pregnancy and throughout the first two years of life. The amount of essential fatty acids in the bloodstreams of multiple fetuses is significantly less than in a single fetus. This indicates that women pregnant with multiples need to consume more essential fats—although the specific amount is not known.[52] See below for some good sources of essential fatty acids.

Good Sources of Omega-3 Fatty Acids

These fatty acids are particularly important for brain and retina development.

Animal Sources:

• Fatty fish, especially cold-water fish like salmon, mackerel, albacore tuna, sardines, and lake trout

- Eggland's Best Eggs
- Meat (Although meat is not high in essential fats, it has been shown to be a significant source when consumed in large amounts.)[53]

Plant Sources:
- Flaxseed oil and flaxseed
- Canola oil
- Soybean oil

Good sources of Omega-6 Fatty Acids
- Sunflower oil
- Safflower oil
- Corn oil

The best approach is to eat cold-water fish like salmon several times a week, cook with canola oil, and use margarines and salad dressings and that are made with canola or sunflower oil.

What about Supplements?

The Institute of Medicine recommends a supplement containing the nutrients listed below. Most prenatal vitamins contain at least these amounts.

Iron:	30 milligrams
Zinc:	15 milligrams
Copper:	2 milligrams
Calcium:	250 milligrams
Vitamin B_6:	2 milligrams
Folate:	300 micrograms
Vitamin C:	50 milligrams
Vitamin D:	5 micrograms

Dr. Luke, however, teaches her clients how to get most of the nutrients above from food. With the exception of calcium, magnesium, and zinc, minerals show promise in reducing preterm birth.[54] Speak with your health-care provider about what supplement is best for you.

A Twin Success Story

At the Montreal Diet Dispensary, a special program called the Higgins Nutrition Intervention Program was used to try to decrease some of the risks apparent in disadvantaged mothers of twins. The program consisted of individualized risk assessment, determination of dietary needs, nutrition education based on clients' eating patterns, and regular follow-up. Women not able to afford the prescribed diet were given a supplement of milk and eggs.

The program, which had previously proven successful with mothers expecting one baby, also produced positive results with mothers of twins. The twin infants of mothers who participated in the program weighed almost 3 ounces more than the infants of nonparticipating mothers. The program infants had a 25-percent-lower rate of low birth weight and a 50-percent-lower rate of very low birth weight. (Babies with very low birth weight are usually the sickest babies, who require intensive care.) Also, the preterm delivery rate was 30 percent less. This intervention program included eating 1,000 extra calories and 50 extra grams of protein above nonpregnant needs after twenty weeks. Women who were underweight before pregnancy and those with special risk conditions, such as a poor outcome of a prior pregnancy, received additional instructions.[55]

What Can the Higgins Program Do for You?

One researcher has found that women who had multiple gestations ate about the same amount as those pregnant with just one fetus.[56] That means you probably need to take a close look at what you're eating. Better yet, seek the services of a registered dietitian, who can give you individualized dietary advice. Increased calories and protein seem to be a significant factor in preventing low birth weight and prematurity in certain groups of women.

To achieve the 35-to-45-pound weight gain, you will need to gain about 1½ pounds per week during the second and third trimesters. This may require an additional 500 to 600 calories per day more than your prepregnant diet. Based on the Higgins research, you could need up to 1,000 extra calories per day.

How Can I Possibly Eat More Food?

While some women enjoy pigging out on healthy foods (plus a few splurges), others have trouble getting all that extra food down. What to do?

First, make sure your diet has all the essentials—especially protein, fruits, and vegetables. (See page 55, "The Eating Expectantly Eating Plan.") Then add extra foods to boost your calorie intake. The foods most concentrated in calories are fat and sugar—the usual no-nos. However, to get all the calories you need with what seems to be an ever-shrinking stomach, you must give yourself permission to eat no-nos.

The easiest extra to add is fat. Concentrate on adding vegetable fat. You may need to eat as much as 40 percent of your calories as fat to gain enough weight. Put nuts, olives, and avocado in your salads and sandwiches. Eat guacamole! Add butter to your vegetables, more salad dressing to your salads, extra oil when cooking, and so on. Eat more salmon; it is high in fat, and the fat is important for your babies' brain and eye development. Another way to add more calories to your diet is by eating high-sugar foods. By that I don't mean you should drink a soda and eat a candy bar every day! Instead, turn to the category of foods I call the "good extras," which includes milk shakes, puddings, peanut-butter cookies, and other foods that are high-calorie but will also provide nutritional basics. (See page 263 for high-energy snack choices.)

Six Ways to Feed Multiples

1. *Eat your way through the day.* Eat three meals and three to four snacks per day. Balanced meals and minimeals that contain protein are best.

2. *Say good-bye to guilt!* Gaining weight is critical for the health of your babies—and that means eating much larger quantities of food (and fat) than you may be used to. Milk shake, anyone?

3. *Where's the beef?* Hopefully in your fridge and freezer. Dr. Luke recommends eating red meat twice a day for the iron. Boost iron absorption more by cooking with an iron or

aluminum skillet and eating a vitamin-C-rich food with each meal. Also, avoid drinking coffee and tea within an hour of a meal.

4. *Drink, drink, drink!* Dehydration can bring on preterm labor, so drink often. Eight 16-ounce glasses of water per day is recommended.

5. *Get in the slow lane.* Since it's important to slow down to allow your body to nurture your babies, you may need to let some things go, such as cooking. Use the quick and easy menus on page 242. Encourage your partner to go crazy in the kitchen. Let your good-hearted friends fill your freezer with ready-to-eat meals. Treat yourself to gourmet takeout or restaurant delivery. (Remember that you may need to fill in some fruits and veggies.)

6. *Drink your snacks from a can.* Some women find nutritional supplements like Sustacal and Ensure drinks to be lifesavers. Often given to people in the hospital who need extra nutrition, these drinks contain balanced nutrition with added vitamins and minerals—plus they have lots of calories. They come in different flavors and are often good over ice or blended with ice cream and fruit.

Resources for Parents of Multiples

Book

Luke, Barbara, and Tamara Eberlein. *When You're Expecting Twins, Triplets, or Quads: A Complete Resource.* New York: HarperCollins, 1999.

On-line Resources

Sidelines (support group for women with high-risk pregnancies)
714-497-2265
www.sidelines.org

The American Dietetic Association (can refer you to a dietitian in your area)
800-366-1655, ext. 1
www.eatright.org

MOST (Mothers of Super Twins)
516-434-MOST
www.mostonline.org

National Organization of Mothers of Twins Clubs
800-243-2276
www.nomotc.org

The Center for Study of Multiple Birth
312-266-9093
www.multiplebirth.com

The Triplet Connection
209-474-0885
www.tripletconnection.org

Twins Magazine On-line
www.twinsmagazine.com

About.com
www.multiples.about.com/parenting/multiples/

American Association for Premature Infants
www.aapi-online.org/

Center for Loss in Multiple Birth, Inc. (CLIMB)
907-746-6123

▼

Coping with Bed Rest

We all dream of having just one day in bed to sleep, watch TV, or catch up on our reading. But spending several weeks in bed may seem more like a nightmare.

Bed rest is prescribed for multiple reasons, including hypertension or preeclampsia, multiple gestation (twins or more), premature labor, or poor growth of baby (also called intrauterine growth retardation, or IUGR). Some women are put on bed rest for several months, which can really give a person cabin fever.

Following is a guide to help you make the most of your rest period. This information was developed by talking with others and also from personal experience. I was on bed rest for eleven weeks for preterm labor. It was all worth it in the end. My son Robert was born healthy and weighed 7 pounds, 7 ounces. My labor even had to be helped along a little!

At first, the days seemed to go on forever. But once I got into a routine and my doctor gave me the okay to get up a little more, time became much more bearable. I wrote most of the following information before I was on bed rest, so I was able to follow my own advice. And it worked! I hope it helps you, too.

Welcome to Club Bed

Setting Up the Room

You will probably want to set up a makeshift bedroom near the place where your family gathers. A family room off the kitchen works nicely. Here are the basic living supplies with which you'll want to furnish your new room:

- Bed with plenty of pillows (Or rent a hospital bed.)
- Phone that will reach to the bed or a portable phone (Think of it as your link to the outside world, and don't forget the phone book.)
- Ice chest or minifridge for your bedside
- Microwave (depending how strict your bed rest is)
- Large bedside table or a hospital-type table that can be raised or lowered to your level (This can be rented from a medical supply company. Several TV trays work well, too.)
- Any medicines you are taking, including those taken occasionally for heartburn, constipation, and so on
- Large pitcher, filled with fresh water daily, and an ice bucket
- Soup cans for doing arm exercises (if your physician approves)
- An intercom system (Invest early in one for the baby; it will save your voice and save your family lots of trips back and forth fetching for you.)

Eating and Dietary Considerations

Yes, eating is a whole new challenge when you spend all your time on a mattress or couch! Keep in mind that you will need fewer calories than usual since you'll be using very little energy for activity. (If you are taking medication to stop your contractions, it may increase your metabolism, and you may need to eat about the same as you did before.) A potential problem is that the lack of activity may increase blood sugar and lead to gestational diabetes. To help control your risk, avoid concentrated sweets and fruit juices. (See page 115 for more about gestational diabetes, and if your appetite isn't good see page 138, "How Can I Possibly Eat More Food?" for tips on adding calories. Following is a guide to bedroom cuisine:

▶ **Make shopping lists and menus so your family or friends can shop for you.**

▶ **Keep snacks next to you:**
- A fruit bowl filled with fresh and dried fruit such as apples, figs, and prunes
- A jar of peanut butter
- Individually wrapped string cheese
- Wheat and rye crackers, graham crackers, rice cakes, baked tortilla chips
- Raw veggie sticks in a plastic container with ice
- Cheese food that doesn't need refrigeration
- Nuts

Note: Beware—convenience foods that need no refrigeration are often high in fat and salt. Eat sparingly!

▶ **If possible, keep a microwave next to you.**
If you have a microwave nearby, you'll also want:
- Low-fat popcorn
- Decaffeinated tea, decaffeinated instant coffee, hot-chocolate mix, and mugs

- Cans of hearty single-serving soups such as split pea, chunky chicken-vegetable, and beans with ham

▶ **If you are allowed to get up briefly to make a meal, the following can be prepared in six to seven minutes from scratch or with leftovers:**
- Scrambled eggs with toast
- Frozen microwave dinners (See page 242 for healthy choices.)
- Refried vegetarian beans, corn tortilla toasted in oven, cheese, lettuce, and tomato
- Chef salad with prepared lettuce in the bag—you just add the tomato, cheese, ham, turkey, and veggies
- Bean soups in a cup
- Chicken salad with pineapple
- Chicken fajitas or burritos
- Chicken curry over bulgur
- Chicken taco
- Chicken-English-muffin melt
- Chicken sandwich
- Pasta with tomato sauce (bottled)
- Pasta salad with tuna
- Pasta primavera
- Turkey tetrazzini
- Quick tuna casserole
- Chinese takeout or delivery
- Pizza delivery (also delivered sandwiches, pastas, and so on)

Bed rest joke: The best and worst thing about bed rest: You aren't the cook and you aren't the cook! (From *Sidelines* newsletter, Winter 1992.)

Entertainment to Keep Handy

You may have to be creative with this!

- Radio or stereo
- TV and VCR with remote control (Be sure you have a *TV Guide.*)
- Minilibrary set up with magazines, books, stationery, and photo albums
- Diary to keep track of your days
- Calendar
- Computer with which to play games, keep track of finances, and write letters (You can also borrow your kid's Nintendo or Game Boy!)
- Large notebook for making all kinds of lists—things to do, things for others to do, things to buy, things to make, bills to pay, what's on sale where, and so on
- Word games
- Crafts such as cross-stitch, embroidery, knitting, and so on
- Books on tape for when you get tired of reading

Eleven Activities to Keep Your Mind Alive

1. *Volunteer by phone.* Have you always wanted to volunteer, but never had the time? Here's your chance. You could do fundraising or check on latchkey kids or elderly shut-ins. Or you could create your own network of bed-bound moms. Check the local paper or the Red Cross for volunteer opportunities.

2. *Enhance your skills.* Take a correspondence course or a class on TV. Learn a new computer program.

3. *Increase your vocabulary.* Several good books are available, such as *30 Days to a More Powerful Vocabulary.* Crossword puzzles and other word games can also help. Keep a dictionary nearby.

4. *Learn a language. Parlez vous Français?* Many language courses are available by mail. Your new language could be the start of a dream trip to Monte Carlo or Madrid.

5. *Interact on-line.* If you have a computer with Internet access next to you, you'll have the world at your fingertips. You can:

- Read the news.
- Invest on-line and track investments.
- Bank and pay bills on-line.
- Chat on-line.
- Play interactive games on-line with people from around the world at:
    www.altavista.com
    www.yahoo.com
    www.aol.com
    www.thehouseofcards.com
- Shop! Most Internet service providers have many links to on-line shopping. This may be particularly useful for buying groceries (www.netgrocer.com, www.priceline.com) or baby clothes, furniture, and other supplies (www.babygear.com).

6. *Learn to cook, craft, or decorate.* Check out shows on PBS, Lifeline, the Food Network, and Home and Garden Television.

7. *Have a makeover.* You may not feel like putting on makeup, but just for a change, you

might have someone come over and give you a new look.

8. *Become a financial wizard.* Plan your retirement. Send for information on all those great-sounding mutual funds. Keep up with the stock market. Plan how you'll pay for your baby's college tuition.

9. *Make a quilt, afghan, or rug.* You can order kits by mail.

10. *Start your Christmas shopping, even if it's March.* Use your TV, computer, or catalogs or start making the presents by hand.

11. *Create new recipes.* No kidding! I met a soldier who was in a national cooking contest. It turns out he developed his recipe while he was stationed in Saudi Arabia during Operation Desert Storm. I was wondering how he ever found access to a kitchen or found time to cook. He thought about cooking and wrote down all his ideas for ingredients. When he got back home, he experimented with a few and sent them to the contest.

Exercise and Activity

Your activity level is a very individual matter that should be discussed with your doctor. However, you should ask about doing isometric exercises and/or arm exercises using light weights or 12-ounce cans. Such exercises will help you keep some muscle tone and help you avoid feeling sore from lack of movement. Remember that you can always practice your Kegels!

Also ask about turning from side to side often during the day. This will help prevent soreness in muscles and skin.

Other Survival Tips

▶ **Make a schedule of what you'll do during the day.**

This will make the day seem shorter and less monotonous.

▶ **Enlist others' help. If you have children, make a poster of chores for them to do.**

This may be a good time for your children to learn to do laundry, dishes, and even cooking–depending on their ages. If you don't have children, you'll need to depend on your partner, family (if they live close by), or friends. Although asking others to do things for you will be tough, make a list of all the little things that need doing and delegate them to different people. Hire a maid service if necessary.

▶ **Remember it's okay to let the housework go. (In your case, it's a must!)**

You have only one priority: for your little one to grow as much as possible for as long as possible. Whether the floor is mopped or the carpet is vacuumed really isn't important. Investigate getting household help from a home-care agency. My insurance covered this benefit, which improved the quality of our life immensely. A home-care assistant can take care of your children, cook, clean, run errands, and so forth.

▶ **Think positive.**

You might want to invest in a "positive thought for the day" type of book. Though the time in bed might be rough, having a premature or sick baby would be much worse. Make the most of your time.

▶ **Find other women in the same boat.**

Ask your health-care provider for names of other women in his or her practice who are on bed rest. When I was on bed rest, Norma, a friend of mine who had been on bed rest, called regularly for support. Get the word out among friends and coworkers or at your place of worship, and folks who have been where you are will likely step forward with a comforting word or a helping hand. You can also call one of the support groups listed below.

Confinement Line
703-941-7183
This organization provides phone support for women on bed rest.

Sidelines
714-497-2265
www.sidelines.org
This organization provides telephone and e-mail support for women with high-risk pregnancies.

▶ **You would be surprised at the number of services that will come to your home!**

I had a massage therapist visit my home weekly because I had a lot of soreness from lying around. I think it improved my circulation and I know it pampered me. You can also find someone who will cut your hair in your home and so forth. Though these are really splurges, it's little things like these that can help you make it through the tough times.

▼

Older Moms

In the past, most women started their families in their early twenties. Now many women are waiting until they are over thirty-five or into their forties. Waiting to start a family can have both advantages and disadvantages. Some women find that thirty-something is the perfect time for them. They are financially stable, have spent time developing a career, and are ready to start on the "mommy track." On the other hand, they may be more set in their ways and may be less physically ready for pregnancy and motherhood.

Barbara never really thought about having children until she was thirty-five years old. Then her biological clock started ticking loudly and suddenly Barbara wanted to join the ranks of moms. She had heard that older moms-to-be had a few more risks compared to their younger counterparts, so she visited her physician, who assured her she was in great physical shape. She worked out five times a week, didn't smoke, had no chronic diseases, and had already cut out caffeine. She did, however, skip meals and often ate on the run.

Her doctor explained that she was on the right track in improving her lifestyle, but that she should work on her diet. He told her that slight nutrient deficits could affect fertility. She then consulted a registered dietitian who, after looking at a three-day food diary, made some suggestions about how Barbara could improve her diet.

The dietitian suggested Barbara continue taking her mulitvitamins (which contained folic acid) and advised her to add supplements of nutrients that were missing in her diet.

Barbara worked a few months to improve her diet and became pregnant eight months later. She delivered a healthy baby boy weighing 7½ pounds! She was so thrilled with motherhood that she became pregnant again when her son Brian was eighteen months old.

Stories like Barbara's are becoming common as more women are putting off having a family until their late 30s or even 40s. But this approach does have its risks, so if you are over thirty-five, it's important to be in the best physical condition possible before you become pregnant.

What Can You Expect?

A large study from Sweden showed that women thirty-five or older are more likely to deliver prematurely, have a baby with low or very low birth weight, and have a baby small for gestational age. Women forty or older were also at increased risk for these complications.[57] However, negative outcomes were more likely with first births than with second births.[58] So you can improve your chances of having a healthy baby if you have your first child before age thirty-five, even if you have more children when you are older. Most of the complications associated with older moms are due to increased rates of fibroid tumors (leiomyomas), hypertension, and diabetes in women as they get older.[59]

The likelihood of a cesarean section increases with age and with increasing pre-pregnancy body mass index (BMI).[60] One reason is that older first-time mothers—especially those over forty—may have a long history of infertility; both patients and physicians may be anxious to avoid a poor outcome and thus may be more likely to resort to cesarean delivery.[61] Older pregnant women also have a higher risk of delivering a baby with Down syndrome and other types of autosomal trisomy (defects caused by an extra chromosome).[62]

Although there is greater risk for pregnancy complications in women over thirty-five, overall outcome can be good.[63]

What You Can Do

The most important thing you can do to reduce your risk of diabetes, C-section, and other complications is to achieve a body weight as close to your ideal weight as possible before you get pregnant. You should be practicing a healthy lifestyle by exercising regularly and eating a well-balanced diet. Start your prenatal care as soon as possible and follow your health-care provider's advice about exercising while you are pregnant.

▼

Teen Pregnancy

Teen pregnancy rates have been dropping since 1992. However, the birth rate for fifteen-to-seventeen-year-olds is similar to the birth rate for women ages thirty-five to thirty-nine.[64] Teen pregnancy is not only psychologically stressful for the teen and her parents, but it is also physically stressful to the teen because she is often still growing. There is some evidence that in pregnant girls who are still growing, the mother and baby may compete for nutrients.[65] Also, teens who are still growing are more likely to have excessive weight gain and deposit more body fat, which may put them at greater risk of being overweight and of developing type II diabetes, cardiovascular disease, and hypertension later in life.[66]

One thing is certain: Teens are not known for having healthy eating habits. A nationwide survey showed that among teens ages twelve through nineteen, only 22 percent ate the recommended two daily servings of dairy, only 19 percent ate the recommended two daily servings of fruit, and only 32 percent ate the recommended 5 to 7 ounces of protein foods each day.[67] Nearly one-fourth of the vegetables eaten by adolescents are French fries.[68] Adolescent girls consume the largest amount of added sweeteners as a percentage of total calories of any age group; one-third comes from soft drinks.[69]

Adolescent girls also tend to practice unsafe weight-loss methods. One study indicated that many white female high school students who smoke report using smoking to control their appetite and weight. A national survey of eighth-grade and tenth-grade students found that 32 percent skipped meals, 22 percent fasted, 7 percent used diet pills, 5 percent induced vomiting after meals, and 3 percent used laxatives to lose weight.[70]

Clearly, many teens may start their pregnancies malnourished.

What Can You Expect?

Infants of teens are twice as likely to have low birth weight and are five times more likely to die in the first twenty-eight days after birth than infants of adults. Among infants born to teens sixteen or younger, 14 percent are born prematurely (before thirty-seven weeks gestation).[71] However, you can give birth to a healthy, normal baby; it all depends on you. By eating the right foods, gaining enough weight, taking a prenatal vitamin, practicing good health habits, and visiting your doctor regularly, you can have the healthiest baby possible.

What You Can Do

Get help. You may be facing problems that you can't solve by yourself. There are many people you and your parents can turn to for help. Your school counselor or nurse can refer you to community programs. Many schools have special programs to help you. Your minister or a close family friend may be able to give you advice. The local health department or community clinic can provide free or low-cost medical care. The Women, Infants, and Children (WIC) program can give you supplemental food and teach you how to eat well. Remember that having social support can mean a healthier baby. A study in Mexico City showed that pregnant teens who received psychological support from the twentieth week (supposedly reducing anxiety levels) gained significantly more weight than pregnant teens who received no support.[72]

Gain enough weight. Weight gain is one of the best predictors of a healthy baby. The suggested weight gain is 25 to 40 pounds; most teens should gain toward the upper end of the recommendation. If you were underweight before pregnancy or are still growing, adequate weight gain is even more important to ensure that you have a healthy baby. It is also critical to gain weight from the very beginning of pregnancy and gain weight consistently throughout pregnancy.[73] Talk about your weight gain goal with your health-care provider.

See your health-care provider regularly. Getting adequate prenatal care is associated with having a healthier baby. The Toronto Healthiest Babies Possible Program showed that nine to eleven visits with a health-care provider throughout pregnancy helped prevent low-birth-weight babies.[74]

Cut back on sweets. High-sugar foods are often zero-nutrient foods and often take the place of healthier foods. One study in New Jersey has shown that pregnant teens with high-sugar diets have a greater risk of having a baby that is small for its gestational age.[75]

Take a prenatal vitamin supplement (or at least a multivitamin supplement containing 400 micrograms of folic acid) as soon as you think you are pregnant. If you eat one serving or less of dairy products (milk, yogurt, cheese) per day, take a calcium supplement containing 600 milligrams of calcium. Tums is an inexpensive choice.

Get ready to eat right. Take the food quiz on page 64. Add up the totals and compare to the Eating Expectantly for Teens Plan below.

Follow the Eating Expectantly for Teens Plan. Make sure not to skip meals and try to eat three snacks every day. Try to make every bite count—for your baby's sake!

Eating Expectantly for Teens Plan

10 or more servings of grains

1 serving is 1 slice any type bread; ½ small bagel, pita bread or English muffin; 1 6-inch tortilla; ½ cup cooked rice or pasta; ½ cup cooked cereal, barley, bulgur, or quinoa; 1 ounce ready-to-eat cereal; 3 to 4 crackers; or 2 cookies.

Note: 3 or more servings per day should be whole-grain.

5 or more servings of calcium-rich foods

1 serving is 1 cup any type milk or yogurt, 1½ ounces natural cheese, 2 ounces processed cheese, or 1 cup calcium-fortified orange juice or soymilk.

4 or more servings of fruit

1 serving is 1 medium fresh fruit; ½ grapefruit, mango, or papaya; ½ cup canned or chopped fruit; ¼ cup dried fruit; or ¾ cup juice.

4 or more servings of vegetables

1 serving is ½ cup cooked vegetables, 1 cup leafy vegetables, 1 small potato, or ¾ cup tomato or vegetable juice.

Note: Be sure to include at least one fruit or vegetable that is high in vitamin C and one that is dark green or orange every day.

3 servings of protein foods

1 serving is 2 to 3 ounces cooked lean meat (the size of a deck of cards); 2 eggs; ½ cup

tuna; ½ cup legumes, tofu, or textured vegetable protein; or 2 tablespoons nuts or nut butter.

Note: Eat a variety of protein foods, including fish at least once a week. Eat an additional ½ protein serving for each cup of milk that you don't drink.

Fats and sweets: Eat sparingly.

If you are having trouble gaining weight, you may need to increase your fat intake. If you are gaining too much weight, you may need to decrease your fat intake. See page 25 for more advice.

Six Ways to Eat Right

1. *Eat three meals and three snacks each day.* This can help you gain just the right amount of weight, while avoiding nausea and heartburn.

2. *If you eat fast food, have a salad and milk (or a milk shake) with it.* Drink water or fruit juice instead of soda. (See page 250 for healthy fast-food menus.) If your diet contains a lot of fast food, make sure to snack on fruits and vegetables between meals.

3. *If you have trouble gaining weight, eat filling snacks.* These include nuts, peanut butter, boiled eggs, cheese, milk shakes, nachos, and guacamole.

4. *If you can't drink milk, try to eat more yogurt and cheese.* Since your bones may still be growing, calcium is very important. (See page 68 for "Twelve Ways to Sneak Calcium into Your Diet.")

5. *Snack on fruits and veggies.* Eat fresh or dried fruit, carrots and broccoli with ranch dip, or a sandwich instead of chips, candy, or soda.

6. *Start the day with a good breakfast.* If you don't have time for breakfast, participate in the school breakfast program at your school or try these on-the-go meals:

> Tortilla with cheese rolled inside
> Bean burrito
> Peanut butter, honey, and banana
>   sandwich
> Granola bar and yogurt
> Leftover pizza

How Much Weight Should You Gain?

The Subcommittee on Nutritional Status and Weight Gain During Pregnancy recommends that you gain 35 pounds if you are considered normal weight for your height. If you were underweight before pregnancy, you should gain about 40 pounds. If you were overweight, you should aim for closer to 25 pounds.[76] Though this may seem like a lot, remember that you have only one chance to make a healthy baby!

Almost as important as *how much* you gain is *when* the weight is gained. Teens who gained little weight in the first six months (less than 10 pounds by the twenty-fourth week) had a higher risk of having small babies, even if their weight gain caught up at the end of the pregnancy. Inadequate weight gain also seems to be a factor in preterm birth (birth of a baby before thirty-seven weeks gestation). Girls who gained less than a pound a week at the end of the pregnancy had more premature deliveries.[77] In a study of pregnant teenagers across the United States, it was found that weight gain of 1.3 pounds per week from week fifteen until delivery resulted in babies that did not have low birth weights and were much less likely to need special care.[78]

The problem with "premies" is that the babies usually aren't quite ready for our world yet. Their lungs may not be developed, and they can have many other problems. Premies are often kept in the special care unit or intensive care unit for infants and aren't able to go home for a while. This is no fun for a baby, who may have to be fed intravenously and have blood taken frequently. Intensive care, if necessary, could cost you and your family a lot of money—tens of thousands of dollars.

Other Nutrient Needs

Calcium

All women need calcium in their diets. A low intake of calcium, especially before the age of thirty, increases your risk of osteoporosis (brittle bones). You've perhaps seen older women slumped over; their curved backs are probably due to osteoporosis. Or maybe you know a relative who fell and broke a hip. This is probably also due to the brittle-bone disease. How does that concern you now?

Your diet now actually affects how thick your bones will be when you become forty years old. The thicker and stronger your bones are, the lower your risk for osteoporosis.

Zinc

Zinc is an important nutrient needed for cell growth, cell division, and brain development. In a study of low-income pregnant teens, low dietary intake of zinc was related to a double risk of having a low-birth-weight baby and a threefold risk of very preterm delivery.[79] In women who had inadequate amounts of zinc in their blood, zinc supplementation increased birth weight and infant head circumference significantly. This underscores the importance of a prenatal supplement containing a balance of nutrients, as well as a diet with zinc-rich foods.[80] See page 33 for food sources of zinc.

Iron

Many pregnant teens start pregnancy with low iron stores. Iron deficiency in early gestation has been associated with a 200 to 300 percent increase in risk of prematurity and stillbirth. It is impossible to get all the iron you need from food; you must take an iron supplement or a multivitamin that contains adequate iron, like a prenatal vitamin. You can also boost your intake of iron-rich foods. See page 33 for more information.[81]

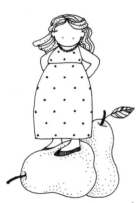

CHAPTER EIGHT

What you will find in this chapter:

- *My Experiences with Breastfeeding*
- *The Feeding Decision: It's Up to You*
- *Why You Should Consider Breastfeeding*
- *Possible Obstacles*
- *A Note to Dad*
- *Preparing for Breastfeeding*
- *Nutrition during Breastfeeding*
- *Nutrients of Special Concern*
- *Drugs and Breastfeeding*
- *Breastfeeding for Special Groups*
- *Tips for Formula Feeding*
- *About Bonding*

This chapter answers such questions as:

- *Who can answer my questions about breastfeeding?*
- *How will I know if I have enough milk for my baby?*
- *What if my husband isn't supportive of my decision to nurse?*
- *Can I drink coffee while breastfeeding? What about alcohol?*
- *Should I try to lose weight while nursing?*
- *What if my baby is premature— can I still nurse her?*
- *What about PCBs in breast milk?*

Considering Breastfeeding

My Experiences with Breastfeeding

When my first son, Nicolas, was born, I never wondered which feeding method I would use. In fact, this decision had been made long before I even met my husband! As a health professional who knew all the physical benefits of breastfeeding and had recommended breastfeeding to thousands of women, I had to breast-feed.

The pressure was on! The most difficult week of my life was that first week after Nicolas was born. I had a long labor and a difficult delivery. Nicolas and I didn't catch on to the fine art of breastfeeding right away. When Nicolas did not breast-feed for twenty-four hours, I felt guilty and gave permission for him to have a bottle. It was a big mistake!

Nicolas continued to receive bottles in the hospital. At home, our breast-feeding attempts failed again; during a feeding, he would latch on and pull away more times than I could count (or bear). As a last resort I called our pediatrician, who referred me to a lactation consultant. She was our savior.

We had two problems, Nicolas and I. He had nipple confusion. (Sounds like the making of a good joke!) That explained his frequent latching on and pulling away. He had gotten used to a plastic nipple in the hospital, so he couldn't get the hang of mine. And I wasn't positioning him correctly. A week or two after seeing the lactation consultant, we started to learn how the special process of breastfeeding works.

If I hadn't known about the benefits of breastfeeding, recommended it to so many women, and been under financial pressure from quitting my job, I would surely have quit breastfeeding that first week. That's why I feel compassion for all the women who want to breast-feed and are having difficulties.

Looking back, I'm so glad I hung in there and nursed Nicolas. The time we spent together was wonderful. And Nicolas was never sick while I was nursing him. One of my most memorable nursing sessions took place at an outdoor jazz concert that my husband Frank, Nicolas, and I attended when Nicolas was three months old. I felt perfectly comfortable feeding him under the privacy of a blanket. Actually I felt proud, because we were enjoying our own little routine. I didn't feel embarrassed about breastfeeding in public, as I had at first, and I liked feeling self-sufficient: no packing up bottles, trying to keep them cold, or looking for a place to warm them.

When my second son, Robert, was born, we had a totally different experience. I nursed Robert very soon after delivery, and he caught on immediately! I made it clear that Robert was not to have any plastic nipples while in the nursery, so he never had nipple confusion. At home, Robert continued to eat very well. Because I felt like a pro, I was comfortable breast-feeding him anywhere—with or without a blanket. Breastfeeding was especially convenient when we traveled overseas to visit our relatives; we didn't have to worry about packing formula.

I would never trade the experiences of nursing my children—both were special. More and more studies are citing the benefits of breastfeeding, so I urge you to give it a try!

▼

The Feeding Decision: It's Up to You

You may have been pondering how you'll feed your baby since the day your pregnancy was confirmed. Or through personal observations, you may have made your decision long ago. In any case, try to ensure that your decision is based on what is best for your baby, you, and your family.

Breastfeeding undoubtedly offers the most benefits for baby and mom. However, whatever method you decide to use, make a decision *you* feel good about.

Keep in mind that you can both breast-feed and formula-feed. Many women find this combination convenient, especially if they are going back to work. Even if you breast-feed for a short time, your baby will still benefit. If you do decide to combine breast- and bottlefeeding, introduce the bottle only after breastfeeding is well established to avoid nipple confusion.

Since this is a nutrition book for moms, this chapter will be primarily devoted to breastfeeding. However, if you decide to combine breastfeeding and formula feeding, I have listed some hints for formula feeding on page 173.

▼

Why You Should Consider Breastfeeding

Breastfeeding has been shown to greatly improve a newborn's short-term and long-term health. Following are just some of the benefits of breastfeeding.

Benefits to Baby

- Breast milk provides superior nutrition matched to your baby's needs. Colostrum, or first milk, is sometimes called "first immunization" because it contains important antibodies. As a result, breast-fed babies have fewer allergies, less diarrhea, a lower risk of serious bowel disorders, and fewer ear infections and respiratory illnesses.
- Research shows that essential fats found in breast milk (but not found in formula) are important to brain development. Studies show that breast-fed children have higher IQs than nonbreast-fed children because of critical brain development during the time of breastfeeding. Breast-fed babies accumulate twice as much docosahexanenoic acid (DHA) in their brains as formula-fed babies.[1]
- Breast-fed babies have a lower risk of sudden infant death syndrome (SIDS).[2]
- Breast milk may exert lifelong protection against insulin-dependent diabetes, cancer (including breast cancer), Crohn's disease (a chronic inflammatory disease of the colon), allergic diseases, and other chronic digestive diseases.[3]

- Breastfeeding promotes good jaw and facial development.

Benefits to Mom

- Breastfeeding helps you and your baby get acquainted and develop a close relationship.
- Women who have breast-fed have a lower risk of premenopausal breast cancer and ovarian cancer and a reduced risk of hip fracture later in life due to improved bone-building in the postpartum period.[4] Breastfeeding may also be related to a small but long-lasting reduction in postmenopausal breast cancer risk.
- Breastfeeding uses many calories and helps moms of newborns lose their "baby fat." Mother Nature designed women to gain a certain amount of fat during pregnancy to be used during breastfeeding.
- Breastfeeding helps your uterus return more quickly to its normal size and can also prevent hemorrhage if you breast-feed right after delivery.[5]
- The time you spend breast-feeding gives you a chance to recuperate, relax, and catch up on your reading. Life is fast-paced; perhaps breastfeeding was intended to slow us down to spend more time with our new little ones.
- Breastfeeding is convenient. You always have food for your baby with you, and it's always at the right temperature—no running to the store to buy formula, no messy mixing, and no worrying about proper refrigeration.

Benefits to the Family

- Breastfeeding saves money. Formula costs for one year can add up to one thousand dollars! Who couldn't use a little extra cash?
- Breastfeeding may give your family a chance to have quiet time together. If you have other children, you can use some of your nursing sessions as a time to read stories to older children.
- Research indicates that breastfeeding might change genetic predisposition to chronic disease, so breastfeeding may improve the health of your family in generations to come!

Breastfeeding for the Nation

Breastfeeding also offers social and economic benefits for the nation, including reduced health-care costs and reduced absenteeism among employees. Because of these benefits, the U.S. government has worked to increase breastfeeding through its "Healthy People" objectives. This effort has helped; the number of mothers who breast-feed their infants in the early postpartum period increased from 52 percent in 1990 to 62 percent in 1997. The number of women breast-feeding their infants at six months increased from 18 percent in 1990 to 26 percent in 1997.[6]

Possible Obstacles

Women who want to breast-feed may encounter obstacles in the people around them. If you plan accordingly, you can remove such obstacles and enjoy a successful nursing experience.

Betty Crase, formerly with La Leche League International, has nursed three out of four of her children. She feels the biggest barrier to breastfeeding is society's attitude. "Society is still prejudiced against breastfeeding," she says. "The breast is still viewed as a sex object instead of for nourishing babies. This attitude can deter a woman from breastfeeding. Women must feel comfortable breastfeeding wherever they are."[7]

Following are some other barriers and some suggestions on how to overcome them:

Unsupportive Family and Friends

▶ **Point out the benefits of breastfeeding that would most interest the unsupportive person.**

For example, your partner might be interested in saving money or in learning about the scientifically proven benefits of breastfeeding. Be assertive in your beliefs.

▶ **Find friends or relatives who have breast-fed and are willing to help you bring your family around to your way of thinking.**

Knowing someone who can share your experience and offer support may also make learning to breast-feed easier.

▶ **Invite your partner, family member, or friend to go to a breast-feeding class or La Leche League meeting.**

Unsupportive Hospital Staff

Unsupportive hospital staff can be quite problematic for women who are still undecided about breastfeeding. If you have some doubt, and your nurse prefers that you bottle-feed, the battle may already be lost!

If possible, find out which hospital in your area is most supportive of breastfeeding. The most supportive hospitals will have:

- Policies that are conducive to breastfeeding, such as rooming-in for the baby. Having your baby room-in with you helps you establish breastfeeding.
- A lactation specialist or consultant on staff who can visit you right after delivery to get you started. Lactation specialists are usually nurses who have extensive knowledge about breastfeeding; they have all the answers! Some hospitals also have lactation specialists who can make home visits to see how things are going. If you receive your prenatal care at a public health department or through a health maintenance organization (HMO), it may have a nurse who can visit you after delivery. Check on this while you are pregnant.
- Classes about breastfeeding for expectant moms and families. These highly informative classes may sell your partner, friends, or family on breastfeeding as well as give you lots of answers.
- Breast pumps for rent. These "industrial" pumps are very efficient and can usually empty both breasts in fifteen minutes. This comes in very handy for women who work.
- A list of community breast-feeding support groups, such as La Leche League, that you can call when you have questions. La Leche League meetings are open to pregnant women, and you may learn quite a lot about nursing just by spending time with nursing women.

Unsupportive Pediatrician or Staff

Before you have your baby, find a pediatrician (or family physician) who supports breastfeeding. This person will probably be the one you will call if you have any problems with or questions about breastfeeding. Do some investigation and call the prospective pediatrician's office. Ask to speak to the nurse and ask him or her a common breast-feeding question such as "How do I know if I'm producing enough milk?" or "What do I do if my baby seems hungry all the time?" or "Do you know of any lactation consultants?" If you plan to interview the doctor, you can ask about breastfeeding during the interview. Another good way to find a doctor who is supportive of breastfeeding is to ask other nursing moms; word usually gets around quickly about who the most supportive doctors are.

Having Enough Milk

Once a mother is breast-feeding her child, her biggest concern may be whether she is producing enough milk. You can make enough milk; it's a simple process of supply and demand. The more often you nurse your baby, the more milk your body makes. Here are some tips to help you make sure your baby is getting enough breast milk:[8]

▶ **Make sure you have positioned your baby properly: tummy to tummy.**

Your baby should be comfortable and should have a good grasp of your nipple to empty your milk glands. When your breasts are emptied, they'll make more milk to fill the demand.

▶ **Let your baby determine the length and frequency of feedings.**

You should nurse eight to twelve times in a twenty-four-hour period during the first week to help establish your milk supply.

▶ **Weigh your baby to ensure adequate weight gain after the first week.**

A breast-fed infant should gain 4 to 7 ounces per week or 1 pound per month.

▶ **Monitor wet diapers and bowel movements.**

These are physical signs that your baby is drinking enough milk. There should be six to eight wet diapers and three to five bowel movements per day in the early months.

▶ **Make a habit of drinking a glass of water or other beverage every time you breast-feed.**

Working While Breast-Feeding

Breastfeeding after going back to work is a great way to provide for your baby while you are away. And it's good for your company, too. Since breast milk protects against infection, women who breast-feed miss fewer days of work due to their babies' illnesses. Breastfeeding while working does take a bit of planning, though. Below are some tips. (See Chapter Nine for more advice on going back to work.)

▶ **Check out breast-feeding support at work while you are pregnant.**

Your supervisor or the personnel department are good places to start.

▶ **If your company has no lactation program, look into starting one.**

Corporate lactation programs are becoming more popular as the business world realizes the benefits of breastfeeding. A lactation program usually includes a mother's room for pumping, an electric breast pump available for use, and attitudes supportive of breastfeeding. Medela, a pump manufacturer, offers tips on starting a lactation program. For more information, visit Medela's website at www.medela.com.

▶ **Investigate flex hours or working part-time temporarily.**

▶ **Find a day-care provider close to your workplace.**

This will enable you to feed your baby during your lunch hour.

► **Rent an electric pump if your workplace doesn't provide one.**

Breast pumps can be rented from hospitals, lactation consultants, and health departments.

► **Be sure to build up a good milk supply before you begin giving your baby breast milk from a bottle.**

You may want to get your baby used to taking a bottle a week or two before you return to work.

► **If your workplace doesn't have a refrigerator, bring a cooler to work so you can store your milk safely.**

Seeking Help

Betty Crase and other promoters of breastfeeding think an early visit to the health-care provider may be a real benefit to nursing moms. Betty says, "An early visit builds the mother's confidence and can answer some of her questions."[9] In fact, the Colorado Breast-Feeding Task Force is encouraging the American Academy of Pediatrics to make a five-to-seven-day postpartum visit standard procedure for breast-fed babies.[10]

Most authorities on breastfeeding agree that the first two weeks are crucial for long-term breast-feeding success. If you have trouble the first few weeks, seek help from your health-care provider, a lactation specialist, or a local La Leche League leader…fast!

You can reach La Leche League International at 800-LA LECHE or www.lalecheleague.org.

A Note to Dad

– from Dr. Steven Nafziger, University Family Medical Center, Pueblo, Colorado

I once fancied myself as much of an expert on breastfeeding as anybody, and I thought that the advice on breastfeeding I gave women was always adequate and well taken. When my wife made the decision to breastfeed our first child, I quickly learned that simplistic advice like "Just keep trying; it will all come together" fell quite short. Every day, I faced some practical but perplexing questions about breastfeeding that made me realize how much I still needed to know about breastfeeding—not only professionally, but also as a father.

I'm sure that most fathers recognize at least some of the merits of breastfeeding. Breast milk is by far the best food for your baby. Breast-fed babies have fewer allergies and fewer illnesses during the breast-feeding period. Breastfeeding is also economical and convenient.

When moms breast-feed instead of bottle-feed, dads do get out of having to feed and mix formula, but they can do other helpful and thoughtful things. Breastfeeding requires a lot of a woman's time, which prevents her from doing other things, especially in the first few weeks. Doing housework and laundry, cooking, caring for other children, answering doorbells and telephone calls, and bringing baby to mom for feeding are only a few examples of what a father can do. Bathing or walking the baby or spending

Words of Encouragement from an Experienced Mom

Helene, the mother of five children, says, "The bond between mother and child while the child is being nourished in the womb is not over when the umbilical cord is cut. The bond continues and grows as the mother breast-feeds and holds that new miracle of life in her arms. It is not just a nutritional need that is being met for the baby. It is a psychological, emotional, and physical need for both as well. No sensation compares with nursing your child. Nothing is as satisfying and fulfilling as nursing. I would tell every new mother who is considering breastfeeding to do it."

time playing with him or her will not only free up time for mom but will also create a bond with the child, which is the best gift any parent can give a child.

Of all the things a father can do to help mom while she's breast-feeding, support is probably the key. Many women will make the decision to breast-feed on the basis of how much they're feeling supported. A woman will be more likely to breast-feed if her partner has an enthusiastic, supportive, and positive attitude rather than an indifferent or negative attitude. A partner's support and willingness to help can ease any reservations or fears a mom might have about breastfeeding. Breastfeeding for the first time is a new experience not only for the father, but also for the mother, and it requires a commitment from both of them. A father who realizes this has taken the first and most crucial step toward the mother's successful breast-feeding experience.[11]

Preparing for Breastfeeding

Before You Deliver

Well before your due date, get ready for breastfeeding by following this checklist.[12]

▶ **Attend a breast-feeding information class or a La Leche League meeting.**

Look in the phone book to find a local chapter, call 800-LA LECHE, or visit www.lalecheleague.org.

▶ **Find someone who has breast-fed whom you can call when you have questions or concerns.**

This person could be a La Leche League leader or member or simply a knowledgeable friend or relative.

▶ **Find a hospital and pediatrician who support breastfeeding.**

Ask whether the hospital where you are planning to deliver meets the Baby Friendly Hospital Initiative of the United Nations Children's Fund (UNICEF) and the World Health Organization (WHO). This policy recommends, among other things, that infants be nursed within thirty minutes of delivery; that no water, formula, or supplements be given to newborns unless medically necessary; and that babies room-in with their mothers twenty-four hours a day.

Surprisingly, not all pediatricians are supportive of breastfeeding. A recent survey of pediatricians showed that only 65 percent recommended breastfeeding to their patients as the exclusive feeding method for the first month. It also showed that 72 percent were not familiar with the Baby Friendly Hospital Initiative.[13]

▶ **Check out on-line resources.**

▶ **If returning to work, find out if your company and boss will support your decision to breast-feed.**

Do whatever you can now to prepare them.

▶ **Prepare yourself for breastfeeding.**

Breast preparation while pregnant is not recommended because it can cause premature labor. (Ask your health-care provider for more details.) Though nipple soreness during nursing is usually a result of incorrect positioning, some soreness may be due to sensitive skin around the nipple. Alleviating the soreness can be as simple as going braless or topless around the house or not washing your nipples with soap.

▶ **Have these things on hand:**

Nursing pads (washable cloth pads or disposable cotton pads) and a breast pump or access to one (useful if you have trouble with engorgement). I found that a battery-operated pump worked much better than a hand pump. Some women prefer to rent an electric pump.

At the Hospital

When you arrive at the hospital, use the following checklist to get off to a good start with breastfeeding.[14]

▶ **In addition to telling the doctors and nurses you plan to breast-feed, write a note ahead of time that states you plan to breast-feed and give the note to the nurse upon your arrival.**

▶ **Ask to room-in with your baby twenty-four hours a day.**

This enables you to feed your baby on demand more easily. However, some moms would rather rest, knowing that their babies are well cared for, and have them brought in frequently to nurse. Ask that your baby not receive any bottles when he or she is away from you.

▶ **Tell the staff to keep anesthesia and other labor medications to a minimum so you and your baby will be alert during breastfeeding.**

▶ **Tell staff you want to breast-feed as soon as possible after delivery–on the delivery table or in the recovery room.**

▶ **Tell staff not to give your baby supplemental water, sugar water, or formula unless medically necessary. Also ask them not to give your baby a pacifier, as this can cause nipple confusion.**

According to Dr. Nancy Krebs, a Denver pediatrician, "Full-term babies don't have to drink very much in the first twenty-four hours or so because most are born relatively well hydrated. Watch for colorless, dilute urine and adequate number of stools, because these are indicators of adequate nutrition. A baby who is very small at birth or who may have had a stressful delivery is more vulnerable to dehydration or low blood sugar."[15]

If your baby doesn't breast-feed much at first, consult your pediatrician or lactation specialist.

▶ Ask a lactation specialist or nurse to help you get started.

Contrary to popular belief, breastfeeding doesn't necessarily come naturally. Most of us need to learn, and some of us need help.

▶ Nurse your baby as often as the baby wants for as long as the baby wants—the sooner the better.

Nurse as often as every one to three hours. You may need to wake your baby for feedings.

What Might Happen and What You Can Do

While you're in the hospital, things may happen that make you question your decisions about breastfeeding. Here's some information to help you stay the course.[16]

▶ The nurses or doctors may tell you that you need your rest.

Tell them you will not sleep well without your baby and that you need all the nursing practice you can get before you go home and are on your own.

▶ Your baby may only nuzzle at the first feeding.

This is okay! It is important for you to get to know each other.

▶ You may wonder why your milk is thick and yellowish.

It's supposed to be! This "first milk," or colostrum, is low in fat and packed with carbohydrates, protein, and antibodies. Feeding your baby as much colostrum as possible will help your baby be as healthy as possible, help you and your baby establish a breastfeeding bond, and help your mature milk come in.

▶ Breastfeeding may be uncomfortable at first.

We all have different tolerances for discomfort. However, breastfeeding should not *hurt*. If it does, ask a nurse to help you get your baby properly positioned and latched on.

▶ The hospital may give you formula or coupons for formula in the discharge packet.

Hospitals do this because formula companies provide the samples free of charge. This does not mean that your baby will *need* the formula. Your body can make all the milk your baby needs.

▶ Before you leave the hospital, be sure to ask for a list of names and phone numbers of people in your area whom you can call if you have breast-feeding questions or problems.

Nutrition during Breastfeeding

The Best-for-Baby Breast-Feeding Eating Plan

While breast-feeding, you actually need to eat more than you ate during your pregnancy. And you should continue to make every bite count. Below is a meal plan that will allow you to meet your nutrition needs during nursing. Your daily diet should contain at least some of the following foods, which add up to about 2,400 calories. Remember that you may need more or less than these.

10 or more servings of grains

1 serving is 1 slice any type bread; ½ small bagel, pita bread or English muffin; 1 6-inch tortilla; ½ cup cooked rice or pasta; ½ cup cooked cereal, barley, bulgur, or quinoa; 1 ounce ready-to-eat cereal; 3 to 4 crackers; or 2 cookies.

Note: 3 or more servings should be whole-grain.

4 to 5 servings of calcium-rich foods

1 serving is 1 cup any type milk or yogurt, 1½ ounces natural cheese, 2 ounces processed cheese, or 1 cup calcium-fortified orange juice or soymilk.

4 or more servings of fruit

1 serving is 1 medium fresh fruit; ½ grapefruit, mango, or papaya; ½ cup canned or chopped fruit; ¼ cup dried fruit; or ¾ cup juice.

4 or more servings of vegetables

1 serving is ½ cup cooked vegetables, 1 cup leafy vegetables, 1 small potato, or ¾ cup tomato or vegetable juice.

Note: Be sure to eat at least one fruit or vegetable that is high in vitamin C and one that is dark green or orange, every day.

3 to 4 servings of protein foods

1 serving is 2 to 3 ounces cooked lean meat (the size of a deck of cards); 2 eggs; ½ cup tuna; ½ cup legumes, tofu, or textured vegetable protein; or 2 tablespoons nuts or nut butter.

Note: Try to eat fish at least once a week to get your share of essential fat for your baby's growing brain. Eat an additional ½ protein serving for each cup of milk that you don't drink. (See pages 25 and 26 for more info on essential fatty acids.)

Fats and sweets: Eat sparingly.

Women who breast-feed for more than six months and have reached their prepregnant weight may need to increase their intake of vegetable fats and other healthy extras to maintain their energy and milk supply.

Sample Meal Plan for Breastfeeding

Breakfast

Corn Bran with blueberries
Whole-wheat bagel with light cream cheese
Milk

Snack

Vegetable juice
Crackers

Carrot sticks

Turkey

Lunch

Grilled cheese sandwich

Sliced tomato

Peach

Sugar cookies

Milk

Snack

Fresh fruit salad

Dinner

Grilled chicken

Grilled vegetables

Spinach salad with red pepper and mushrooms

Whole-wheat roll

Fresh orange

Milk

Snack

Peanut butter and graham crackers

Yogurt with dried fruit

Calorie Needs

Your breast-feeding diet should be similar to your pregnancy diet, except now you need about 200 calories more (or 500 calories more than the amount you ate before you were pregnant). A good way to get the extra calories is to eat an additional snack or higher-calorie snacks. (See Chapter Thirteen for snack ideas.)

The suggested calorie intake for lactation takes into consideration the 100 to 150 calories a day that come from fat stored during pregnancy. For this reason, breastfeeding can help you lose weight; what a wonderful

way to do it! The average weight loss for breast-feeding women is 1 to 2 pounds per month, after the first month postpartum. If you breast-feed longer than that, you will probably continue to lose weight, but at a slower rate.[17]

While research has shown that the extra 500 calories are needed for successful breast-feeding, you may be less active during your first month or so postpartum.[18]

Therefore, after breastfeeding has been well established, you should evaluate your energy needs based on weight gain during pregnancy, weight loss per week during breast-feeding, and your activity level. You may need more or less than 200 calories above pregnancy needs, but it's a good place to start.[19] To ensure you have a nutritious and adequate milk supply, make sure that your calorie intake does not go below 1,800 calories.

If you breast-feed longer than six months, if you didn't gain much during pregnancy, or if you drop below your usual weight, you may need up to 650 calories per day (or even more) over your nonpregnant calorie needs. Also, if you are very active, you will need more calories than the average woman. If you find that you are losing weight too quickly or are having trouble eating the recommended amount of food, you should visit with a registered dietitian for some individualized advice.

Protein Needs

Your protein needs also increase during breastfeeding. You'll need 65 grams of protein per day (or 5 grams more than during pregnancy) during the first six months of breastfeeding. If you nurse longer than six months, you will need about 62 grams of protein per day because your baby will start eating solids and so will drink less milk.[20]

If you can drink or eat the recommended four daily servings of dairy products, you can meet your protein needs by eating just 2½ ounces of protein per day (including the amount of protein in six servings of grain products.) This is because each cup of milk contains the same amount of protein as 1 ounce of meat. The Best-for-Baby Breast-Feeding Eating Plan contains a protein boost to ensure that you get enough of the important nutrients like zinc, iron, and vitamin B_6 that are found in some protein foods.

If you prefer not to eat much meat, you will need to choose the rest of your diet wisely. (See pages 72, 73, and 85 for good food sources of iron and zinc.)

Nutrient Needs

Most of your nutrient needs stay the same during lactation; some decrease and some increase. You will need slightly more thiamin, riboflavin, vitamin B_{12}, and magnesium. You will need significantly more vitamin C, vitamin E, niacin, zinc, and selenium. You will need less folate and iron than during pregnancy. However, many physicians will recommend that you continue to take an iron supplement to help replace iron deficits from pregnancy or blood loss during delivery.

Be sure to continue getting plenty of fiber in your diet. (See page 53 for "Focus on Fiber.") When I experienced some constipation during the first few weeks of breastfeeding, my doctor explained that the hormones associated with breastfeeding can slow down the digestive process.

Don't forget fluids! Although in the past it was thought that women needed to drink a lot of extra fluid to produce breast milk, it now appears that drinking to your thirst will provide you with adequate fluid. However, if you live in a dry climate or exercise in hot weather, your thirst may lag behind your actual fluid needs.

If you were to eat very poorly while breast-feeding, your body would draw from stored pools of nutrients. If you breast-fed for six months and depended entirely on stored nutrients to feed your baby, you would deplete 19 percent of protein stores, 4 percent of calcium stores, 14 percent of iron stores, 46 percent of vitamin A stores, and close to 100 percent of folate stores. Most of us get more than enough protein. But if your diet does not include adequate amounts of calcium, iron, vitamin A, and especially folate, your own nutritional status could be in danger. Since pregnancy and breastfeeding are such physically demanding jobs, make sure that your own diet is as good as it can be so you'll have all the energy you possibly can.[21]

Calcium Needs

During pregnancy, women are often reminded about their need for calcium. After delivery, calcium in the diet may not seem that important. It is. First, the calcium in bone is often used as a calcium source during breastfeeding, especially if you do not have enough calcium in your diet. Heavy metals (like lead) accumulated in your bones over your lifetime can be released into your bloodstream—and to your baby—if you lose too much calcium from your bones during breastfeeding. Calcium loss during breastfeeding also puts women at risk for developing osteoporosis later in life.[22] The Dietary Reference Intake (DRI) for calcium during breastfeeding is 1,000 milligrams—the same as during pregnancy.[23] However, the National Institutes of Health recommends 1,200 to 1,500 milligrams per day for pregnancy and lactation. (See pages 70 and 71 for calcium contents of your favorite foods.) If you cannot obtain the recommended amount of calcium through your diet, ask your health-care provider about a calcium supplement.

Nutrients of Special Concern

When we compare average vitamin and mineral intakes of women in the United States to the needs of breast-feeding women, we find that intakes of several nutrients are below the DRIs. When a woman eats 2,700 calories per day, only zinc and calcium may fall below the DRI. However, if the diet contains less than 2,700 calories (and the average nursing woman's probably does), intakes of calcium, magnesium, zinc, vitamin B_6, and folate will likely fall well below the DRI.

Improved food choices are better than taking a nutrient supplement for several reasons. Most nutrients are absorbed better from foods than from supplements, and foods may contain unidentified nutrients not found in supplements. Also, taking a supplement can give you a false sense of security; you may be tempted to make poorer food choices, thinking that your vitamin will make up the difference.

If you do choose to take a supplement, take one that contains a broad spectrum of vitamins and minerals and contains no more than 100 percent of the DRI for any of them. Some doctors recommend that you continue taking prenatal vitamins. This is fine, but be aware that their high iron content may worsen constipation. Remember that after pregnancy, a woman's need for iron generally decreases—unless she has lost a lot of blood during delivery or is anemic. Ask your physician.

Best Food Sources

Calcium

Milk, cheese, yogurt, canned or small fish with edible bones (salmon, mackerel, sardines), tofu processed with calcium, bok choy, broccoli, kale, molasses, collard, mustard, and turnip greens.

Zinc

Oysters, seafood, lean red meats, poultry, eggs, wheat germ, nuts, dried beans and peas, yogurt, and whole grains.

Magnesium

Bran cereal, wheat germ, Swiss chard, spinach, nuts, seeds, beans and peas, whole grains, dried fruit, shrimp, and scallops.

Vitamin B$_6$

Mustard greens, bananas, poultry, meat, fish, potatoes, sweet potatoes, spinach, prunes, watermelon, some legumes, soybeans, lentils, chickpeas, pinto beans, fortified cereals, and nuts.

Folate

Spinach, leafy green vegetables, asparagus, black-eyed peas, lentils, kidney beans, fortified cereals, legumes, broccoli, Brussels sprouts, and orange and grapefruit juices.

Drugs and Breastfeeding

If you must take a medication during breast-feeding, you don't necessarily have to stop nursing. The safety of the medication depends on the drug and its dosage. For example, if you are taking an antibiotic for a breast infection, you are actually encouraged to breast-feed. However, some drugs pose a risk for your baby, including antiprotozoal compounds, antineoplastic drugs, some antithyroid drugs, and synthetic anticoagulants. Make sure your physician knows you are breast-feeding before he or she prescribes a medication.

If you must take one of the above drugs, pump your milk temporarily to keep your milk supply up. Discard the pumped milk

and resume breast-feeding several days after you stop the medication. Ask your health-care provider or pharmacist when the medication will leave your system so you can start breast-feeding again. If you take a lactation-suppression drug to stop breast-feeding, don't give your baby any of your milk while your milk supply is dwindling.

Some over-the-counter drugs should not be taken while you are breast-feeding. For example, acetaminophen (such as Tylenol) is usually recommended for pain instead of aspirin. Consult your health-care provider about which over-the-counter medications he or she recommends before the need arises.

Breastfeeding for Special Groups

Moms of Multiples

If you have given birth to multiple babies, can you still breast-feed? The answer is an enthusiastic "Yes!" As you may have guessed, breast-feeding multiples is a bit more complicated than nursing a single baby. But since multiples are often born smaller than single babies, your breast milk is even more important to give your babies a healthy boost.

Mothers of single babies need more energy while they are nursing, but according to Dr. Barbara Luke at the University of Michigan Multiples Clinic, mothers of multiples need about 300 calories less.

Some on-line resources for nursing multiples

are parentingweb.com/lounge/multiples.htm and www.lalecheleague.org. Books are listed in the Recommended Resources at the back of the book.

Vegetarians

Vegans (vegetarians who eat no animal products) need to plan their diets a little more carefully to make sure their breast milk contains everything their babies need. Vitamin B_{12} must be consumed from a reliable source; the DRI for breastfeeding is 2.9 micrograms. Vitamin D, calcium, and zinc may also be harder to find in a vegan diet. Please see pages 31, 71, and 85 for food sources of these nutrients.

Another factor that could affect your baby's development is the type of fat in your diet. Amounts of DHA (an essential fat) are lower in the blood of breast-fed infants whose mothers are vegetarian. DHA is not found in vegetarian diets, although alpha-linolenic acid, a fatty acid found in vegetable oils, can be converted to DHA in small amounts. It has been suggested that excess linoleic acid be avoided to support the production of DHA.[24] For more information, visit the Vegetarian Resource Group's website at www.vrg.org. (See also Chapters Six and Seven for more information on vegetarian eating and multifetal pregnancy.)

Teens

You can give your baby the best possible start by breast-feeding him or her. Breastfeeding has many benefits that may be especially important to you: It is less expensive, it is all-natural, it can help you get your body back in shape, and it can help you bond with your baby. There are also many health benefits, as described earlier in this chapter. One important one is a reduced risk of breast cancer—this applies to teens, too![25] Just remember to continue eating as well as you can, and take a multivitamin/mineral supplement.

Moms of Premies

If your baby was born prematurely, breast-feeding can give him or her a vital boost. And breast-feeding a premature infant can be even more rewarding for you than nursing a full-term infant, because you'll know that you are doing all you can to help your baby grow.

New research indicates that breast-feeding the premature infant may provide even more health benefits than feeding a full-term infant; it has been shown to improve short-term and long-term health (by decreasing risk of infections), gastrointestinal function, and neurological development. However, preterm infants often have higher nutrient needs than breast milk can satisfy. A premie's special nutritional needs may be met by the use of multinutrient supplements during the time the infant is being tube-fed. A human milk fortifier like the one made by Enfamil can also add nutrients to your milk so that your baby gets the nutrition he or she needs while still getting the benefits of breast milk.[26]

Your baby may have to stay in the neonatal intensive care unit so he or she can be monitored closely. If so, you will probably be pumping milk to be fed to your baby through a tube. However, skin-to-skin contact (also called kangaroo care) is encouraged to help increase milk production. While you are pumping, it may be helpful to keep a picture of your baby (or babies) next to you. While it may be disappointing not to be able to nurse your baby "in person," just remember what a special gift you are giving.

Because your baby is extraspecial, your milk should be extraspecial, too. Besides following all the dietary advice in this chapter, you should look at your intake of essential fatty acids and make sure you eat a good source of them on a daily basis. While exact requirements for these fats have not been determined, eating foods rich in them may help your baby's brain and eye development. Please see page 26 for sources of essential fatty acids.

For more information on parenting premies, see *Your Premature Baby and Child: Helpful Answers and Advice for Parents* by Amy E. Tracy. On-line resources include www.lalecheleague.org and the websites for parents of multiples listed on page 139.

On-Line Breast-Feeding Resources

La Leche League
www.lalecheleague.org

Nursing Mothers Association of Australia
avoca.vicnet.net.au/~nmaa/

Breastfeeding.com
www.breastfeeding.com

? Questions You May Have

Q: I've heard that if I eat gassy foods such as broccoli, onions, and even milk and chocolate, my baby can get gas. Do I have to stop eating all my favorite foods?

A: No. Although strongly flavored vegetables and spices may give your milk a different flavor or may cause your baby gas, to stop eating such foods is not necessary for everyone. After talking to many women, I have learned that baby's reaction to mom's diet seems to be an individual matter. One friend of mine continued eating plenty of garlic while nursing, and her baby had no problem with it. Another friend loved to eat hot peppers, and her baby apparently liked them, too.

Keep in mind that a lot of gas can simply be a result of the baby's immature digestive system. Both my children had problems with gas pains. I altered my diet in every way possible, but nothing seemed to help. I chalked it up to their own digestive systems and used a lot of over-the-counter infant gas medicine. They finally outgrew it.

If your baby has gas, you might try changing your diet for several days to see if the change makes a difference. Sensitivity to flavors and gas-causing foods seems to vary from baby to baby. If your baby has no problem with gas, you should be able to eat any food in moderation.

Q: We have a lot of food allergies in my family. Can breastfeeding help prevent them in my baby?

A: It's possible, but it hasn't been proven conclusively. Some studies suggest that components of food eaten by the mother can pass into the breast milk and cause allergic reactions in the baby. While avoiding certain foods during breastfeeding is sometimes recommended, one study has shown that there is no difference in the number of allergies among people whose mothers followed restricted diets.[27]

Evidence does show that breastfeeding lowers the risk of both asthma and eczema. A whey-hydrolysate formula (made for infants with allergies) showed similar results.[28]

Probably the best advice for women who have allergies or a family history of allergies is to breast-feed as long as possible and to eat a large variety of foods so that no one food will be passed in large amounts to the baby through the milk.[29]

Q: Can I start drinking coffee again?

A: Your baby will receive about 1 percent of the caffeine kick that you get in your coffee or other caffeinated beverage. The equivalent of one or two cups of coffee per day is not likely to have a negative effect on baby.[30] However, caffeine can accumulate and cause your baby to be irritable and to have trouble falling asleep. So go easy.

Q: I have gone into premature labor. Though I am now on bed rest and medication to stop the labor, I am concerned that I won't be able to breast-feed if my baby arrives prematurely. Any advice?

A: Breast-feeding a premature infant can be even more rewarding than nursing a full-term infant. One study shows that feeding an infection-prone premature infant with colostrum (first milk) may have even more significant anti-infective effects than feeding it to full-term infants.[31] Another study reports that preterm infants who were tube-fed breast milk in their early weeks of life had significantly higher IQs at seven-and-a-half to eight years of age than those who did not. This difference was still significant after allowing for the mother's education and social class.[32]

If your baby comes very early, he or she may have to stay in a special area of the nursery to be monitored closely and to have the environment kept at a precise temperature. You may have to express milk so that it can then be fed to your baby through a special bottle or tube. In this case, you will need to pump your breasts.

The fact that you are thinking ahead is wonderful; you can arrange to rent a good-quality breast pump (such as Medela) or find out whether you can use one while you're at the hospital. Taking pictures of your baby and keeping them near you while pumping may help you express milk. Not being able to breast-feed in person may be disappointing, but think of the benefits you are still able to provide for your baby.

Q: My mother says I should drink a beer before I breast-feed to increase my milk supply. Will it? And is it safe for my baby?

A: This old wives' tale has not been scientifically proven. On the other hand, we do know that alcohol is released in the milk and that excessive drinking can cause problems with letdown, high alcohol level in breast milk, and lethargic babies. There has been one report of lowered psychomotor development scores in babies with increased alcohol exposure.[33] Since fetal brain development continues to occur during the first year of life, avoiding alcohol or drinking only limited amounts makes sense.

A recent study showed that the smell of alcohol could be detected immediately in the breast milk of moms who had drunk the equivalent of the amount of alcohol in one can of beer. The smell was strongest at thirty to sixty minutes after the mom imbibed. The babies drank less milk during the feeding, possibly due to the change in taste and smell of the milk. Another theory is that alcohol could decrease the mom's milk supply.[34]

Alcohol in breast milk can also significantly change an infant's sleep pattern, causing him or her to sleep less.[35]

If you'd really like to go out on the town and have more than one or two drinks, just pump your breast milk afterward and discard it. You can give your baby some previously pumped milk. Or if you'd just like an occasional drink, use common sense. Don't drink on an empty stomach, as this will speed the flow of alcohol into your bloodstream and your breast milk. Ask your health-care provider for more information.

Q: I still smoke. Can this somehow affect my milk?

A: Nicotine and cotinine (another component of cigarette smoke) have been found in breast milk. No symptoms of exposure to the chemicals have been seen in infants, but nicotine can affect how much milk you are able to produce. Some researchers advise that if you do smoke, you should not smoke for two-and-a-half hours before nursing and avoid smoking while near your baby.[36]

For information on kicking the habit of smoking, call 800-4CANCER.

Q: If I breast-feed, will my baby have a smaller risk of being overweight when he gets older?

A: Yes. Breastfeeding does seem to decrease your baby's chances of becoming overweight or obese as he or she gets older. The longer you breast-feed, the less your child's risk of becoming overweight.[37]

Q: Should I try to lose weight while breast-feeding?

A: You will probably lose weight without even trying. Instead, you need to focus on eating a well-balanced diet so that your breast milk continues to contain a good supply of the nutrients your baby needs. Losing 1 to 2 pounds per week is generally safe. However, you should not eat less than 1,800 calories per day. Monitoring the growth and general health of your baby is also a good way to check the quality of your milk.

Most women lose the first 20 pounds quite easily; it's the last 5 or 10 pounds that may hang on. This is when you should bring in the reinforcements: aerobic exercise and weight resistance. These exercises help you lose more body fat while keeping muscle. More muscle means burning more calories all the time![38]

Q: I want to have another baby right away. Should I still breast-feed if I get pregnant?

A: In developing countries, mothers commonly continue to breast-feed well into the second trimester of another pregnancy. However, breastfeeding during pregnancy can take its toll on you. Pregnancy and lactation are nutritionally and physically demanding. One study showed that moms who breast-fed while pregnant had babies that weighed slightly less than the babies of mothers who did not.

Much depends on your nutritional status. If you breast-feed while pregnant, you must meet the nutritional demands of your growing fetus, your growing baby, and yourself. These demands can add up to as much as 900 extra calories a day, depending on the age of your baby. If you aren't able to consume all those extra calories, protein, vitamins, and minerals, you could wind up nutritionally depleted.

Although breast-feeding while pregnant is possible, you may want to wait at least a few months after weaning your baby before conceiving again.[39]

Q: I've heard that women who breast-feed could have a lower risk of osteoporosis later in life. Is that true?

A: Research shows breastfeeding can affect osteoporosis. While it appears that some calcium stored in bone is used during breast-feeding, when you stop nursing, the bone is rebuilt, sometimes with even more calcium. For this reason, your calcium intake during nursing is important, but it may be just as important to have a calcium-rich diet afterward, when bone rebuilding is taking place.[40]

Q: Does my diet really affect my breast milk?

A: Yes. Breast milk is a constantly changing fluid. It changes from the beginning to the end of a feeding and it changes as an infant gets older. It also can vary according to your diet.

The most variable component in breast milk is fat. The amount of body fat you have can affect the fat in milk. Dietary fat also affects the amount and types of fat in breast milk. Essential fats (necessary for brain and retina development) in your breast milk are related to the amounts of those fats in your diet. So are trans fats. (See page 26 for more info about trans fats.) The amount of vitamins in your breast milk is also related to the vitamins in your diet; vitamins D and K may not always be adequate. On the other hand, minerals in breast milk (except selenium and iodine) do not vary according to diet.[41]

All these facts should motivate you to eat well while you are breast-feeding!

Q: I've heard that PCBs can be in breast milk. Can this affect the safety of my breast milk?

A: Over a lifetime, a person is exposed to environmental pollutants that accumulate in small amounts in the body—mostly in fat. The chemicals of greatest concern are organochlorines, a group of synthetic compounds persistent in the environment. Examples of these are polychlorinated biphenyls (PCBs), a family of industrial chemicals, and dichlorodiphenyl trichloroethane (DDT), an insecticide. Chemical treatment for termites is often associated with these residues. Although some of these chemicals have been banned in the United States for years, they persist in the environment and are still used in other parts of the world.

Infants are exposed to these environmental pollutants during pregnancy and through breast milk. In one ongoing study, infants whose mothers' breast milk contained PBB, a chemical related to PCBs, were followed. At ages two to four, children who had higher exposure to the chemical had lower scores on development tests; however, by ages four to six, these differences had disappeared.[42] A study of Dutch children found lower test scores among children exposed prenatally to dioxin (another environmental chemical) and PCBs. However, exposure to these compounds during breastfeeding was not related to forty-two-month cognitive performance.[43]

During pregnancy, a fetus's exposure to chemicals is much higher than during breastfeeding, but since body fat stored during pregnancy is used during breastfeeding, your diet during pregnancy can affect the amount of pollutants in your breast milk.

Should this information affect your decision to breast-feed? No. Betty Crase, former Director of Scientific Information at La Leche League International, says, "Unfortunately, we live in a contaminated world. However, the known and documented benefits of breastfeeding still outweigh the risks of contaminants that may be found in breast milk. What many people don't realize is that artificial infant formula can also contain environmental contaminants, especially if the water used to prepare it contains lead or other chemicals."[44] And the foremost researcher of PCBs in breast milk says, "Breastfeeding is recommended despite the presence of chemical residues."[45]

Chemicals in our environment are an unfortunate reality. The commonsense solution is to try to limit your present and future exposure to chemicals by following the tips below.

▶ **Avoid recreationally caught fish not caught by you (fish that is caught by friends or sold at a roadside stand). Also, avoid fish from areas you know are polluted.**

These fish are more likely to come from contaminated water or from water with specific state health department consumption recommendations for breast-feeding women. Friends who give you leftovers from their fishing trip may not know you are breastfeeding or may not have paid attention to the sign that says "Pregnant and breast-feeding women should avoid fish A." If you or your family catch fish, be sure to read any posted signs regarding recommended consumption or call your local health department. (See page 210 for more information on food safety.) You should definitely still eat fish; the omega-3 fatty acids found in fish are important to your baby's brain, which continues to develop during the first year of life.

▶ **Avoid quick weight loss while breast-feeding.**

Toxins from the environment are stored in body fat. If you go on an extreme weight-loss diet, some of these accumulated chemicals can enter your milk in larger amounts as your body fat is released from storage.[46]

▶ **Avoid using pesticides, herbicides, and insecticides (especially chemicals for termite extermination) in your home–even those that claim to be nontoxic.**

▶ **Avoid eating the skin and fat of poultry, meats, and fish. Drink skim or 1-percent milk. Eat more plant sources of protein.**

Q: I just had a case of food poisoning. Can the bacteria that caused my illness be passed to my baby in breast milk?

A: According to Dr. Steven Nafziger of the University Family Medical Center in Pueblo, Colorado, "The bacteria that cause most common types of food poisoning do not pass through the breast milk. However, some rarer forms of food poisoning involve bacteria that make toxins. These toxins can directly affect the baby through the mother's breast milk. I encourage a breast-feeding mom who is experiencing flu-like symptoms to come into the office so I can evaluate her condition and make a specific recommendation."[47]

Q: I'd like to start a vigorous exercise program. Can I still successfully breast-feed?

A: Yes. One study showed that among women who did aerobic exercise forty-five minutes per day, five times per week, for twelve weeks, their exercise had no effect on the amount of milk they produced or how much weight their babies gained.[48]

Q: I am a total vegetarian. Is there anything that my milk will be missing?

A: People who eat no animal protein or dairy products sometimes need another source of vitamin B_{12}, since it is found naturally only in animal products. You need to consume foods fortified with vitamin B_{12} or take a B_{12} daily supplement of 2.6 micrograms.[49] (See page 30 for more information about vitamin B_{12}.)

The calcium requirement for vegetarians is thought to be less than for meat eaters because vegetarian diets are lower in protein than the diets of meat eaters.

If you consume no dairy products, you may need to plan your diet carefully to include high-calcium foods or take a calcium supplement. Zinc and iron are other nutrients that may require you to work at getting sufficient amounts. (See page 85 for vegetarian sources of zinc, pages 70 and 71 for calcium, and pages 72 and 73 for iron.) If you have concerns about your diet, discuss them further with your baby's health-care provider or ask a registered dietitian to help you analyze your diet.

Q: Can breastfeeding lower my risk of breast cancer?

A: Yes. Several studies indicate that breast-feeding has a protective effect against breast cancer.[50] Breastfeeding can also cut your child's breast cancer risk when the child grows older.[51] What a special gift!

Q: Does my baby need any special vitamins while I am nursing?

A: Your breast milk contains nearly everything your baby needs. However, a few nutrients are not contained in adequate amounts in breast milk, and some moms have special dietary considerations that are discussed under "Breastfeeding for Special Groups."

Vitamin D and vitamin K have recently been reported not to appear in sufficient amounts in breast milk. If your water does not contain fluoride, or if your family drinks bottled water, your baby may need a fluoride supplement at six months. Ask your pediatrician if he or she recommends a supplement for breast-fed babies, like Tri-Vi Fluor.

By six months, your baby will have depleted his or her iron stores. This is the right time for introducing iron-rich foods like fortified cereals and teething crackers.

▼

Tips for Formula Feeding

If you decide to feed your baby formula or to combine breastfeeding and formula feeding, the following information may be useful:

- If formula is your baby's sole source of nutrition for the first four to six months, the American Academy of Pediatrics recommends you choose one that is iron-fortified to prevent iron-deficiency anemia.[52]

- If you use powdered or concentrated formula that needs to be mixed with water, make sure your water contains adequate fluoride. You can call your local water department to find out. If your water does not contain enough fluoride, your baby's health-care provider will need to prescribe a supplement.

- Whether you feed your baby breast milk, infant formula, or a combination of the two, you should not give your baby cow's milk or products containing cow's milk until your baby is one year old. The American Academy of Pediatrics recommends this because, among other effects, the protein in cow's milk may trigger the development of insulin-dependent diabetes.[53]

- If you use formula that has to be mixed with water, make sure that your water doesn't contain too much lead. Three common preparation practices that can increase lead in formula are:

–Using water that is drawn from the faucet first thing in the morning. If your pipes contain lead, water that has been sitting in the pipes for several hours will have a high concentration of lead.

–Excessive boiling. In just five minutes of boiling, the amount of lead is concentrated threefold.

–Using a lead-based kettle for boiling.[54]

(See page 40 for more information on lead.)

▼

About Bonding

Bonding is a term often used when discussing breastfeeding. Bonding refers to touching, cuddling, and holding and can be acheived regardless of the feeding method. The long-term effects of bonding are very positive and are thought to affect a child's self-esteem as well as the mother's attitude toward the child.

A breast-feeding mom must remain with the baby while feeding, unless she expresses milk into a bottle. Bottle-fed babies can also bond with whoever is feeding them. However, some parents learn that the bottle can be propped by a blanket, which allows them

More Information on Infant Feeding

For more information on infant feeding, see *Healthy Food for Healthy Kids*, the follow-up book to *Eating Expectantly*. *Healthy Food for Healthy Kids* is written in the same easy-to-read style, contains information about feeding kids from birth to school age, and also contains delicious kid-tested recipes. To review an excerpt from *Healthy Food for Healthy Kids*, visit www.healthyfoodzone.com.

to go about doing other things. This hands-off feeding is not recommended because of choking danger and also because it does not promote bonding, or developing a close relationship with the baby. Furthermore, if a baby falls asleep with a bottle in his or her mouth, the milk remaining in the baby's mouth can cause tooth decay.

Whatever method of feeding you choose, feeding your baby will be enjoyable–but it can also be stressful. Since babies can't talk to you, figuring out what they need is sometimes difficult. Some great advice about infant feeding can be found in *Child of Mine: Feeding with Love and Good Sense* by Ellyn Satter, R.D., M.S. (Bull Publishing). Ms. Satter is a dietitian and a social worker who gives advice about eating and tips on how to encourage a positive feeding relationship with your child.

CHAPTER NINE

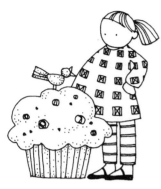

Now That You Can See Your Feet Again, or...

The First Weeks with Baby

What you will find in this chapter:

- *What to Expect after Delivery*
- *Menus for the First Week with Baby*
- *Going Back to Work*
- *Your Body Is Changing*
- *Losing That Baby Fat Sensibly*
- *Weight-Loss Plans*
- *Preparing for Your Next Pregnancy*

This chapter answers such questions as:

- *When will I be able to eat if I have anesthesia during delivery?*
- *How can I possibly eat balanced meals if I'm too tired to cook?*
- *What is the difference between breast- and bottlefeeding?*
- *What's a good weight-loss diet?*
- *How can I tell a good weight-loss program from a bad one?*
- *How long should I wait before I get pregnant again?*

What to Expect after Delivery

The first few days of postpartum life will likely be spent oohing and aahing over your new arrival and recovering from a very tiring event. You'll need to eat especially well those first few days at the hospital to muster as much strength as possible before you go home.

You may be too tired after delivery to eat a meal; that's normal for some women. You may just feel like drinking some juice or a decaffeinated soda for quick energy. Mary never drank sugared sodas, but after eighteen hours in labor, she drank 18 ounces of 7-Up in just five minutes! Some women are so hungry after delivery that they call out for pizza.

High-carbohydrate snacks that might be available at the hospital include English muffins, bagels, toast, bran muffins, raisin toast, canned or fresh fruit, graham crackers, milk, yogurt, milk shakes, sherbet, angel food cake with fruit, fruit juices, and sodas.

When you do feel like eating, these tips will help you get back on your feet:

▶ **If you select from a menu in the hospital, pick as many high-fiber foods as possible to get your digestive tract back to normal.**

Labor and anesthesia slow down your digestion immensely. You may also have hemorrhoids from pregnancy or from the pushing stage of labor. Eating high-fiber foods will make your bowel movements softer and easier.

Some high-fiber foods you are likely to see on a hospital menu are Raisin Bran cereal, All Bran, 100% Bran Flakes, wheat bread, wheat rolls, apples, oranges, bananas, strawberries, prunes, raw vegetables, salad, baked potatoes, legumes, peas, corn, and sliced tomatoes. Be sure to drink plenty of liquids when eating high-fiber foods.

▶ **Those first few days, eat as much as you want and drink plenty of fluids.**

If you had a long labor, you probably didn't drink much and you'll need to rehydrate. If you are planning to breast-feed, you will need to continue drinking 8 to 10 cups of fluid per day.

▶ **Concentrate on getting your strength back and taking care of your baby those first few weeks.**

Hopefully you cooked some meals ahead of time and froze them. If not, let your partner or other family members cook. Or send them out for fast food or convenience foods. (See Chapter Twelve for healthy, fast, and convenient menus.)

▼

Menus for the First Week with Baby

Those first few days will probably be too hectic to plan menus. Here is a week's worth of quick meals; some include takeout, and some can be made quickly at home.

Day 1
Takeout chicken and Snow Peas, Moo Shoo Shrimp
Steamed rice
Fresh fruit
Milk

Day 2
Canadian bacon pizza on whole-wheat crust
Tossed salad
Raspberry sorbet

Day 3
Garden Chef Garden Burger on whole-wheat bun
Grated carrots with mayo and raisins
Frozen yogurt with strawberries

Day 4
Minute steaks
Mixed vegetables
Easy Microwave Potatoes (page 342)
Cantaloupe or canned peaches

Day 5
Broccoli Quiche (page 350)
Sourdough rolls
Sliced tomatoes with basil
Tropical Pudding (page 288)

Day 6
Bean tostadas
Mexican rice
Avocado-and-tomato salad
Frozen bananas

Day 7
Pasta with Quick Alfredo Sauce (page 276)
Garlic bread
Mixed green salad
Fig bars

▼

Going Back to Work

Because of economic necessity or for personal fulfillment, most women go back to work when their babies are six weeks old. Going back to work can affect your feeding decisions. Unfortunately, many women view going back to work as an insurmountable obstacle to breastfeeding.

During my counseling sessions with pregnant women, I often found that if a woman knew she was going back to work, she threw the idea of breastfeeding right out the window. However, more and more companies are supporting breastfeeding. There's a compelling reason: One study showed that illnesses in breast-fed infants were reduced by 36 percent and women who breast-fed missed 27 percent fewer days due to their sick children.[1] You can continue to nurse *and* return to work. Here are three examples of how working women handled their feeding decisions:

• Barb was determined to breast-feed Joshua. Her company supported breast-feeding. She rented a breast pump from the hospital and used it at work. (She used the Medela Double Pumping Kit, which allowed her to empty both breasts at the same time and still have time to run errands or eat lunch. For more information on electric pumps, contact your hospital, a lactation consultant, or www.medela.com.) During her lunch break, she came home and fed Josh. Barb found that breast-feeding

Josh was just the contact she needed after being away most of the day. I admired Barb for her determination. She carried on this routine for nine months, until she started daycare in her home. She continued to nurse Joshua thereafter.

• Sarah had a high-stress job. Her boss and company were not very supportive of motherhood. Yet Sarah wanted to breast-feed. She learned that breastfeeding didn't have to be done full-time. She established a good milk supply while she was home with Erin, then she gradually figured out the routine that worked best for her family. She nursed Erin in the morning, Erin's daycare fed Erin two bottles of formula in the early afternoon, then Sarah nursed Erin in the late afternoon while her husband prepared dinner and again before she went to bed. Sarah's milk supply adjusted to Erin's feeding schedule. On the weekend, Erin's dad helped out with the midday bottles to give Sarah a break from feeding.

• Nicole didn't want to have to pump at work, but she wanted to breast-feed. By planning ahead, she and her husband saved some money so that she could work part-time after Sean was born. While at home for ten weeks after her delivery, she built up her milk supply and arranged her schedule to be away four hours each morning. By working part-time, Nicole had the best of both worlds.

If you will be returning to work, your environment at work will influence your feeding decision. Consider the following:

Parental leave time. If your company allows an extended maternity leave, this will give you more time to be with your baby. And if you decide to breast-feed, additional time off will allow you time to increase your milk supply. Even if you decide to breast-feed for just a month, your baby will still receive colostrum, which contains important disease-fighting agents.

Required travel. If your job requires you to travel frequently, you might want to cut your travel time to a minimum whether you breast-feed or not. If you can't cut your travel time, nursing still won't be impossible–but it will require diligent planning. Kristen arranged daycare with a national franchise when she traveled so she could take Katie with her. Not everyone can make such a commitment, but Kristen is a good example of creative problem solving!

Flexible hours. Many companies offer flexible hours, which are useful in many ways. For example, some couples work four ten-hour days instead of five eight-hour days. If both partners can arrange this type of schedule, they would need daycare only three days a week and would both gain time with their baby. Flexible hours can also help a breast-feeding mom. For example, if you can take a long lunch and work later, you might be able to breast-feed your baby at lunch. (On-site daycare makes this even easier.)

Supportive boss and coworkers. Going back to work while your child is an infant may be emotionally difficult. Seek out supportive coworkers–perhaps those who also have children. A supportive boss will understand if you need to take breaks to pump your breasts or take a little extra time off to feed your baby.

▼

Your Body Is Changing

Welcome to the "fourth trimester," the twelve weeks after you have your baby. This often-neglected period is important to understand. You are now adjusting from having been pregnant to being a mother. Life is different in many ways, and you are facing many new experiences and emotions. It is important that you take care of yourself physically and mentally. Proper diet and a gradual return to exercise can help you adjust. Listed below are the different changes that will be occurring in different parts of your body.

Uterus

Immediately after delivery, your uterus weighs about 2 pounds and is the size of a grapefruit. In the next six weeks, it will shrink down to normal–around 3 inches long and 2 ounces in weight. Nursing your baby will help your uterus contract and reduce in size. You may feel these contractions for two or three days, especially if this is your second or third baby.

Lochia

Lochia is the vaginal discharge that occurs the first few weeks after delivery. It is your body's way of getting rid of leftover debris from pregnancy. Lochia is a combination of red blood cells, skin cells, mucus, white blood cells, bacteria, and occasionally some of your baby's stool or hair.

Your blood flow will be red and plentiful for the first few days following delivery. Remember that your body generated a greater volume of blood during your pregnancy, and now the excess is being reduced. The amount of blood flow is an individual matter, but within two to three weeks many women return to having a whitish discharge.

If you revert to bright red bleeding, you are being too active. Slow down and enjoy the simple first days of your newborn's life. If your flow remains bright red or has a foul odor, please contact your physician. Remember that ovulation can occur within weeks after delivery, even if you are breast-feeding. However, ovulation may not occur in the breast-feeding mom until after weaning. The first periods may be heavy and irregular for several months.

Discuss contraception with your doctor if you want to resume having sex within three to four weeks after delivery.

Perineum and Vagina

The area between your vagina and rectum is called the perineum. This area will feel sore due to the tremendous stretching it has undergone, even if you did not have an episiotomy. Ice will be applied in the first twelve hours after your delivery to reduce swelling. After this time, heat will promote healing. Many women take sitz baths (sitting for a short time in warm water).

Kegel exercises will help tone muscles in the perineum. You should have learned how to do Kegels in your childbirth education class or prenatal exercise class. If not, consult your health-care provider.

If you had an episiotomy, your stitches will dissolve by themselves. Your vagina will have decreased mucus until ovulation returns to normal, and intercourse might need additional lubrication. Please note that if you are nursing, ovulation may be delayed for a while, so you may continue to have reduced mucus.

Abdomen

After the birth of your baby, your abdomen will still look very much pregnant, but flabby. This may be one of your biggest disappointments after delivery, unless you are prepared for it. You can start doing exercises to help tighten your abdominal muscles. Remember that good muscle tone will take time and discipline; diet, good posture, and exercise are important. If you have no energy or time to think about exercise in the first few months, tighten your perineum (do a Kegel) and abdomen every time you turn on a water faucet.

▼

Losing That Baby Fat Sensibly

Are you ready to get rid of the extra pounds you gained during pregnancy? Not so fast! Remember that it took nine months to gain the weight; it's not going to come off in a week or two. The key to long-term weight control is a healthy diet combined with exercise.

However, you'd better not exercise vigorously the first six weeks. (Personally, I didn't have to worry about that; I was too tired!) Remember those hormones discussed in Chapter Five: The Third Trimester (the ones that caused your joints and pelvis to become more elastic)? Well, they haven't quite returned to normal yet, so take it easy for a while or you could damage some joints or ligaments. A simple walking regimen is a good start. It's a great way to show off your new baby to the neighbors or meet other new moms at the mall.

Chances are, if you were at your ideal weight before your pregnancy, you won't need any "diet" at all. And if you are nursing, you shouldn't reduce your calorie intake below 1,800 calories. You may just need to consciously cut back on extras and fat intake (no more middle-of-the-night snacks!) and start moving more. The weight will come off gradually.

Many women want a program to follow even if they have just 10 pounds to lose. Some women were overweight when they became pregnant; they may need something more structured. Later, we will review steps to help you evaluate a weight-loss program.

Regardless of your situation, my advice is to lose as much of your excess weight as possible before you become pregnant again (that is, if you are planning to have another child). Many of the women I see for weight loss are in their fifties and explain that they never lost all their weight between pregnancies or after their last baby. By the time they see me, they are often forced to lose weight for a medical reason: diabetes, high blood pressure, or heart disease. Avoid these problems now by controlling your weight sensibly.

I believe many people suffer from yo-yoing weight because they are in a hurry. I've seen this situation over and over in my weight-loss classes. Mary has been overweight for fifteen years, but now she has a class reunion to attend, and all of a sudden she wants to lose her weight *now*. It's human nature.

When we're motivated, we'll do anything to reach our goal quickly. The problem in applying this mindset to weight loss is that most people are easily discouraged and lose the battle before it really begins.

According to some experts, people need almost six months to truly change their habits. Yet Mary expects to do a major overhaul of her diet and lifestyle in two weeks!

When people change their diets drastically, they may at first lose weight quickly because much of it is water. Then, when weight loss tapers to 1 pound or less per week, people feel they're failing and give up. What they forget is that 1 pound per week adds up to 52 pounds per year! That's a lot of pounds!

The key to losing weight permanently is determining which diet or lifestyle habits need changing, and then gradually altering eating habits, setting realistic goals, and adopting an exercise program that you can stick with for life. Remember: Temporary changes may result in temporary weight loss.

Following are some of the characteristics I've observed in people who are most successful in losing weight. People who lose weight successfully . . .

- exercise regularly.[2]
- set realistic goals. When they don't meet their goals, they learn from their experiences instead of giving up.
- have social support from family, friends, coworkers, or support groups.[3] People who complete a weight-loss program with friends or family lose more weight and are more likely to keep it off.
- work on liking themselves (or already do).
- are motivated to lose weight for internal reasons rather than external reasons.[4] For example, Judy used to lose weight to fit into her old size-six jeans. Now she is losing weight to improve her health.
- concentrate not on the bathroom scale, but on some positive outcome, such as lowered cholesterol or being able to walk further without becoming tired.
- have conquered emotional eating (eating when bored, angry, depressed, or stressed) or are working on it.[5]
- have learned to eat sensibly at restaurants, at parties, while traveling, and so on.
- work at self-monitoring. This may mean keeping a food diary, tracking the amount of fat eaten in a day, or logging those exercise hours each week.
- control their diet; they don't let their diet control them! They make educated, conscious choices about the food they eat. If they want to splurge for a special occasion, they do. They are honest with themselves about the reasons they eat.

Weight-Loss Plans

Diet plans and diet books are abundant, but beware! Many of them promote quick weight loss, which is unhealthy. Others may recommend unbalanced diets, which leave out one or more foods or food groups. Some can be downright dangerous. Virtually all diets work—for the short term. However, many diets fail over the long term. Repeated weight loss and weight gain, often called weight cycling or yo-yo dieting, can be harmful to the body and devastating to the self-esteem.

Evaluating Weight-Loss Plans

The steps below can help you evaluate a weight-loss plan.

1. *Does the plan promote a balanced diet, allowing all foods in moderation? Does it omit certain foods or food groups?*
A balanced plan should allow all foods, even the so-called "bad" ones, at some point in the program.

2. *Does the plan include exercise?*
Exercise is so important to weight loss. Most people who lose weight lose some muscle along with fat. However, if you exercise, you will lose little or no muscle mass. Maintaining muscle mass helps you lose more weight, since muscle uses more calories than fat—even when you are sitting in front of the TV! A combination of aerobic and weight resistance exercise is very effective for losing weight and shaping up.

3. *Does the plan include behavior modification (changing current behaviors)?*

For long-term weight loss, you must identify your problem behaviors so you can work to change them. Some tools used for behavior modification might include self-monitoring (keeping a diet record) or exercises that promote an awareness of eating patterns.

4. *Does the plan use trained professionals as counselors or people whose only qualifications are that they have lost weight?*

Many plans use people who have lost weight or are good salespeople as counselors. Though these people may be good motivators, they may give out inaccurate information unintentionally.

There are lots of quacks out there trying to make a quick dollar. Beware of anything that sounds too good to be true; it probably is. Look for counselors who are licensed, registered, or have a degree from an accredited college or university.

5. *Does the plan involve buying special foods or supplements?*

Personally, I feel that learning how to eat "real" food is better for long-term weight loss. However, some people like the convenience of packaged foods.

6. *Does the plan provide a foundation for good future eating habits?*

Hopefully, the plan teaches you how to cook healthfully, plan menus, and eat sensibly in social situations.

The Moderate Approach

The recommended postpregnant weight loss is about 1 pound or less per week. You're probably thinking, "A pound a week! I'll never lose this weight!" Consider the importance of long-term success, which means keeping the weight off. People who lose weight slowly seem to keep it off the longest.

To lose 1 pound per week, you can cut your food intake by 500 calories per day, use more calories by exercising, or combine eating less and exercising more. For example, Colleen walks about 2 miles every evening, which uses approximately 200 calories. She has also cut 300 calories of extras out of her diet. Colleen's diet-and-exercise approach works best for long-term weight maintenance. Besides being good for muscle tone, cardiovascular health, and endurance, exercise is also good for your mental health! Following is an example of a good fitness program. Most of these activities can be done with a baby nearby or in a front pack. Postnatal exercise programs often encourage baby participation. As you can see, fitness doesn't have to be boring!

Suggested Activity Program for Colleen

Height: 5'4"

Weight: 160 pounds

Goal Weight: 120 pounds

Activity Goals: Aerobic activity 5 hours per week, strength training ½ hour twice per week

Monday: 1 hour of postnatal exercise class

Tuesday: 30-minute walk at lunch, 30 minutes of strength training after dinner

Wednesday: 1 hour of postnatal exercise class

Thursday: 30-minute walk with baby in front pack, 30 minutes of strength training

Friday: Colleen's day off

Saturday: 1-hour hike with baby in front pack

Sunday: 1 hour of gardening

By following this activity program, Colleen burns over 1,700 calories! To lose 1 pound per week, she also needs to reduce her diet by 1,800 calories per week or about 250 calories per day. (Please note that the numbers of calories burned are calculated specifically for Colleen.)

The chart below lists a few of the extras Colleen eats that she can easily cut from her diet. These changes add up to a reduction of over 700 calories per day. Colleen will only need to follow half the proposed changes to lose 1 pound per week.

Depending on your weight, height, and activity level, you will probably want to eat between 1,200 and 1,800 calories per day to lose 1 pound per week. Eating under 1,200 calories is usually not advised unless you have a petite build.

Lose Weight by Leaning toward Vegetarianism

Cutting down on animal protein is one good way to cut calories and fat, which can lead to weight loss. Leaning toward vegetarianism, or even becoming vegetarian, might be a good idea. While testing meatless recipes for the book *Make the Change for a Healthy Heart,* I was losing weight without even trying. I had to consciously eat extra snacks to avoid losing weight! (See Chapter Six for more on vegetarian eating.)

Here are two good sources to help vegetarians with weight loss: *Simple, Low-Fat, and Vegetarian* by Suzanne Havala, M.S., R.D.

Low-Fat Food Substitutions			
Food	**Calories**	**Action**	**Calories Saved**
1 tablespoon margarine	100	Substitute Butter Buds or Molly McButter	100
1 cola drink	150	Substitute diet soda	148
2 chocolate-chip cookies	140	Substitute 1 peach	100
1 cinnamon roll	230	Substitute 1 Quaker Caramel Corn Cake	180
3 cups whole milk	450	Substitute 2% milk	90
3 tablespoons blue cheese dressing	180	Substitute Wish Bone Healthy Sensation Chunky Blue Cheese	120

(Vegetarian Resource Group, 1994) and *Vegetarian Weight Loss Guide* by Suzanne Havala, M.S., R.D., published in *Vegetarian Journal Reports* (Vegetarian Resource Group, 1990).

Lose That Baby Fat Eating Plan

This meal plan has about 1,500 calories and is meant to be a rough guideline for healthy weight loss. While some women prefer a structured plan, many women do well just concentrating on eating more fruits and vegetables and cutting back on extra fats. This meal plan does not contain enough calories or nutrients for breast-feeding moms.

7 servings of starches/grains
1 serving is 1 slice any type bread, 1 flour tortilla, ½ cup pasta, ⅓ cup rice or legumes, 6 crackers, or ½ cup potato.

3 servings of fruits
1 serving is 1 medium piece fresh fruit, ½ banana, ½ cup canned fruit in its own juice, 1 cup melon or berries, 2 plums, or 2 nectarines.

3 or more servings of vegetables
1 serving is ½ cup any nonstarchy vegetable or 1 cup lettuce.

5 protein equivalents
1 protein equivalent is 1 ounce lean meat, 1 ounce reduced-fat cheese, ¼ cup cottage cheese, ½ cup tofu, 2 tablespoons peanut butter, ½ cup cooked dried beans, or 1 egg.

2 to 3 servings of dairy products
1 serving is 1 cup skim or 1% milk or low-fat yogurt.

If you have just stopped breast-feeding, aim for 4 servings per day to help boost bone mineralization.

3 servings of fat
1 serving is 1 teaspoon margarine or butter or 2 teaspoons reduced-fat margarine, 1 teaspoon mayonnaise or 2 teaspoons reduced-fat mayonnaise, 1 slice bacon, ½ ounce cream cheese, 1 tablespoon sour cream, ⅛ avocado, 10 peanuts, or 5 olives.

For more information about weight loss or healthy eating, see the Recommended Resources in the back of this book for weight-loss books and low-calorie cookbooks.

? Questions You May Have

Q: I've never been much of a breakfast eater, but I've heard that it's good for you. Is it?

A: You may have heard that breakfast is the most important meal of the day. In many respects, that's true. A recent study showed that people who skipped breakfast had trouble working on tasks that required concentration. Diane Odland, nutritionist at the U.S. Department of Agriculture Human Nutrition Information Service, says, "When you consider it's been eight or nine hours since you've had a meal, it's obvious that refueling at breakfast will make you feel and perform better during the day."[6]

Eating breakfast can also help you lose weight. People who skip the first meal of the day often make up for it later by eating larger meals or snacking on high-fat, high-sugar foods. Whether you stay home with a child or work outside the home, eating breakfast will definitely improve your energy level.

Q: Will I lose all my pregnancy weight without really trying?

A: It depends on how much you gained. In one study, women who gained more than 20 pounds retained from 5 to 10 pounds between pregnancies. Those who gained over 40 pounds were an average of 17 pounds heavier at the start of their next pregnancy. Since the current recommendation for weight gain is over 25 pounds, you will probably have to make an active effort to lose the weight.[7]

Q: How long will it take me to lose my baby fat?

A: Again, it depends on how much you gained, how much you eat, and how active you are. A lucky few fit into their prepregnancy clothes right after delivery, though that wasn't the case for me or any of my friends.

The amount of time needed to lose the weight and get your old body back is probably a big surprise to every mother. Much to my disappointment, I needed almost nine months to return to my normal weight. I thought I'd be back to my old self within a few months. Doing aerobics three times a week made the biggest change in the way my body looked and helped me lose those stubborn last 5 pounds.

When I surveyed other dietitians about this book, several suggested that I outline some realistic expectations for weight loss and body size after pregnancy. Here are some things you should expect:

- Very few people go back to wearing their "skinny" clothes right after delivery. Expect to wear your maternity clothes for a few more months–even though you probably feel like burning them!
- You may need to buy a few outfits one size bigger than you wore before pregnancy to wear until you get your shape back.
- Your body may have reproportioned itself. For example, Kate weighs the same as she did before pregnancy, but her hips are a few inches wider. Most of us continue to have a little tummy unless we diligently practice abdominal exercises. Some women find their rib cages permanently expanded and need to wear a larger bra size. Believe it or not, some women even wear a larger shoe size after pregnancy.
- If you are breast-feeding, you may feel as though you are bursting out of your blouses. Judy was exasperated because, for the first few months of breastfeeding, the only shirts she could wear were her husband's T-shirts and her old maternity shirts. Sandy, however, was glad to have an excuse to buy new clothes!
- Many women lose the last few pounds after they stop breast-feeding.
- Exercise can't be emphasized enough. It will help you lose baby fat and tone up some of the muscles you haven't used in quite a while.

• Overall, be patient. I clearly remember asking my aerobics teacher how fast I could get into shape after the baby came, if I worked out regularly. I wanted *real* numbers. She said it could be done in six to eight weeks, but I might need time for recovery. "Not me," I thought. I was going to be Supermom! Well, after a tough labor and delivery and a long adjustment to motherhood, months passed before I had the time and energy to restart my exercise program. After my second son was born, I didn't have a problem losing the weight. I breast-fed him longer and I was much more active chasing two kids around.

▼

Preparing for Your Next Pregnancy

Sometime after your labor anesthesia wears off and before you send out birth announcements, someone will ask, "So when are you going to have another baby?" You may not be ready to answer that question for a long time. On the other hand, you may want another baby right away. I recommend waiting at least eighteen months before you become pregnant again. A study of nearly 300,000 infants showed that women with less than eighteen months between pregnancies were 14 to 47 percent more likely to have very premature and moderately premature infants than women with intervals of one-and-a-half to five years.[8] In the meantime, consider getting back to your ideal body weight and following the advice on page 213 for reducing environmental pollutants in your diet. Most importantly, enjoy that baby of yours! The time passes quickly! When you are ready to think about getting pregnant again, turn to Chapter One: Contemplating Pregnancy to learn what you can do for a healthy pregnancy *before* you conceive.

No matter when you decide to have another baby, or even if you decide not to, don't lose the good habits you established during pregnancy. A healthy diet is one of the most important things you can do to ensure good health for you and your children, and teaching your children good eating habits is one of the most precious gifts you can give them.

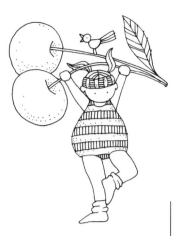

CHAPTER TEN

Fitting Fitness In

What you will find in this chapter:

• *Benefits of Exercise*
• *What Every Pregnant Woman Should Know about Exercise*
• *Fitting Fitness into Your Busy Lifestyle*
• *Exercise after Pregnancy*
• *Tips for Getting with the Program after Your Baby Is Born*

This chapter answers such questions as:

• *What if I don't have time for exercise?*
• *Should I exercise differently while I'm pregnant?*
• *How can I relieve back pain?*
• *How does exercise fit in for those on bed rest?*
• *How can I get back in shape after I have my baby?*

Benefits of Exercise

Throughout this book I've mentioned exercise over and over. I'm hoping repetition will bring home the message that exercise is one of the most important things you can do for your present and future health. Regular exercise can bring you numerous benefits from a small time investment.

While you are pregnant, exercise offers even more benefits:

• Exercise helps battle the fatigue many women feel during pregnancy.
• Exercise makes you physically fit and helps your body get ready for labor.
• Exercise helps you feel better about your expanding body.
• Once you've established a fitness routine, resuming exercising after you have your baby (when you're trying to lose weight) will be easier.
• If you have diabetes, exercise can help you control your blood glucose. But always check with your doctor for exercise advice.
• Exercise classes for pregnant women can help you find interaction and support from a group that understands what you're experiencing.
• Regular exercise will help you sleep better. You may need all the sleep you can get during those last few weeks of pregnancy!
• Exercise will probably help you feel better all over. You'll have a better emotional outlook and you may have improved immunity.

A former couch potato says, "I was never interested in exercising, but when I became pregnant, my doctor suggested I get involved in an exercise program for pregnant women at the YWCA. I went to an aerobics class mostly for my baby, and much to my surprise, I began to really enjoy it. I shared labor and delivery stories with other moms-to-be and began a mommy network. Toward the end of my pregnancy, exercise really helped me sleep better. Also, I felt much less tired than I did with my first pregnancy. I had more energy and felt vivacious."

If you didn't exercise before you were pregnant, you should ask your health-care provider about exercising. He or she may have some special guidelines for you, depending on your current situation. If you exercised routinely before pregnancy, you can probably continue your exercise program with some modifications.

▼

What Every Pregnant Woman Should Know about Exercise

Note: For the most part, these guidelines also apply to the postpartum period.[1]

▶ Don't do too much at first.

Have you ever watched the Olympics and gotten so inspired that you wanted to jump up, drive to the gym, and work out for an hour—even though you hadn't done any exercise in months? Don't! Start out slowly and exercise as little as five minutes per day, and don't forget to warm up and cool down.

▶ Be kind to your joints.

The hormones of pregnancy make joints very elastic, which prepares them for childbirth. Exercise that involves lots of bouncing, jerky movement, jumping, or quick changes in direction could cause joint pain or injury. You should also avoid deep flexing or extending your muscles. Use gentle stretches to cool down instead of stretching to the limit.

▶ Avoid ironman marathons and other rigorous events unless you are already an athlete and you have your health-care provider's permission.

Stay away from competitive sports. Stick to walking, swimming, or low-impact aerobics (preferably aerobic classes developed just for pregnant women).

▶ Do kinder, gentler exercise.

The extra weight gain in pregnancy changes your body's center of gravity, so you should avoid sports like downhill skiing, skating, and skateboarding that involve a high risk of falling. Exercise on a wooden floor or a securely carpeted surface to reduce shock and to provide sure footing.

▶ Be consistent.

Regular exercise is best, even if it's only a few minutes per day. Thousands of people are would-be exercisers with good intentions. Their homes are full of treadmills, stationary bikes, rowing machines, and weight sets. Unfortunately, many collections of exercise paraphernalia serve as dust collectors and clothes racks. Their owners would be much better off if they simply set aside fifteen minutes a day to go for a walk.

▶ Warm up and cool down.

Always begin with a five-minute warm-up period of low-intensity exercise, such as slow walking, cycling, or water walking for swimmers, to warm up your muscles, followed by ten minutes of stretching. Strenuous exercise should last fifteen minutes, unless you were exercising before you were pregnant; in that case, check with your physician. Follow a period of intense exercise with ten to fifteen minutes of cool-down and stretching.

▶ Exercise at least three times per week.

Exercising just twenty minutes a day, three times per week, is much better for you than being a weekend athlete.

▶ Measure your heart rate during exercise.

Exercising too intensely can increase your body's internal temperature and harm your fetus. Measure your pulse at the peak of your activity and also before cool-down. To measure your pulse, place your index finger at your carotid artery on your neck. Keep moving. Count your heart rate for either six or ten seconds. A pregnant woman's heart rate should not exceed 140 beats per minute (fourteen beats in six seconds or twenty-three beats in ten seconds). Check with your health-care provider for alternate guidelines.

▶ Take your time.

Get up from the floor slowly to avoid dizziness or fainting caused by a sudden drop in blood pressure.

▶ Drink, drink, drink!

Drink water before, during, and after exercise to prevent dehydration. Drinking will also help cool you off. Take a squirt bottle filled with water on your walk or to aerobics.

▶ Stay out of the heat.

Don't do any vigorous exercise in hot, humid weather or when you have a fever.

▶ Watch out for danger signs.

Stop your activity immediately and call your doctor if any of these symptoms occur: pain, bleeding, dizziness, shortness of breath, rapid heartbeat, back pain, pubic pain, and/or difficulty walking.

▶ Be kind to yourself.

Think of exercise as a special time for you. You may not always agree, but exercise is a way to pamper yourself!

▶ Eat enough food.

During pregnancy, blood sugar levels are usually lower than nonpregnant levels, and your body uses carbohydrates at a greater rate. So you might have low blood sugar during strenuous exercise. Make sure you don't exercise on an empty stomach. You may want to have some crackers, fresh or dried fruit, or juice before your workout for more energy.

If you worked out regularly before pregnancy and continue to have a vigorous workout schedule, keep in mind that you will need to increase your calories accordingly.

Your weight gain will let you know if you're eating enough.

Following are some reasons why exercise should be toned down during pregnancy.

- Your resting heart rate is higher than a nonpregnant woman's, and it also rises more quickly during exercise. So watch the intensity of your exercise.
- Your body temperature may rise more rapidly than a nonpregnant woman's. And since your baby's body temperature is always 1°F warmer than yours, elevating your body temperature could mean trouble for your baby. Be careful of how hard and how long you exercise.
- After your fourth month, your uterus may compress your inferior vena cava—the main blood vessel returning blood to your heart. This could interfere with blood flow to your baby. (After your fourth month, don't do any exercise while lying flat on your back.)
- Some hormones relax joints and connective tissue in preparation for delivery and can make joints susceptible to injury. Treat your joints gently by doing slow stretches daily and don't forget to warm up and cool down!
- Some studies have shown that vigorous activity can cause contractions, which may lead to premature labor. One study done with women who had gestational diabetes showed that the safest exercises were those that used mostly the upper body or those that applied little stress below the waist. Researchers found that walking on a treadmill was fine, but jogging was likely to cause contractions.

Exercising on a conventional stationary bike caused contractions in half of the women, and exercising on a recumbent bicycle (one in which you sit back with your legs in front of you, not under you) caused no contractions. The upper-arm ergometer proved to be the safest exercise machine. It is similar to a stationary bicycle but is pedaled with the arms.[2]

For more specific information about exercise, ask your health-care provider or childbirth educator. Always check with your health-care provider before starting an exercise program, especially if you haven't recently exercised.

When You Shouldn't Exercise

According to the American College of Obstetricians and Gynecologists, several conditions totally restrict you from exercising vigorously.[3] If any of these conditions apply to you, consult your health-care provider before exercising.

- History of three or more miscarriages
- Ruptured membranes
- Premature labor
- Diagnosed multiple gestation (twins, triplets, or more)
- Incompetent cervix
- Bleeding or a diagnosis of placenta previa
- Diagnosed cardiac disease

Some conditions may require you to limit strenuous exercise.[4] If any of these conditions apply to you, be sure to talk with your health-care provider before starting an exercise program.

- High blood pressure
- Anemia or other blood disorder
- Thyroid disease
- Diabetes
- Cardiac arrhythmia or palpitations
- History of premature labor
- History of intrauterine growth retardation (slowed growth of fetus)
- History of bleeding during current pregnancy
- Breech position of baby in last trimester
- Excessive obesity
- Extreme underweight
- History of extremely sedentary lifestyle

▼

Fitting Fitness into Your Busy Lifestyle

Some people don't exercise regularly because they don't think they have time. It's true: We live in a very fast-paced society. Yet most of us probably have fifteen minutes a day that we waste. Here are a few ideas for fitting fitness into your lifestyle:

▶ **Take a walk every morning before work.**

If you happen to have a treadmill, you can walk while watching the morning news.

▶ **Make more trips up and down the stairs.**

For example, you could unplug the downstairs phone so that every time the phone rings, you need to go up and down the stairs once. Tricks like this will give you more

activity, but remember that such activity uses only short bursts of energy and won't improve your overall fitness much.

▶ **Use half your lunch hour to take a walk.**

I did this on the days I didn't go to aerobics. The funny part of it was that I had to turn down many rides. Everyone must have felt sorry for the big pregnant woman walking down the street!

▶ **Write your exercise dates on your calendar and keep them!**

▶ **Exercise with your partner or a friend.**

▶ **Walk the dog; your pooch will love you for it!**

▶ **Sign up for an exercise class just for pregnant women.**

Sometimes, if you pay for a class, you are more motivated to go.

▶ **On the weekend, take a drive to the country where you can walk while admiring scenic views.**

▶ **Get the whole family into exercising!**

Take walks or hikes together.

▶ **Rent or purchase an exercise video just for pregnant women.**

These videos follow the pregnancy exercise guidelines of the American College of Obstetricians and Gynecologists: *Kathy Smith's Pregnancy Workout, Buns of Steel Pregnancy Workout,* and *Denise Austin's Pregnancy Plus.* You can order them by calling Collage Video at 800-433-6769.

Your Personal Exercise Schedule

Take a moment to write your exercise plan below.

My goal is to exercise _____ **times per week, for** _____ **minutes each time.**

My Exercise Schedule:

Monday _____
                                    (time)

Tuesday _____

Wednesday _____

Thursday _____

Friday _____

Saturday _____

Sunday _____

Ten Sneaky Ways to Exercise

Not everyone truly enjoys exercising. If you cringe at the idea of a daily workout, you can increase your physical activity without a planned exercise routine.

▶ **Walk the dog.**

▶ **Shop 'til you drop.**

Or you can walk around the entire mall and window-shop.

▶ **Go dancing!**

Ballroom, country-western, or even square dancing will do. Or put on your favorite music at home and cut a rug!

▶ **Take a stroll around a scenic place like a lake, a tree-lined avenue, or a forest trail.**

▶ **Go canoeing or paddleboating.**

▶ **Do arm exercises using 1-pound weights or cans of soup while watching your favorite show.**

▶ **Go to the pool and just walk from side to side.**

Bring a friend. You won't notice the time passing as you chat away.

▶ **Try aerobic lawn mowing.**

Cut your grass with a push mower and start a fad in your neighborhood.

▶ **Plant a garden.**

A bonus of gardening is enjoying the fruits of your labor. If you don't care for gardening, clean your house often; vacuuming *can* be aerobic.

▶ **Set a walking date with a neighbor or coworker.**

Once you get to talking, you'll hardly notice the time or the exercise.

Exercise after Pregnancy

Women often face weight problems after having children. Those last 5 pounds just don't seem to come off. If you add another 5 pounds with another pregnancy, before you know it, you're 15 or 20 pounds overweight.

Research has shown that people who

exercise regularly lose more weight and have the best odds of keeping it off. Other benefits of exercising include improved cardiovascular fitness, lowered heart rate, lowered blood pressure, decreased blood lipids, decreased blood sugar, toned muscles, less body fat, improved immunity, and more!

After you have your baby, it may be a while before you feel motivated to exercise. That's okay. You have just gone through one of life's biggest events. You may need some time to get used to having a baby in the house and to set up a new routine. (I needed four months to adjust!) Remember those hormones that made your joints more elastic so that your pelvis could stretch for childbirth? Weeks will pass before those hormones drop to their normal levels. Most physicians will approve an exercise program after the six-week checkup. Until then, walking is generally fine.

A new mom says, "I was one of those people who thought I would be out of the house and back to exercising within days after delivery. Surprise, surprise! After a week, I still had trouble walking! My neighbor had a C-section, and she was taking her baby on a walk in the stroller when he was just four days old! I was jealous!"

Women have unique labor experiences. Some breeze through labor in a few hours. Other labors last a day and a half. If you had a long labor, it may have taken a lot out of you. If you had stitches, hemorrhoids, or both, it may be even longer before you'll feel okay walking and sitting. Be prepared for the best or worst situation, and remember that this, too, shall pass.

You Don't Have to Be a Race Walker to Lose Weight!

One study compared the effects of low-intensity and high-intensity exercise. Women who walked four days a week for twelve weeks lost 5 pounds of body fat, whether they exercised slowly or vigorously. Women in both groups burned 300 calories during each workout. Low-intensity walkers lost more body fat in the abdomen and buttocks, so if those areas are a problem for you, you may want to exercise at a slower rate.[5]

▼

Tips for Getting with the Program after Your Baby Is Born

▶ **Start at your own pace, no matter how slow it seems.**

▶ **Stretching is important, even if you don't feel like exercising.**

▶ **Find activities you enjoy and include other family members if possible.**

▶ **Join a fitness class for moms and babies.**

You won't feel as though you are the only one out of shape in such a class. You can meet other moms there, and you won't have to find daycare. Call your local YMCA.

▶ **Schedule your time.**

While you are at home the first six weeks, the days seem to drift by. A schedule that includes some activity will give you a sense of purpose.

▶ **When you have time during baby's naps, pop in an exercise video.**

Thousands of exercise videos are now available. How can you tell which are best? A company called Collage Video does the research for you. It sells only videos rated for effectiveness and technique by fitness instructors with American Council on Exercise (ACE) certification. The videos are also rated for motivation, interest, and fun by "regular" people. Here is a list of beginner or beginner/intermediate and aerobic or aerobic/toning videos that I've selected from Collage Video's recommendations. The first two are specifically for post-pregnancy fitness. All can be ordered by visiting www.collagevideo.com or by calling 800-433-6769.

Baby and You: Workout for Two

Buns and Abs of Steel: Post Pregnancy Workout

Kathy Smith: March to Fitness

Chuck Norris: Private Lessons

Richard Simmons: Sweatin' to the Oldies

Richard Simmons: Sweat and Shout

Richard Simmons: Get Down the Pounds

Leslie Sansone's Walk and Firm 2-Mile Fat Burner

Linda Evans: The New You

Denise Austin: Anti-Aging Baby Boomers Workout

10-Minute Solution

The most important aspect of exercising is simply doing it. Do whatever it takes to get started, but as that sports-shoe commercial says, just do it! (See the Recommended Resources section at the back of this book for more fitness resources.)

▶ **Check out these on-line fitness resources:**

Fit Pregnancy Magazine
www.fitpregnancy.com

American College of Sports Medicine
www.acsm.org

American Academy of Family Practice
www.aafp.org

? **Questions You May Have**

Q: Won't exercise make me more tired?

A: At first you may feel a little more tired after exercising while pregnant. This tiredness is a result of the extra weight you are carrying and the extra blood that must be pumped through your heart. (During the first trimester, hormonal changes can also cause fatigue.) However, since exercise increases endurance, you will gradually feel less tired as your body gets accustomed to exercise. Of course, if you are already exercising, you shouldn't feel as tired. If you do, you may not be eating enough foods or the right foods.

Q: How will I know if I'm eating enough while exercising during pregnancy?

A: The rule of thumb here is to eat when you're hungry and to watch your weight gain. If you're not gaining enough, you need to eat more. If you have a busy schedule and just can't seem to eat enough, you may need to slow down. (See page 263 for high-energy snack ideas.)

Q: I'm on bed rest. How can I prevent my body from turning into flab?

A: Pregnancy often causes us to make changes in our lifestyle and habits. Bed rest takes this to the extreme. You *will* lose your level of fitness while on bed rest. However, by stretching and doing isometric exercises (if approved by your health-care provider), you can retain some of your muscle tone. Ask your health-care provider for a list of suggested exercises to keep yourself limber and for permission to do arm exercises. And remember that after you have your baby, your endurance for exercise will be very low. You'll need to start out slowly. I thought I would need practically *forever* to get back into shape after I was off bed rest. In just a few weeks, my endurance returned to normal. Your body *will* bounce back, and you *can* become fit again, so think of your situation as a temporary one.

Q: My back hurts all the time lately. What can I do?

A: I can sympathize with you. During the last two months of my pregnancy, I couldn't sweep and mop the kitchen floor in the same afternoon because my back hurt so much. I finally wised up and gave that job to my husband.

Your back undergoes a great deal of stress during pregnancy. Most traditional back-strengthening exercises are not recommended during pregnancy because you perform them lying on your back. One that is recommended is the pelvic tilt. If you are attending an exercise class for pregnant women, you probably already know this exercise. If not, here's a quick tutorial:[6]

How to Do a Pelvic Tilt

1. Stand with feet shoulder-width apart and knees slightly bent.

2. Contract the muscles of the buttocks and abdomen and gently thrust your pelvis forward, rotating your pubic bone upward. Hold this position for ten seconds and release.

3. The pelvic tilt can be done while lying or squatting on your hands and knees.

You should try to do the pelvic tilt as often as possible during the day. Keep in mind that after your delivery, lifting and carrying can still be painful. Continue doing pelvic tilts and other back-strengthening exercises to improve your back health. Keeping your stomach muscles strong will support the back muscles and will prevent back strain. Stomach crunches (or half sit-ups) are a great tummy exercise for the postpartum period.

For more information on exercise, I recommend *Essential Exercises for the Child-bearing Year*, an excellent book by Elizabeth Noble.

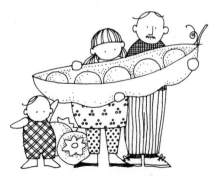

Section II

Shopping, Cooking, and Eating Out

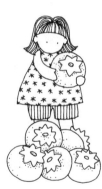

CHAPTER ELEVEN

Stocking the Pregnant Kitchen

What you will find in this chapter:

- *Check Out Your Kitchen*
- *A Peek in My Kitchen*
- *Reading Food Labels*
- *Eating on a Budget*
- *Stocking the Kitchen Toolbox*
- *Keeping the Vitamins in Your Vegetables*
- *The Essential Guide to Food Safety*
- *How to Lower Your Risk*
- *Food Safety Reports: Whom to Believe?*
- *Food Safety in a Nutshell*

This chapter answers such questions as:

- *How can I start shopping more healthfully?*
- *What do "lite" and "low-fat" mean on a food label?*
- *Is homemade eggnog safe to drink?*
- *Should I avoid fish?*
- *Why is a variety of foods so important?*
- *How can I eat well if I have a limited food budget?*
- *How can I avoid food poisoning?*

So, now you're motivated to eat well! If your diet is already good, you may not need much help. But if you're turning over a new leaf nutritionally, you may be thinking, "Where do I begin?"

The best place to start improving your diet is, of course, your own kitchen. First, you need to identify your shopping and eating patterns so you can change them if necessary.

Check Out Your Kitchen

1. What takes up the bulk of room in your freezer? Frozen vegetables? Ice cream? Frozen juice? Fish, chicken, or meat? Fish sticks? Frozen dinners? Frozen pies or cheesecakes? Pizza?

2. Does the top shelf of your fridge hold milk or soda?

3. Are your produce drawers bulging with fresh fruits and veggies, or do they contain only a few lonely, shriveled carrots?

4. Does your pantry hold many convenience foods? Canned vegetables and fruits? Potato chips? Candy?

5. Do you keep on hand a mix of grains, such as brown rice, pasta, bulgur, quinoa, whole-wheat flour, wheat germ, oats, and barley, or just white flour, rice, and pasta?

6. Do you keep a variety of vegetables in the house or do you regularly eat your two favorite vegetables and fruits?

▼

A Peek in My Kitchen

People are always curious about how I, a registered dietitian, eat at home. I think they envision my family eating perfectly all the time. They don't realize that we are just like any other family; we have our habits, our likes, and our dislikes. To show you how my family eats and shops, I'll let you take a peek in my kitchen.

In My Cupboards

Canned tomatoes, tomato sauce, tomato paste

Jarred spaghetti sauce without meat

Canned corn, peas, sweet potatoes, pumpkin

Canned black beans, vegetarian refried beans, kidney beans

Fantastic Foods Soup-in-a-Cup (usually Jumpin' Black Bean or Leapin' Lentils)

Dried lentils, split peas, twelve-bean mix

Canned tuna, salmon

White and whole-wheat flour

Skim evaporated milk

Yeast, sugar, brown sugar, molasses, honey

White rice, brown rice, bulgur, barley, and lots of pasta

Sun-dried tomatoes

Raisin Bran, All Bran, economy-size old-fashioned oatmeal, grits, Product 19, Multibran Chex, low-fat granola

Raisins, mixed dried fruit

Canola oil, olive oil, soy sauce

Many miscellaneous spices

Apple cider vinegar, red wine vinegar, tarragon wine vinegar

Boboli bread

Graham crackers, popcorn cakes, pretzels, Fig Newtons, Le Petit Beurre

Toblerone or Cadbury chocolate (My motto: Buy the best, but eat one piece at a time!)

Lay's Baked BBQ Potato Chips, Tostitos Baked Tortilla Chips, Guiltless Gourmet Oil-Free Tortilla Chips

In My Freezer

Miscellaneous frozen juices

Nutri-Grain waffles

Healthy Treasures Fish Sticks, regular fish sticks

Trout, salmon, sole, shrimp

Chicken, turkey breast

Top or bottom round, ground buffalo

Mashed bananas (to use in banana bread or pancakes)

Chopped spinach or broccoli, mixed vegetables, peas

Budget Gourmet Light & Lean Pockets, Michelina's Frozen Entrees

In My Refrigerator

1% milk, eggs, part-skim mozzarella string cheese, regular American cheese, part-skim mozzarella or farmer's cheese, reduced-fat or fat-free Cheddar, fresh Parmesan cheese, light Velveeta

Juice, Diet Coke, decaffeinated iced tea

Miscellaneous meat, fish, or chicken, thawing

Yoplait flavored low-fat yogurt, Land O' Lakes fat-free sour cream

Ham or turkey breast deli meat

Brummel & Brown Yogurt Spread,
   I Can't Believe It's Not Butter! (light)

Natural-style peanut butter

Mayonnaise, fat-free mayonnaise, homemade vinaigrette dressing, homemade
   Hidden Valley Ranch dip or dressing
   (almost fat-free), Good Seasons fat-free
   Zesty Herb dressing, barbecue sauce,
   teriyaki marinade, ketchup, hoisin
   sauce, grated ginger, chopped garlic in
   a jar, Dijon mustard, capers, horseradish, lemon juice, wheat germ and
   wheat bran (to prevent rancidity)

Various leftovers

In My Produce Drawers

Summer: all kinds of berries, cantaloupe,
   watermelon, apricots, nectarines,
   peaches, mangos, pineapple, lemons,
   tomatoes, carrots, cucumber, zucchini,
   eggplant, red and green peppers, alfalfa
   sprouts, ready-to-eat spring salad mix,
   romaine, leaf, or Boston lettuce

Winter: apples, bananas, pears, grapes,
   oranges, grapefruit, dates, figs, eggplant, acorn squash, butternut squash,
   carrots, leeks, cabbage, broccoli, cauliflower, tomato, lettuce, cucumber

▼

Reading Food Labels

Chances are, you are more concerned about
what you eat now than you were just a few
months ago. Your favorite new pastime may
be studying food labels. Why should you
read labels? It's the perfect way to put your
nutrition knowledge into practice and make
informed purchases.

What Can You Learn from a Label?

In 1990 Congress passed the Nutrition
Labeling and Education Act, and in 1991
the Food and Drug Administration (FDA)
proposed label revisions in accordance with
the new law. According to Dr. David
Kessler, then Commissioner of the FDA,
the old food labels placed consumers at a
disadvantage. The new labels "take the
guesswork—and the element of chance—out
of food labeling."

Food labels now contain a gold mine of
information. For example, by looking on
my box of Raisin Bran, I can see how many
calories, how many grams of fiber, and how
much sugar or sodium a serving contains. I
can find how much protein and fat it has
and see how all these numbers compare to
a standard 2,000-calorie diet called Daily
Value. I can also check out how vitamin A,
vitamin C, calcium, and iron in a serving of
Raisin Bran stack up to the Daily Value.
Suppose I'm allergic to milk protein. I can
look for it on the list of ingredients.

Following is a list of everything required
on a food label:[1]

- Total calories
- Calories from fat
- Total fat
- Saturated fat
- Cholesterol
- Sodium

- Total carbohydrate
- Dietary fiber
- Sugars
- Protein
- Vitamins A and C, calcium, and iron (listed as a percent of Daily Value)
- Nutrient information (listed in customary serving sizes using household measures)

It has been proposed that the amount of trans fat be included on food labels and in defining nutrient content and health claims. Trans fats are formed when liquid oils are hydrogenated to form solids like margarine and shortening. Trans fats can raise serum cholesterol the same way saturated fat does and can increase the risk of coronary heart disease.

You'll also find that certain terms have standard meanings:[2]

Fat-free: Less than ½ gram of fat per serving and no added fat.

Low-fat: Contains 3 grams of fat or less per 3½-ounce serving.

Light: Has at least ⅓ fewer calories than or ½ the fat of a comparable product. Can also mean that a low-calorie, low-fat food has had its sodium reduced by 50 percent. May mean light texture or color.

Reduced: Has at least 25 percent less of a nutrient or calories than the regular product.

Low in saturated fat: Contains 1 gram or less of saturated fat per serving.

Lean: Has less than 10 grams of fat, 4½ grams of saturated fat, and 95 milligrams of cholesterol per serving.

Extra lean: Contains less than 5 grams of fat, 2 grams of saturated fat, and 95 milligrams of cholesterol per serving.

Cholesterol-free: Has less than 2 milligrams of cholesterol and 2 grams or less of saturated fat per serving.

Low in cholesterol: Contains 20 milligrams or less of cholesterol and 2 grams or less of saturated fat per 3½-ounce serving.

Percent fat-free: Can only be used on low-fat or fat-free products.

Low sodium: Has less than 140 milligrams of sodium per 3½-ounce serving.

Very low sodium: Contains less than 35 milligrams of sodium per 3½-ounce serving.

Calorie-free: Has fewer than 5 calories per serving.

Sugar-free: Contains less than ½ gram of sugar per serving.

High in: Has 20 percent or more of the Daily Value for a particular nutrient.

Good source of: Contains 10 to 19 percent of the Daily Value for a particular nutrient.

Nutrition and Health Claims

Health claims describing the relationship between a food or nutrient and the risk of a disease or health-related condition are allowed on food labels. The health claim must meet certain requirements and must be phrased so that consumers can understand the food-disease relationship. Some such relationships are:

- Folate—neural tube defects
- Calcium—osteoporosis
- Sodium—hypertension
- Dietary saturated fat and cholesterol—risk of coronary heart disease
- Fruits, vegetables, and grain products that contain fiber (particularly soluble fiber)—risk of coronary heart disease
- Dietary fat—cancer
- Fruits and vegetables—cancer
- Fiber-containing grain products, fruits, and vegetables—cancer
- Dietary sugar alcohols—dental caries (cavities)
- Whole-grain foods and other plant foods—heart disease and cancer
- Soy protein—reduced risk of coronary heart disease

The Ingredient List

Every food label carries a list of ingredients arranged in descending order by weight. The new labeling law requires that even standardized foods, such as mayonnaise and ice cream, have a list of ingredients. In addition, all FDA-certified color additives must be listed by name. Another helpful requirement is that beverages that claim to contain juice must declare the total percentage of juice present: for example, "Juice blend—2 to 7 percent juice."

Sugar Is Sugar by Many Names

Some ingredients have many names, which makes deciphering food labels tricky. Corn syrup, high-fructose corn syrup, dextrose, glucose, corn sweetener, sucrose, sugar, brown sugar, fructose, maltose, sorbitol, mannitol, honey, and fruit-juice concentrate are all types of sweeteners.

There are also artificial sweeteners, sometimes called nonnutritive or noncaloric sweeteners, that are widely found in diet products: NutraSweet (the sweetener in Equal), saccharin (found in Sweet 'n Low and Sugar Twin), acesulfame K (found in Sweet One), and sucralose (found in Splenda). Several other nonnutritive sweeteners are currently awaiting FDA approval. (See page 123 for information on using these products during pregnancy.)

Let's find out how looking at a food label can help you make a healthier food choice. To most people, jam is jam. You may look at the price per ounce and pick up the cheapest. Or you may be partial to a particular brand and not look twice at the others. After all, jam is jam...right? Let's see.

Jam #1

Ingredients: High-fructose corn syrup, strawberries, pectin, natural flavoring.

Jam #2

Ingredients: Strawberries, high-fructose corn syrup, pectin, natural flavoring.

The better choice would be Jam #2, which ounce for ounce contains more strawberries than sugar.

Other Ingredients to Look For

Hey, what are all those funny words on food labels? You may have noticed there are many other things on ingredient lists besides food; these other ingredients are called food additives. An additive is a substance other than a basic foodstuff that is in food as a result of production, processing, storage, or packaging.

The media has given a lot of attention to food additives—so much that the word *additive* may have negative connotations to you. In truth, additives often protect our food from spoilage (and therefore keep us from getting sick) and bring clear benefits. For example, many foods are fortified with vitamins and minerals, which are considered additives. Many new fat-free products contain plant gums or seaweed derivatives that have been used safely for centuries. These are also considered additives.

Listed below are the main categories of additives and what they do.

Preservatives: Help give food a longer shelf life by retarding spoilage.

Antimicrobials: Prevent food spoilage from bacteria, mold, or fungus. For example, calcium propionate is used to keep bread from molding.

Antioxidants: Prevent oil-containing foods from going rancid and also delay browning. Vitamin C (ascorbic acid) is commonly used in meats as an antioxidant.

Curing agents: Prevent spoilage in meats. Sodium nitrate is a curing agent often found in smoked meats.

Flavoring agents: Directly or indirectly add flavor to a product.

Sweeteners (including natural and artificial): Make foods taste sweeter. Many new artificial sweeteners are awaiting FDA approval.

Flavor enhancers: Enhance flavor without leaving flavors of their own. Monosodium glutamate (MSG) occurs naturally in food and is sometimes added to food to bring out natural flavors.

Artificial flavoring: Adds flavor lost in processing or increases natural flavor.

Coloring agents (natural, nature-identical, and synthetic): Most foods we eat have some added coloring—even Cheddar cheese! Color is often added to a product because consumers expect it to be a certain color.

Texturizing Agents

Emulsifiers: Help evenly distribute tiny particles of liquid; keep oil and water mixed, as in creamy salad dressings.

Stabilizers or thickeners: Provide body or texture. Gums and other thickeners are used in fat-free salad dressings to give them the consistency of regular dressing.

Fat replacers or fat substitutes: Replace the properties of fat. They may be added to provide moisture or the taste or texture of fat. Fat replacers include natural plant substances, such as guar gum, xanthan gum, and carageenan, or they may be products developed specifically for replacing fat, such as Simplesse (found in Simple Pleasures ice cream) or Olestra (a fat substitute used for frying snack foods). Olestra should be avoided during pregnancy.

Nutrients: Vitamins, minerals, and fiber are often added to replace nutrients lost in processing or to improve nutritional value.

Miscellaneous: Other types of additives include leavening agents, propellants, pH control agents, humectants, dough conditioners, and anticaking agents.

Are Food Additives Safe?

Yes, the vast majority of food additives are safe. Some are uniformly beneficial; others may cause reactions in sensitive individuals. Questionable additives continue to undergo evaluation. Keep in mind that overconsumption of any one food or food component can have consequences. Lack of variety in the diet causes an excess of some dietary elements and a deficit of others.

For example, sodium nitrate, which is found in cured meats, can be converted to nitrosamines, which may cause cancer. Vitamin C is often added with nitrates to prevent their conversion to nitrosamine. Sulfites, used as antibrowning agents, are another type of additive. They are most often found in dried fruits and in some beer and wine. Up to 10 percent of the population is sensitive to sulfites–particularly people with asthma. If a food contains sulfite, it is listed on the nutrition label.

If you have questions about food additives, below are some good places to begin searching for answers:

www.cfsan.fda.gov/~lrd/foodadd.html
www.cspi.org
www.ificinfo.health.org

If You Are Concerned about Food Additives

▶ **Make sure to eat a wide variety of foods.**

▶ **Eat as many "whole foods" as possible, limiting mixes and convenience foods.**

▶ **Use fresh meat more often than cured or smoked meats.**
There has been some association between childhood cancer and eating cured meats during pregnancy.

▶ **Eat fresh fruits, vegetables, milk, and whole grains for snacks instead of packaged snack foods.**

▼

Eating on a Budget

Let's face it: Raising children is expensive. If you are pregnant with your first child, you may be discovering that just furnishing a nursery can cost a bundle! You may be looking for ways to cut costs on food. You *can* eat a nutritious diet and limit your food costs. But eating nutritiously on a budget does take some advance planning and investing in the long term.

Investing in the Long Term

Buy a Deep Freezer

Deep freezers aren't cheap, but owning one can allow you to buy food in bulk and stock up on sale items. A grocer in my city often has buy-one-get-one-free sales with no limit on the number of items one can buy. If one could buy enough chicken for six months and get it for half-price, that would be quite a bargain. If you live near a cattle ranch, you can invest in a side of beef (or split it with a friend) and get a great deal on very lean cuts of meat.

Try making a double pot of beans or lentil soup and freezing half. This ready-made meal will be wonderful on a cold winter night. You can also freeze leftovers instead of keeping them in the refrigerator and eventually throwing them away or feeding them to the dog when everyone is tired of them. Consider freezing small portions in microwaveable containers for homemade frozen dinners.

Buy Food in Bulk

This only works if you will actually use the food. If half of it spoils before you use it, bulk food is no bargain! A friend of mine makes homemade granola and lots of other homemade goods. She buys 50 pounds of oatmeal at a time from a health-food store and saves lots of money.

Plant a Big Garden

Fresh produce can be expensive. Growing your own and canning or freezing what you can't eat right away can save you a bushel of money, especially during the winter.

Plant Fruit Trees

Can you imagine stepping out in your back yard and picking a fresh grapefruit? My cousin in Florida does. Or how about some fresh apples to make a pie? Ask a local horticulturist which fruit trees grow well in your area.

Smart Shopping

► **Clip coupons and shop the sales.**

Many stores offer double and triple coupons. One Saturday I went to three stores, buying up all the great bargains. This storehopping was tiring, but I saved at least 30 percent on my groceries that week!

► **Shop alone. Or if you must take children shopping with you, make sure they are not hungry or tired.**

Reducing distractions will help you concentrate on reading labels and comparing products. It'll also help you avoid buying extra treats to keep the kids happy.

► **Don't go shopping when you are tired or hungry.**

► **Always shop with a list.**

► **When using coupons, compare the discounted price of each food with the store or generic brand.**

I often find that couponed items are still more expensive than other brands.

► **Go to farmers' markets.**

In the summer, farmers' market prices are often cheaper than supermarket prices. Again, if you can buy in bulk, you can save money. For example, we bought a large box of tomatoes for just five dollars and made homemade tomato sauce, which we then froze for future soups and sauces.

► **Buy your bread at a thrift store.**

I prefer a brand of bread that is one of the most expensive on the market. But by buying it at a thrift store, I can afford it. I also buy fat-free cakes, cookies, and ready-to-make pizza crusts at reduced prices.

▶ **If you buy staples such as beans, cereals, dried fruit, and oats from bulk containers, you not only save money, but you also reduce packaging to help the environment.**

Ditto for buying large-size snack foods instead of single-serving packages.

▶ **Get the best per-pound value.**

Fruit sold in 5-pound bags is often cheaper than bulk fruit, but packaged vegetables are not always cheaper. Mushrooms and tomatoes are good examples of this. And packaged ready-to-eat produce such as salads are more expensive than the individual ingredients. However, if you don't have the time to make salads and the ingredients end up spoiling in your fridge, then buying packaged food is a much better value for your money and your body!

The Cost of Convenience

We Americans want our food fast and easy, and we pay for it. When you compare the costs of homemade foods to various types of convenience foods, you may be shocked!

- Frozen pancakes are 18 cents each; pancakes from a mix are 4 cents each.
- A popular Italian salad dressing costs $1.65 for an 8-ounce bottle. A dry mix plus oil and vinegar costs $1.52. By adding your own herbs and spices to oil and vinegar, you pay only 55 cents, (plus pennies for spices) for 8 ounces of dressing.

- Packets of instant oatmeal cost 36 cents each. Old-fashioned oatmeal, which offers the best nutrition, costs only 8 cents per serving–and that's for Quaker, a name brand.
- Ready-to-eat muffins from the bakery cost 69 cents each. A Jiffy Banana Muffin Mix muffin, including added ingredients, costs only 9 cents! For the cost of one ready-to-eat muffin, you could feed the whole family with muffins from the easy-to-make mix.

When Menu Planning

- Plan menus with your budget in mind. Make less-expensive foods like grains, beans, and vegetables the main course, with more expensive foods like meats as side dishes. Not only is a meatless or almost-meatless diet good for your food budget, it can save you the pain, anguish, and cost of having a diet-related chronic disease such as heart disease or cancer many years down the road. (See page 327 for vegetarian meal ideas.)
- Plan your menus around what's on sale at the store.
- When cooking, use powdered milk. You can double your calcium by using canned evaporated milk, which is cheaper than fresh milk.
- Fresh fruit may seem more expensive than a conventional dessert, but it's usually not!
- Plan your menus with leftovers in mind. Think of different menus you can do with one dish. For example, you could make beef fajitas the first night and fiesta

salad with beans and beef strips the second night, or your could freeze the leftover fajita fixings in individual containers for future lunches or quick dinners. Most people end up throwing a lot of food away because they forget about it, get tired of it, or just don't like leftovers. (See page 323 for leftover menus.)

- Are you eating out or buying vending machine snacks often because of a busy schedule? Frozen waffles or pancakes, though expensive, are still cheaper than a drive-through meal. Frozen sandwiches such as Lean Pockets are still cheaper than a burger meal. If you can plan ahead a bit and use leftovers for lunch, you'll probably see the greatest savings.

▼

Stocking the Kitchen Toolbox

To make tasty, nutritious meals with minimum hassle, you need to have the tools of the trade! I consider the following tools essential for a cook who wants to eat well but doesn't have lots of time to waste in the kitchen:

Essential Items

Blender or food processor. One of these is essential for making quick soups, low-fat cheese dips, stuffings, and meal-on-the-go drinks.

Meat thermometer. Using a meat thermometer is the most reliable method of determining whether your meat is cooked to the right temperature. If you like your meat rare, you definitely need a thermometer to make sure you have cooked your food enough to kill bacteria.

Microwave. I didn't realize how much I used mine until I started writing down the recipes for this book. Though most people use microwaves just for warming leftovers or heating water, using them for cooking can be a real timesaver. Microwave cooking can also preserve nutrients.

Nonstick pans. You don't have to add fat when you use nonstick cookware. I also like the fact that cleanup is a breeze.

Plastic cutting board. Use a plastic or acrylic cutting board instead of a wooden one (at least for raw meats). Wooden boards are harder to sterilize and can harbor bacteria from uncooked meats.

Microwave-safe cookware. Many people use leftover margarine containers for cooking in the microwave. This is risky because some of the chemicals in the plastic (also in plastic wrap) have been shown to migrate into food. Until further research is done on this, use Pyrex cookware or plastic containers made especially for the microwave.

Miscellaneous utensils. A few good-quality knives, nylon spatulas and spoons for nonstick cookware, measuring cups and spoons, and a wire whisk should be part of every kitchen. These few utensils will make life much easier for the cook!

Nice-to-Have Items

Minichopper. This little food processor holds only about 1 cup and is great for chopping onion, garlic, or other vegetables to a fine consistency. It's a great gadget for pregnant women who are sensitive to cooking smells in the first trimester. Another nice-to-have item is a hand-held slicer/chopper with several blades. With it you can chop an onion in about thirty seconds or slice a potato paper-thin in a minute.

Rotating platter for microwave. This item ensures that your food is cooked evenly to the correct temperature without having to be turned manually every few minutes.

Salad spinner. I love salad, but I hate washing and drying lettuce leaves. We received a salad spinner as a wedding gift, and now salad making is much easier.

Luxury Items

Add these to your wish list after you have a nice college fund going.

Ice-cream maker. This gadget is great for making frozen yogurts and sorbets that can satisfy your sweet tooth without a lot of fat.

Bread maker. Imagine waking up to fresh bread every morning! Making your own whole-grain bread may help you increase the fiber in your diet.

Hand-held blender. These are the type you see advertised on TV. Some of my clients have told me these gadgets really *do* whip skim milk and they really *can* grind meat, crush ice, and make milk shakes.

▼

Keeping the Vitamins in Your Vegetables

Which are better—frozen, canned, or fresh vegetables? Nothing beats freshly picked food straight from your garden. However, in some cases, frozen vegetables can actually have a higher nutrient content than fresh.

Fresh vegetables may not be very fresh by the time you buy them, and they're even less fresh if they stay several days (or weeks) in your refrigerator. Recently, a University of Illinois researcher found that "fresh" store-bought beans had lost 50 percent of their vitamin C since leaving the farm seven days earlier. After three days in a home refrigerator, they had lost 10 percent more. However, frozen beans had lost only 30 percent of their vitamin C after four months in the freezer. In this case, the frozen vegetables were a better choice.[3]

Canned vegetables are not as nutritious as fresh vegetables, but eating canned vegetables beats eating no vegetables at all! If you look in my cabinets, you will find a multitude of canned beans, tuna, and tomato sauce. Because I rarely can (or want to) take the time to cook beans from scratch, buying canned beans makes sense for me.

Caring for Vegetables

▶ **Store veggies in your refrigerator crisper in their bags.**

Ziploc makes special vegetable bags with air vents that let the right amount of moisture out to keep your veggies fresh.

▶ **To keep lettuce and other greens fresh, wrap in paper towels, then store in their bags.**

▶ **Don't cut, peel, or wash vegetables until you are ready to cook or eat them.**

An exception to this might be keeping carrot and celery sticks cleaned, cut, and ready to eat. Having them ready to eat will increase their chances of being eaten. Eating vegetables with reduced nutrient content is better than eating none at all!

▶ **If possible, avoid soaking vegetables to wash them; soaking depletes water-soluble vitamins.**

Healthiest Cooking Methods

1. No cooking

2. Steaming or microwaving

3. Stir-frying

4. Baking

5. Boiling

When foods are cooked to death, they taste bland, have the consistency of baby food, and lose water-soluble vitamins like B vitamins and vitamin C.

Cooking Tips for Healthy Vegetables
• To cook vegetables in the microwave, add 1 or 2 tablespoons of water and cover tightly. After the microwave cycle is finished, let the vegetables stand a few minutes while covered to continue cooking. This method is wonderful for cooking cubed potatoes, which wind up so moist, they taste great without any added fat. (See page 342 for variations on this recipe.)

• When stir-frying, put the more dense vegetables in the pan first. For example, start with onion, garlic, and spices for flavor, then add carrots, celery, cabbage, and broccoli. At the end, add softer vegetables such as peas, mushrooms, and greens.

• Steaming vegetables on a rack in a pressure cooker is almost too fast! Watch the time carefully to avoid overcooking.

• When boiling, use just enough water to prevent scorching. Some vegetables, such as potatoes, need to be covered with water. Cut large vegetables in pieces to shorten cooking time.

▼

The Essential Guide to Food Safety

You may be so busy cooking all the right foods, exercising, and preparing for your baby's arrival that you don't stop to think about making your kitchen safe. And I don't mean just making sure no pot handles are sticking out. Many other dangers lurk in kitchens, and they are related to how you select and handle your food.

The dangers I'm referring to usually can't be seen, smelled, or tasted. They are hidden in the forms of bacteria, fungi, and molds. The Centers for Disease Control and Prevention estimate that food-borne bacteria caused 76,000,000 illnesses; 325,000 hospitalizations; and 5,000 deaths in the United States in 1998. Pregnant women have more at risk; fetuses can be severely harmed by some bacteria. A bout of food poisoning reduces mom's nutrition intake, which could also slow baby's growth.

Even if you don't read the rest of this chapter, make sure to read the summary on page 230.

Making Your Kitchen Safe

When You're Preparing Food

▶ Wash your hands.

Wash your hands in hot, soapy water before preparing food and after using the bathroom, blowing your nose, petting the dog, changing a diaper, and so on. This advice is common sense, of course, but hands are the most common spreaders of bacteria to food.

▶ Keep raw meats and produce away from each other.

Use a separate cutting board for raw meats and uncooked foods. Wash the meat board in the dishwasher after use. Use a plastic cutting board instead of a wooden one; wood can't be cleaned as well and may harbor bacteria. Use paper towels instead of a reusable sponge or rag to wipe away juices from meat, fish, or poultry. Wash your hands well with soap after handling meat and before handling other foods, especially raw produce.

▶ Wash sponges, towels, and kitchen rags often.

Bacteria can survive quite well in used sponges and fabrics. Wash sponges in the washing machine with bleach or in your dishwasher or soak them in a weak bleach solution daily. Replace sponges every few weeks.

▶ Thaw food in the microwave or refrigerator—NOT ON THE KITCHEN COUNTER.

When Eating Away from Home

▶ Don't eat anything that has been sitting out for hours without proper refrigeration or heat.

Cantaloupe once caused an outbreak of salmonella. The person who cut the cantaloupe did not wash the outside, and bacteria got onto the edible portion. After the cantaloupe was out of the refrigerator for a while, the bacteria multiplied enough to cause illness.

▶ If meat, fish, or chicken doesn't look as though it is cooked well enough, ask to have it cooked more thoroughly.

Be assertive. (Keep in mind that smoked foods will still look pink, even when they're done.)

▶ If food that should be cold isn't, don't eat it.

Recently, my husband and I ordered a piece of cream pie to share. After eating almost half of it, I realized that the pie wasn't cold at all and alerted the waitress. She found out that the refrigerator was broken, and no one had noticed it!

▶ Avoid restaurants that don't practice good sanitation.

People who handle food should wear hair coverings and should have clean hands. Employees who take money should not also be touching food. People who work with food must wash their hands after using the restroom, blowing their noses, smoking, or eating before they handle food again. Workers who don't follow these rules should be reported to your local health department.

Is It Still Good?

Do you find yourself asking this question often? On pages 217–222 you'll find guides from the U.S. Department of Agriculture (USDA) about how long you can safely refrigerate and freeze various foods.

According to Dee Ann Whitmire, a registered dietitian and communications specialist with the Western Dairy Council, "A good rule of thumb is that you can keep a dairy product one week after the date printed on the package. When in doubt, throw it out, since how you handle a product can affect its freshness."[4]

When Is It Done?

Don't be impatient when you cook meats; thorough cooking is necessary to kill harmful bacteria, and cooking meat thoroughly takes time.

When checked visually, red meat is done when it's brown or gray inside; poultry is done when juices run clear; and fish is done when it becomes opaque and flakes with a fork.

If you're using a meat thermometer, cook beef, pork, and lamb to an internal temperature of 160°F, whole chicken or turkey to 180°F, and fin fish to 145°F for at least five minutes. In general, fin fish should be cooked ten minutes per inch of thickness.

Cook eggs until whites are firm and yolks are no longer runny. This reduces the likelihood that an egg is harboring salmonella.

Microwave Cooking Tips[5]

▶ Choose only microwave-safe containers.

Chemicals from packaging and from containers not deemed microwave safe can leach into food at high temperatures.

▶ Cover the dish with a lid, paper towel, or wax paper. Avoid using plastic wrap in the microwave unless it is labeled polyethylene.

If you do use plastic wrap, don't let it touch the food. The trapped steam will help regulate the food's temperature throughout.

▶ Rotate the dish halfway through cooking time.

Even if the dish is on a turntable, repositioning it is still a good idea. Turn over large food items. These practices help food cook more evenly and safely.

▶ Let microwaved food stand for an additional third of the cooking time.

Food continues cooking after being removed from the microwave. This helps equalize its temperature throughout.

▶ **Take care when cooking raw chicken or ground beef in the microwave.**

Even cooking is critical to killing food-borne bacteria in these vulnerable foods. It may be best to use an alternate cooking method. However, reheating these foods thoroughly in a microwave should be fine.

Other Hidden Risks in Your Food Supply

Recent research shows that exposure to some chemicals before and during pregnancy could be linked to infertility, spontaneous abortion, birth defects, and developmental problems.[6] While the verdict is still out on the specific chemicals and the amounts that could cause problems, it is prudent to learn what you can do to avoid being exposed to chemicals that could harm your baby. It's perfectly okay to be picky about what you eat; your baby will thank you for it! And it's especially important to eat a variety of foods to decrease your exposure to individual pollutants and pesticides and to increase your intake of a variety of nutrients.

Endocrine Disruptors

The scientific community has recently voiced concerns about environmental contaminants called endocrine disruptors. Endocrine disruptors are hormonally active agents that have been associated with reproductive and developmental problems in wildlife. It is known that exposure to high amounts of endocrine disruptors can affect humans as well as wildlife, but the effects of smaller exposures is debated. Scientists fear that endocrine disruptors do the most damage during times of rapid growth: the prenatal period, infancy, early childhood, and puberty. While further research is being conducted, you can try to avoid endocrine disruptors by following these tips:

Selection

Some pesticides—not only those found on food, but also the ones used on plants and in insecticides—are endocrine disruptors. Endocrine disruptors are also found in certain types of plastic, including plastic wrap.[7] Environmental pollutants can be stored in the fat of meats, fish and poultry. Read the next few pages for more information on these topics.

Storage

Don't store high-fat food such as cheese, meat, pie, and cake in plastic wrap. Some chemicals in plastic wrap can migrate into high-fat foods. It's better to store such foods in plastic bags or microwave-safe plastic or glass containers. Plastic containers bearing a recycling code of "2" or "5" on the bottom are considered free of potential endocrine disruptors. If food is sold in plastic shrink-wrap, stretchy plastic wrap, or a foam container, repackage it at home.

Cooking

Use microwave-safe plastic, glass, or ceramic to cook or reheat foods in the microwave. To cover food while microwaving, use wax paper, paper towel, or plastic wrap labeled "polyethylene" and leave an inch between food and wrap. Avoid plastic wraps labeled "PVC" (polyvinyl chloride).

Pesticides

In 1996, the Food Quality Protection Act was signed into law. Its purpose is to keep Americans safe from pesticide residues in food. The act takes special care in evaluating pesticides that infants and children might consume. The Environmental Protection Agency (EPA) will probably be banning some harmful pesticides; however, it may take years to complete its evaluation. Because your unborn baby may be particularly vulnerable to some pesticides, it is best to be safe and follow the advice on the next few pages to decrease your pesticide exposure.

Consumers Union, a nonprofit group devoted to consumer product safety, has done toxicity testing on milk and common fruits and vegetables. It found that some products contained as many as twenty different pesticide residues, while others contained few.[8]

Fruits and Vegetables with Most Pesticide Residues

- Fresh peaches (both domestic and imported)
- Frozen and fresh winter squash grown in the United States
- Domestic and imported apples, grapes, spinach and pears
- U.S.-grown green beans

Among the foods listed above, U.S. peaches and frozen winter squash contained pesticide residues much higher than the other produce.

Fruits and Vegetables with Least Pesticide Residues

These foods contained the lowest amounts of pesticides:

- Frozen and canned corn
- Milk
- U.S. orange juice, broccoli, bananas, and canned peaches

Other relatively "clean" foods were:

- Frozen and canned sweet peas
- U.S. and imported apple juice
- Frozen winter squash from Mexico
- Tomatoes from Canada
- Brazilian orange juice
- U.S. wheat

What's Organic?

Eleven states now have standards for organic produce, and a national standard is coming soon. The Organic Foods Production Act of 1990 requires the establishment of national standards governing the marketing of certain agricultural products as organically produced. The National Organic Program is now being formed to carry out the terms of the act. The program would create national standards for the organic production and handling of agricultural products, which would include a national list of synthetic substances approved for use in the production and handling of organically produced products.

According to a proposed rule,[9] an organic product is defined as one that:

- has been produced and handled without the use of synthetic chemicals;
- has not been produced on land to which any prohibited substances, including synthetic chemicals, have been applied during the three years immediately preceding the harvest of the products; and
- has been produced and handled in compliance with an organic plan agreed to by the producer and handler of the product and the certifying agent.

Until the rule is finalized, the organic produce available at grocery stores is usually certified using state or private certification methods.

▼

How to Lower Your Risk

This section provides tips on selecting and handling foods so that you can eat the safest food possible.

Fruits, Vegetables, Grains, and Nuts

In recent years, bacteria that were once found mostly in animal products have made their way into fruits and vegetables. *Escherichia coli* (commonly known as E. coli), for example, has been found in alfalfa sprouts and unpasteurized apple cider. Because of this, you must be more careful about washing your produce well. Your risk of illness due to pesticide exposure is less than your risk of illness from inadequate fruit and vegetable intake, but you should still take steps to ensure the safety of the fruits and vegetables you eat.

Safety Tips

▶ **Grow your own produce without using pesticides.**

▶ **Consider buying certified organic produce.**

Consider buying organic produce or produce labeled "no detectable residues"—especially when buying produce that is more likely to contain pesticide residues. (See page 214.) Remember that organic produce may not look as perfect as produce to which pesticides have been applied.

▶ **Buy locally grown produce.**

Such produce is fresher, picked closer to its peak ripeness, and probably isn't coated with wax or sprayed with post-harvest pesticides. Usually, a local farmers' market or roadside stand is a great source. But be inquisitive. Last summer when I asked where the produce came from at my local farmers' market, I found that some of it had been shipped from four states away!

▶ **Wash off pesticide residues.**

If you'd like a little help in removing pesticide residues, use a few drops of dish soap or Fit Fruit and Vegetable Rinse, a product made by Procter and Gamble. It's usually found in or near the produce department.

▶ **Buy domestically grown produce (this is also good for local farmers).**

Ironically, pesticides that are banned in the United States are still produced in the U.S.

for export. Some of those pesticides find their way back into our country on imported foods.

▶ Buy fruits and vegetables in season.

If you live in the north and buy a cantaloupe in the dead of winter, you can be sure it was grown pretty far south of you. That means it had to be picked early and was likely sprayed with post-harvest pesticides and wax to make sure it arrived at your store looking just picked.

▶ Exercise caution with nut products.

The large national brands of peanut butter probably have the highest quality standards in terms of aflatoxins, a naturally occurring carcinogen. Throw away any moldy, discolored, or shriveled peanuts, pecans, walnuts, almonds, Brazil nuts, and pistachios—they can also contain aflatoxins.

▶ Store potatoes in a cool, dark place.

Trim away any green or damaged parts; they contain glycoalkaloids, toxins that can affect the nervous system.[10]

▶ Avoid unpasteurized juices.

▶ Avoid eating sprouts, such as alfalfa and mung bean sprouts, unless you cook them first.

Peeling and Washing Produce

To peel or not to peel? It's a tossup: Peeling does completely remove all surface pesticides (whereas washing might not), but peeling can also mean losing valuable fiber and nutrients. As a general rule, if your diet is otherwise rich in fiber, peel produce—especially

Questions about Pesticides?

Contact the National Pesticide Telecommunications Network, funded by the EPA's Office of Pesticide Programs, by calling 800-858-PEST from 6:30 a.m. to 4:30 p.m. Pacific time (except holidays) or by visiting nptn.orst.edu. You can also contact the National Antimicrobial Information Network by calling 800-477-6349 or by visiting ace.orst.edu/info/nain.

produce that is obviously waxed—to remove the wax and any other surface pesticides.

Always wash produce. Adding a few drops of dish soap to a pint of water is more effective than plain water in removing many pesticides. Choose a soap that doesn't contain dyes and perfumes. Don't use salt water or vinegar; these won't help. Salt is something we get more than enough of in our diets. No evidence shows that specially formulated pesticide and wax washes are more effective than regular dish detergent—and they can cost up to eight times as much! Scrub with a vegetable brush, and be sure to rinse food completely.

Here are some tips for cleaning specific types of produce (instead of buying organic):[11]

▶ For leafy vegetables such as lettuce and cabbage, discard outer leaves and wash inner leaves.

▶ Wash celery after trimming off the leaves and tops.

▶ For recipes that need grated peel, buy organic fruit if possible.

▶ **Peel carrots. (You won't be losing fiber, since carrots contain fiber throughout.)**

▶ **Peel cucumbers if they're waxed.**

▶ **Wash eggplants, peppers, tomatoes, potatoes, green beans, cherries, grapes, and strawberries.**

▶ **Peel apples, peaches, and pears if you get plenty of fiber from other sources, since the peels of these fruits likely contain risky residues.**

▶ **Cut up cauliflower, broccoli, and spinach before you wash them, since pesticides may otherwise be hard to wash off.**

Dairy Products

The biggest potential risks from eating dairy products come from drinking raw or unpasteurized milk and from bacterial contamination due to improper handling.

Like all perishable foods, dairy products are very safe foods if handled properly. One issue that has gotten recent media attention is the use of the hormone bovine somatotropin (BST) on dairy cows.

Dairy cows produce this hormone naturally. Scientists have found a way to produce the hormone synthetically, and when given to cows, it can increase the cows' milk production by 10 to 30 percent.

The National Institutes of Health (NIH) have concluded that milk from BST-treated cows is safe for humans.[12] The medical community generally regards the use of supplemental BST as safe.[13]

So why all the fuss? Much of the controversy surrounding this issue is unrelated to human health. Some people feel that an increased milk supply may take jobs away

Dairy Products Storage Guide		
Food	Refrigerator at 40°F	Freezer at 0°F
Milk	8–20 days	
Buttermilk	2–3 weeks	Not recommended due to reduced quality of product after thawing
Eggnog	1–2 weeks	
Parmesan cheese	Almost indefinitely	
Sour cream	3–4 weeks	
Ultrapasteurized cream	6–8 weeks	
Yogurt	3–6 weeks	
Processed cheese food in jars, unopened	12 months	
Grated cheese in moisture-proof packaging, unopened	12 months	6–8 weeks
Swiss and Cheddar cheese	1 month	6–8 weeks

Note: Storage time begins at processing, not purchase.

Sources: *Newer Knowledge of Milk*, National Dairy Council, 1988, and *Newer Knowledge of Cheese*, National Dairy Council, 1986.

from dairy farmers. Some people are concerned that BST injections may adversely affect dairy cows. Others are just opposed to biotechnology in general.

Safety Tips

▶ **Buy only pasteurized milk products. Avoid any raw milk, including goat's milk.**

▶ **Avoid cheeses that have been known to have been contaminated with the dangerous listeria bacteria.**

These include Brie, Camembert, feta, blue cheese, and Mexican-style soft cheeses (queso blanco, queso fresco, queso de crema, and queso Asadero).

▶ **Keep your refrigerator at or below 40°F and keep milk refrigerated.**

If you like to put milk on the table for meals, don't keep it out long. Leaving milk out at room temperature, even briefly, can allow bacteria to grow and hasten spoilage.

▶ **Never return unused milk to its original container after it has been sitting out for a while.**

▶ **See chart on page 217 for storage times for dairy products.**

Eggs

The number-one food safety problem with eggs is salmonella bacteria. Though salmonella poisoning is rarely fatal, it is dangerous to people with weak immune systems, such as pregnant women, infants, children, people with chronic disease, and the elderly.

Unfortunately, salmonella poisoning is on the rise, especially in the northeastern states. You don't have to entirely avoid eggs, which is fortunate because the protein in eggs is of very high quality. But do use the following tips to keep your eggs safe:

Safety Tips: Buying and Storing

▶ **Buy only eggs that have been refrigerated.**

▶ **Store eggs in their own container to keep them from cracking.**

▶ **Don't wash eggs; they are usually washed, sanitized, and coated with mineral oil to keep out bacteria.**

▶ **Buy eggs that aren't cracked; bacteria can seep through the cracks.**

Buy AA or A eggs, which are required by law to be clean and uncracked.

Safety Tips: Eating

▶ **Avoid any food containing raw egg or egg white.**

According to Dr. Pat Kendall, Food Science Specialist with Colorado State University, most of the salmonella bacteria in an egg are found in the yolk.[14] When you eat out, you may want to avoid health shakes, caesar salad dressing, and cold mousses or soufflés, which may contain raw eggs. Also avoid unpasteurized eggnog and eggnog made with raw eggs, homemade ice cream, and lightly cooked egg products such as meringue and French toast.

► **Cook your eggs until yolk and white are firm or at least until yolk thickens.**

If you prefer your eggs runny, you might consider an egg substitute, which contains pasteurized eggs. Avoid the temptation to taste cake batter or cookie dough that may contain raw eggs.

Beef and Pork

The food safety risks associated with eating beef and pork are bacterial contamination and the presence of parasites.

Eating raw and undercooked beef can increase your chances of getting toxoplasmosis, a disease caused by parasites. E. coli is a dangerous bacteria mostly associated with ground beef.

The danger of contracting trichinosis is much reduced from past generations. Trichinosis is an illness caused by eating raw or undercooked pork infected with a type of worm. It is completely destroyed at 138°F.[15]

The Facts about Drugs and Hormones

Drugs

One of the main concerns regarding consumption of animal meat is drug residues.

About forty years ago we discovered that small, preventive doses of certain antibiotics improved livestock growth. The National Cattlemen's Association recommends against routine use of antibiotics in cattle feed, and most beef producers are following the recommendation. When antibiotics are used to treat illnesses in cows, the cow goes to the market only after a specified quarantine period.

Hormones

"Growth hormones have been used safely and successfully for almost thirty years to increase lean production and feed efficiency," says Lowell L. Wilson, Animal Science Department, Pennsylvania State University.[16]

Hormones improve animal growth. Beef cattle given a small amount of growth hormone grow faster, go to market sooner, and are leaner. According to the beef industry, if hormone implants were not used, the supply of beef would shrink and prices consumers pay would rise.

A Texas A & M University report concluded that the scientific community now agrees that the proper use of certain hormones is harmless to the consumer and may

Estrogen Levels in Food		
Food	Serving Size	Estrogen (in nanograms*)
Beef, from a cow implanted with estrogen	3 ounces	1.85
Beef, from a cow not given estrogen	3 ounces	1.01
Egg	1	1,750
Cabbage	3 ounces	2,016

*One nanogram is one billionth of a gram. If a gram were a football field, a nanogram would be equal to one blade of grass.
Source: Inter-American Institute for Cooperation of Agriculture. *Report on Use of Hormonal Substances in Animals*, December 1986.

enhance animal growth performance by as much as 20 percent.[17] The University of California Wellness Letter, March 1989, reported, "At the prescribed dosages used in feedlots, these hormones have been certified safe by numerous scientific studies."

Surprisingly, hormones are present in nearly all the plant and animal foods we eat.

In fact, the estrogen in many common foods far exceeds the estrogen found in beef given supplemental estrogen. (See the chart on page 219.)

Men, women, and children also produce estrogen in their bodies at levels thousands and millions of times greater than the levels found in beef. In the third trimester of

Eggs, Meat, and Poultry Storage Guide

Cooked

Food	Refrigerator at 40°F	Freezer at 0°F
Chicken, fried	3–4 days	4 months
Chicken nuggets or patties	1–2 days	1–3 months
Chicken pieces, plain	3–4 days	4 months
Chicken pieces with broth or gravy	1–2 days	6 months
Corned beef (in pouch with pickling juice)	5–7 days	1 month drained and wrapped
Egg, chicken, tuna, ham, or macaroni salad (deli or homemade)	3–5 days	Don't freeze
Ham, canned, unopened package	6–9 months	Don't freeze
Gravy and meat broth	1–2 days	2–3 months
Ham, cooked, half	3–5 days	1–2 months
Ham, cooked, slices	3–4 days	1–2 months
Ham, cooked, whole	7 days	1–2 months
Hard sausage (such as pepperoni)	2–3 weeks	1–2 months
Lunch meats, opened package	3–5 days	1–2 months in freezer wrap
Lunch meats, unopened package	2 weeks	1–2 months in freezer wrap
Meat and meat dishes, cooked	3–4 days	2–3 months
Pork and lamb chops, prestuffed, or chicken breast, stuffed	1 day	Don't freeze
Poultry dishes	3–4 days	4–6 months
Smoked sausage	1 week	1–2 months
Soups and stews (vegetable- or meat-based)	3–4 days	2–3 months
Store-cooked convenience foods (ready-to-eat)	1–2 days	Don't freeze
TV dinners, frozen casseroles		3–4 months

pregnancy, your body will produce thirty-seven million times the amount of estrogen found in a 3-ounce serving of beef.

Poultry

The greatest risks from eating poultry are illnesses caused by the food-borne bacteria *Salmonella typhimurium, Salmonella enteritidis,* and *Campylobacter jejuni.*

Chicken is the most popular meat among my clients because it is a low-fat dish that can be prepared quickly. However, chicken is also a common carrier of campylobacter and salmonella bacteria. Campylobacter

passes among chickens during processing. Salmonella is found in chicken feces and spreads to other parts of chickens during processing. Improper handling of raw chicken in the kitchen adds to the risk of contracting salmonellosis and campylobacterosis.

Most people are aware of salmonellosis, but campylobacterosis is a different story. Because campylobacterosis symptoms (cramps, diarrhea, and fever) are flu-like and can occur up to five days after eating a contaminated food, it is estimated that only one in a hundred cases is reported. Two to six million people in the United States are thought to contract

Eggs, Meat, and Poultry Storage Guide (continued)		
	Fresh	
Food	**Refrigerator at 40°F**	**Freezer at 0°F**
Bacon	1 week	1 month
Beef roast	3–5 days	6–12 months
Beef steaks	3–5 days	6–12 months
Chicken or turkey, pieces	1–2 days	9 months
Chicken or turkey, whole	1–2 days	1 year
Eggs, in shell	3 weeks	Don't freeze
Giblets	1–2 days	3–4 months
Ground turkey, veal, pork, or lamb	1–2 days	3–4 months
Hamburger and stew meats	1–2 days	3–4 months
Hot dogs, opened package	1 week	1–2 months in freezer wrap
Hot dogs, unopened package	2 weeks	1–2 months in freezer wrap
Lamb chops	3–5 days	6–9 months
Lamb roast	3–5 days	6–9 months
Mayonnaise, commercial	2 months	Don't freeze
Pork chops	3–5 days	4–6 months
Pork and veal roast	3–5 days	4–6 months
Sausage, raw	1–2 days	1–2 months
Variety meats (tongue, brain, kidney, liver, heart)	1–2 days	3–4 months

Food	Purchased Commercially Frozen for Freezer Storage	Purchased Fresh and Home-Frozen	Thawed, Never Frozen, or Previously Frozen and Home-Refrigerated at 32°F
Seafood Storage Guide			
Fish Fillets/Steaks			
Lean:			
Cod, flounder, haddock, halibut	10–12 months	6–8 months	36 hours
Pollock, ocean perch, sea trout, rockfish, Pacific Ocean trout	8–9 months	4 months	36 hours
Fat:			
Mullet, smelt	6–8 months	N/A	36 hours
Salmon (cleaned)	7–9 months	N/A	36 hours
Shellfish			
Blue crabmeat, fresh	N/A	4 months	5–7 days
Blue crabmeat, pasteurized	N/A	N/A	6 months
Clams, shucked	N/A	N/A	5 days
Cocktail claws	N/A	4 months	5 days
Dungeness crab	6 months	6 months	5 days
King crab	12 months	9 months	7 days
Lobster, live	N/A	N/A	1–2 days
Lobster, tail meat	8 months	6 months	4–5 days
Oysters, shucked	N/A	N/A	4–7 days
Shrimp	9 months	5 months	4 days
Snow crab	6 months	6 months	5 days
Surimi (imitation seafood)	10–12 months	9 months	2 weeks
Breaded Seafood			
Fish sticks	18 months	N/A	N/A
Portions	18 months	N/A	N/A
Scallops	16 months	10 months	N/A
Shrimp	12 months	8 months	N/A
Smoked Fish			
Herring	N/A	2 months	3–4 days
Salmon, whitefish	N/A	2 months	5–8 days

Notes:
- N/A–not applicable
- These storage guidelines indicate optimal shelf life for seafood refrigerated or frozen properly. Temperature fluctuations in home refrigerators will affect optimal shelf life, as will frequent opening and closing of refrigerator and freezer doors.
- Although the above storage times ensure a fresh product for maximum refrigeration storage life at 32°F, the consumer should plan on using seafood within 36 hours for optimal quality and freshness.
- To determine approximate storage time for species not listed, ask your retailer which category (lean, fat, shellfish, breaded, or smoked) they fall within and refer to the guide.

Source: National Fisheries Institute, 2000 M Street NW, Suite 580, Washington, D.C. 20036

campylobacterosis each year.

Sanitary kitchen procedures are your best defense against campylobacter and salmonella bacteria. Follow the safety tips below to protect your family:

Safety Tips

- Salmonella bacteria multiply at room temperature. Keep hot foods hot (above 140°F) and cold foods cold (below 40°F). Thaw poultry in the microwave instead of on the countertop. At a picnic or buffet dinner, keep cold poultry dishes in a cooler or on ice.
- *Campylobacter* can live in your refrigerator for weeks! Clean up any juices that spill from a defrosting chicken. If juice falls on food that will be eaten raw, such as vegetables, fruit, or cheese, throw that food away.
- Because microwave ovens cook unevenly, they may not completely kill campylobacter or salmonella bacteria. Traditional methods like baking, broiling, or boiling are preferred for poultry.
- Research shows that most of the reported cases of campylobacterosis occur during barbecue season—a hint that perhaps people are undercooking their grilled chicken! A combination of microwaving and grilling would ensure thorough and quick cooking. (An internal temperature of 180°F ensures that chicken is thoroughly cooked.)
- Since campylobacter does not survive freezing, buy frozen chicken or freeze chicken for a few days before using.

For more information about poultry, call the USDA Meat and Poultry Hotline at 800-535-4555 (toll-free nationwide), 202-720-3333 (Washington, D.C.), or 800-256-7072 (TDD/TTY).

Seafood

Ben Franklin said, "Fish and house guests begin to smell after three days." He should have said "two days"—at least for fish—because it's unwise to keep fresh fish longer than that.

People are eating more fish these days, probably because they are realizing how healthy it can be. It's low in fat and saturated fat and high in protein, and it contains significant amounts of omega-3 fats. Omega-3 fats can have very beneficial effects on your health. Research suggests that omega-3 fats may prevent blood platelets from sticking to the walls of arteries, thereby lowering the risk of atherosclerosis and heart attack.

The greatest potential risks from eating fish are food poisoning from bacteria or parasites and consumption of environmental pollutants. Proper handling and cooking can reduce or kill bacteria and parasites. If you are considering becoming pregnant, are already pregnant, or are breast-feeding, you should limit your tuna consumption to once or twice per week and your shark and swordfish intake to once a month.

Bacteria

Fish are among the most perishable foods; they have a shelf life of seven to twelve days once they're out of the water. Some fish stay on fishing boats for several days, so by the time they arrive in stores, they may have little shelf life left. If fish get warmer than 32°F, their shelf life decreases; at 42°F, the shelf life is cut in half. Fattier fish and cold-water fish spoil even faster. Poor sanitation practices, such as using unwashed knives and cutting boards and leaving fish at room temperature, can increase bacterial growth. So can some display procedures. For example, if a fish is kept under a hot light, it gets warm, and bacteria in it can multiply quickly. If raw fish is kept next to cooked fish, the cooked fish can be contaminated.

Pollutants

The environmental pollutants found in fish (as well as in other animal products) cannot be reduced or destroyed by cooking. You can, however, limit your risks by choosing fish with the least pollutants.

Organochlorines and dioxins are persistent organic pollutants (POPs), chemicals that persist in the environment. While you are pregnant, the POPs your baby is exposed to come mainly from what is already stored in your body (mostly in body fat). Large amounts of POPs accumulated in a pregnant woman's body are thought to affect neurological and cognitive development in a growing fetus.[18]

Mercury is a heavy metal that is a potent neurotoxin; it affects brain and nervous system development. Predatory fish generally have higher mercury content than bottom feeders. Fish with above-average mercury content include king mackerel, various bass, orange roughy, pike shark, swordfish and freshwater fish from contaminated waters.[19]

The FDA recommends limiting your consumption of shark and swordfish to once a month, due to its mercury content.

Since the body fat stored during pregnancy is used during breastfeeding, your diet during pregnancy can affect the amount of POPs your baby receives in breast milk. (See Chapter Eight for more information.)

Which Fish Are Safe for Pregnant and Breast-Feeding Women?

Given the complex and sometimes conflicting reports on environmental contaminants, this question isn't easy to answer. After consulting with toxicologists and government organizations and doing an extensive search of the literature, I advise the following:

- Limit consumption of shark and swordfish to once a month.
- Limit tuna consumption to twice a week.
- Choose smaller fish; they contain less stored pollutants.
- Avoid fish from polluted waters, especially the Great Lakes and Boston Harbor. Many other lakes and rivers are also polluted. In general, fish caught the farthest from land have smaller amounts of POPs.
- Avoid recreationally caught fish, unless you know where they come from and what fish advisories are posted there. (Most lakes and rivers have signs posted that recommend which fish, if any, are unsafe for pregnant or breast-feeding women to eat.) Contact your local health or wildlife department to check on fish advisories. For a national listing of fish and wildlife advisories, visit www.epa.gov/OST.

Listeriosis and Toxoplasmosis: Bad Bugs for Babies

Listeria, a kind of food-borne bacteria, and *Toxoplasma gondii*, a parasite, can both be bad bugs for babies.

Listeria is most often found in soft cheeses, unpasteurized milk products, hot dogs, deli foods, and undercooked poultry, meat, and seafood. Listeriosis causes flu-like symptoms in pregnant women, but if listeria is passed on to a fetus, it can cause miscarriage, premature birth, blood poisoning, and birth defects. Listeriosis can be treated with antibiotics, but play it safe and avoid soft cheeses and unpasteurized milk products, cook ready-to-eat meat and seafood products, and cook raw meat, poultry, and seafood products thoroughly.

Toxoplasma gondii is carried by cats and can also contaminate food. Toxoplasmosis may cause mild flu-like symptoms in pregnant women, but if the parasite is passed on to a fetus, it can cause miscarriage, disability, and retardation. Toxoplasmosis can result from eating undercooked meat and poultry or unwashed fruits and vegetables, from cleaning a cat litter box, or from handling contaminated soil. Severity of the disease may be reduced with antibiotics, but prevention is best. Avoid cleaning cat litter boxes or wear gloves while doing so, wash fruits and vegetables well, and cook meat and poultry thoroughly.

For more information on these food-borne illnesses and their effects on pregnancy, contact:

March of Dimes Birth Defects Foundation
Resource Center
888-MODIMES
www.modimes.org

American College of Obstetricians and Gynecologists
800-762-2264
www.acog.org

Organization of Teratology Information Services (OTIS)
Pregnancy Riskline
888-285-3410
orpheus-1.ucsd.edu/otis/

United States Department of Agriculture
Food Safety and Inspection Service
202-720-7943
www.fsis.usda.gov

Sources: Center for Science in the Public Interest. Protect Your Unborn Baby: Important Food Safety Information to Help Avoid Miscarriage.

U.S. Department of Agriculture Food Safety and Inspection Service. Expectant Mothers and Food-Borne Illness, revised May 1999.

U.S. Department of Agriculture Food Safety and Inspection Service. Listeriosis and Food Safety Tips. May 1999.

- Do not eat the fat or fatty parts of fish. Cook fish without the skin if possible. When making fish broth, remove the head and skin first.
- Remember, you should not avoid eating fish during pregnancy. On the contrary: You should try to eat fish every week. Just limit or avoid the high-risk fish and eat a variety of others.

Did You Have Your Omega-3 Today?

Omega-3 fats, a type of oil found primarily in fish, shows great promise in controlling blood pressure, reducing heart disease, and improving the symptoms of rheumatoid arthritis. We also know that developing fetuses need omega-3 fats—especially docosahexanenoic acid (DHA)—for building brain tissue, for nerve growth, and for development of the retina. Omega-3 fats are so important that some scientists think that a lack of them could result in delays or deficiencies in nervous tissue development and possibly in impaired vision.[20] Before birth, your baby gets DHA from you—especially if you eat your share of fat-rich fish. After birth, your baby gets DHA from breast milk.

The omega-3 fats found in the foods below are particularly important for brain and retina development.

Fish

These fish are listed in descending order according to omega-3 content.[21]

- Atlantic salmon
- Anchovy
- Sablefish
- Chinook salmon
- Mackerel
- Herring
- Canned pink salmon
- Coho salmon (wild)
- Tuna (light, in water)
- Blue mussels
- Imitation crab made from surimi

Other Animal Products

- Eggland's Best Eggs
- Meat (Although meat does not have a high content of omega-3 fats, it has been shown to be a significant source because of the popularity of meat in the diet.)[22]

Plant Products

These plant products contain omega-3 fats (linolenic acid) which can be converted to DHA and eicosapenaenoic acid (EPA) in small amounts.

- Flaxseed oil and flaxseed
- Canola oil
- Soybean oil

While some physicians (such as those at the University of Michigan Multiples Clinic) recommend fish oil supplements, these should only be taken under close medical

---

Buyer Beware

Labels that say "USDA Inspected" or "U.S. Govt. Inspected" are sometimes incorrectly found on fish. The USDA inspects beef, pork, and chicken, but not fish.

---

supervision. While there does not seem to be harm in fish oil supplementation, more research needs to be conducted before it can be recommended for pregnant women.[23]

Safety Tips: Buying Seafood

▶ **From a food safety standpoint, frozen fish is often the best choice.**

Frozen fish is usually quick-frozen (frozen right on the boat where it's caught), resulting in fish that is actually fresher than "fresh." Look for and avoid freezer burn, ice crystals, and broken wrappers. Don't buy fresh salmon, bluefish, or catfish and freeze it when you get home. According to Clare Vanderbeek of the National Fisheries Institute, "Fish with a higher fat content will deteriorate more quickly than low-fat fish. Consumers should buy those fish already commercially frozen, which will ensure a higher-quality product."[24]

▶ **If you choose to buy fresh fish, learn how to recognize freshness.**

Fish gills should be bright red and moist, not brown and covered with mucus. Eyes should be bright, clear, and bulging. Avoid fish with cloudy or slime-covered eyes. The skin should have a translucent, varnished look. Fish with skin that is starting to discolor or has tears or blemishes should be left at the store.

▶ **Watch for troubling display habits.**

Do not buy fish in stores where fish is stacked in large piles (harder to keep at coldest temperatures), where raw fish is displayed next to cooked fish, where you smell a strong fishy odor (means more bacteria), or where fish is displayed under bright, hot lights.

▶ **Find out, if possible, where your fish came from–the farther from shore, the better.**

You can also ask to see a tag for shellfish, which indicates when the shellfish was caught and shipped. But be warned: This information may require some real "fishing."

▶ **The National Fisheries Institute recommends avoiding recreationally caught fish.**

Fish caught recreationally are more likely to be from contaminated waters or handled improperly. It's also wise to avoid buying shellfish at roadside stands; they may be from polluted waters.

▶ **Good choices for pregnant women and women who breast-feed include flounder, cod, pollock, orange roughy, squid, clams, rockfish, Alaskan salmon, shellfish, and sole.**[25]

Variety is important!

Safety Tips: Storing and Handling Seafood

▶ **Before refrigerating, remove fish from its package, rinse under cold water, and pat dry with paper towels.**

To keep cleaned fin fish more than twenty-four hours, place the fish on a cake rack in a pan, fill with crushed ice, and cover tightly with plastic wrap or foil. Rinse the fish daily, cleaning the rack and changing the ice.

▶ **Keep fish stored at 32 to 38°F or in the coldest part of your refrigerator and use within one day if possible.**

Keep frozen fish at 0°F and use within six months.

▶ **Store live oysters, clams, and mussels in the refrigerator.**

Keep live shellfish damp by covering them with a clean, damp cloth or moist paper towel. Do not place them on ice or allow fresh water to come in contact with them. Never store live shellfish in an airtight container; this will kill them.

▶ **Keep freshly shucked oysters, scallops, or clams in their shells and store them in the coldest part of the refrigerator, preferably packed with ice.**

▶ **Keep live lobsters, crawfish, and crabs in the refrigerator in moist packages (use seaweed or damp paper strips), but not in airtight containers, fresh water, or salt water.**

Lobsters should remain alive for about twenty-four hours.

▶ **Be sure to discard any fish juices and marinade used for raw fish, and do not reuse sponges, utensils, or cutting boards used for raw fish.**

Don't forget to wash your hands well after handling raw seafood.

► **Throw out fish that smells fishy or like ammonia.**

► **Discard any shellfish that die during storage.**

For more information, see *Consumer Reports Magazine,* February 1992, pages 103–120; *FDA Consumer* 91-2246; and *Seafood A to Z,* by Janis Harsila, R.D., and Evie Hansen, National Seafood Educators.

Safety Tips: Cooking Seafood

► **Avoid raw and undercooked fish and shellfish at all times!**

► **Don't leave raw or cooked seafood out of the refrigerator for more than two hours (including preparation time and time on the table).**

► **Cooking fish well will destroy most or all bacteria present.**

Fish is done if the flesh is opaque and flakes easily when tested with a fork at its thickest part. You can also check doneness with a thermometer. Fish is ready when its internal temperature reaches 145°F.

Fin Fish

Although you don't want to undercook fish, overcooking it will make your fish less tasty. National Seafood Educators suggest the following for perfectly cooked fish every time:

► **For baking (400 to 450°F), broiling, grilling, poaching, steaming, and sautéing, measure fish at its thickest part. Cook ten minutes per inch, turning halfway through cooking time.**

If the fish is stuffed, measure after it's stuffed. Pieces that are less than ½ inch thick don't need to be turned.

► **Add five minutes to cooking time if fish is cooked in foil or sauce.**

► **Double the cooking time for frozen fish that hasn't been thawed.**

Shellfish

► **One pound of medium shrimp in the shell needs three to five minutes to boil or steam.**

► **Shucked oysters, clams, and mussels become plump and opaque when done.**

Overcooking causes them to shrink and toughen.

► **Oysters, clams, and mussels in the shell will open when cooked.**

Remove them one by one as they open.

► **Sea scallops take three to four minutes to cook through.**

Smaller bay scallops may take as little as thirty to sixty seconds.

► **Sautéed or deep-fried soft-shell crabs take about three minutes each.**

Steamed hard-shell crabs or rock crabs take about twenty-five to thirty minutes for a large pot.

► **If you poach or steam fish, let liquid come to a boil first, then add fish and cook as described above.**

Microwaving

▶ **Split-second timing is important when cooking fish in the microwave.**

Fish will continue cooking after it has been removed from the microwave, so take it out before it looks done–when the outer edges are opaque and the center is still slightly translucent. Allow the fish to stand covered for a few minutes before serving.

▶ **Use a shallow microwave-safe dish.**

▶ **Arrange fillets with the thicker parts pointing outward and the thinner parts toward the center of the dish.**

Rolled fillets cook more evenly than flat fillets.

▶ **Cover the dish with plastic wrap and lift one corner to vent.**

▶ **Cook three to six minutes on high per pound of boneless fish.**

▶ **Cook thawed, shucked shellfish two to three minutes per pound, stirring and rotating half a turn during cooking.**

Allow to stand for a third of the cooking time.

▶ **Place clams, mussels, or oysters in the shell in a single layer in a shallow dish.**

Cover with plastic wrap, venting one corner. Cook two to three minutes on high. Check and remove shellfish as they open.

The above information comes from *Seafood: A Collection of Heart-Healthy Recipes*

by Janis Harsila, R.D., and Evie Hansen, National Seafood Educators.

▼

Food Safety Reports: Whom to Believe?

In 1989 two stories about food safety hit the headlines, and people all over the country lingered at their plates, wondering whether anything was safe to eat. First there was the Alar scare. Alar is the brand name of the pesticide daminozide, which was banned by the EPA in 1989 because it was carcinogenic. It took Washington apple growers almost ten years to recover from this scare. Soon after the Alar scare, a story about two cyanide-tainted grapes made the news. As a result, the purchase of all imported foods from Chile dropped off, causing economic hardship in that country.

Food safety reports appeal to our emotions because they often imply that our families are in danger. But when we react with our hearts instead of our minds, our decisions are likely to be based on feelings, not facts.

Many activist groups are involved in food safety issues, and for the most part their claims are valid. However, scientific information is sometimes taken out of context and blown out of proportion to its real effect on our health, needlessly misleading, confusing, and frightening people.

Regardless of your position on a particular issue, you can probably find a scientific study to back you up. Frankly, we don't know all the answers about nutrition and health, which is why you may hear one story today and hear a completely different story tomorrow. When a nutrition or health report hits the headlines, you should ask yourself these questions:

1. *Who is reporting the information?*

Is it a neutral group or someone with something to gain from the information? For example, someone who is selling vitamin supplements may cite this or that convincing study. Though the facts may be true, they may be incomplete, or the person's opinions may be biased—so try to separate facts from opinion.

Keep in mind that large companies commonly fund research by well-respected universities. But don't assume this means the research is biased or of lower quality. Let's face it: Who else would want to put up millions of dollars for research on oatmeal?

2. *If the study is scientific, was it done on animals or humans?*

Though many effects are the same in animals and humans, you can't assume that this is always true.

3. *How large was the sample size?*

Research using a group of ten people won't be as reliable as research on a group of a thousand people.

4. *How many studies have been done on the subject?*

Many studies are usually necessary to prove a theory. However, in some cases one large, well-designed, multicenter study (such as the study that showed the benefits of folic acid) is enough to change the thinking of the scientific community.

5. *How old is the study?*

While some studies are still used as benchmarks of knowledge, others are outdated because of newer statistical methods or better study designs.

To check out the latest news in food safety, you can visit the websites listed below:

National Food Safety Database
www.foodsafety.org

Database of food safety topics from the North Carolina State University
www.ces.ncsu.edu/depts/foodsci/agentinfo

Gateway to government food safety resources
www.foodsafety.gov

Food and Drug Administration
www.fda.gov

Seafood safety at the University of California
www.seafood-ucdavis.edu

Food Safety in a Nutshell

Choosing Foods

▶ **Choose a variety of foods.**

This limits your exposure to too much of one pesticide or pollutant.

▶ **Avoid raw or unpasteurized juices.**

Food labels should indicate whether juices are pasteurized.

▶ **Avoid raw sprouts such as alfalfa, clover, or mung bean sprouts.**

▶ **Avoid eating deli food.**

▶ **Buy foods with as little pesticides as possible.**

Buy organic foods or foods with no detectable residues—especially those foods that tend to contain the largest amounts of residues.

▶ **Choose low-fat fish, meats, and milk.**

Pesticides, chemicals, and metals accumulate in fat.

▶ **Do not eat raw fish or shellfish.**

▶ **Avoid foods that may contain environmental pollutants.**

The FDA recommends that women of child-bearing age limit eating shark and swordfish to once a month. People living in the Great Lakes or Hudson River areas should eat as little as possible of locally caught swordfish, shark, bluefish, and salmon. These fish can be contaminated with heavy metals or chemicals that can harm a fetus. (See page 224 for more details.) While there is no official advisory regarding eating canned tuna, it may be advisable to eat it no more than once or twice per week.

▶ **Avoid eating unpasteurized soft cheeses.**

These include Mexican-style cheeses (queso fresca, queso blanco, queso de crema and queso Asadero), feta, Brie, blue-veined cheeses, and Camembert.

▶ **Do not use water with high lead content for drinking or cooking.**

The only way to know for sure if your water contains lead is to have it tested. If you have lead pipes or lead-soldered pipes, let the water run for a few minutes before using it to decrease lead content. Avoid using warm tap water for drinking or cooking. (See page 40 for more information on lead exposure.)

If you are concerned about the quality of your tap water because of bacteria, lead, or other contaminants, consider getting a water purification system. According to Consumers Union, publisher of *Consumer Reports Magazine*, federal regulations for city water systems appear to be getting weaker, not stronger.

Kitchen Sanitation

▶ **Wash your hands often.**

Wash your hands before touching food and after blowing your nose, using the restroom, changing a diaper, or handling an animal. You should also wash your hands after handling raw meat or fish. To wash your hands thoroughly, scrub them with soap under running water for at least twenty seconds. Use gloves to change cat litter boxes and don't allow animals on food preparation areas.

▶ **Handle raw meat and fish with care.**

Use paper towels to wipe up juices from raw meat or fish on counters. Then follow with a paper towel soaked with a weak bleach solution (1 teaspoon bleach to 1 quart cool water), disinfectant, or antibacterial kitchen cleaner. Wash hands and utensils with hot, soapy water after contact with raw meats.

► **Clean your sink regularly with disinfectant or antibacterial kitchen cleaner.**

In a recent study, the kitchen sink was shown to harbor more bacteria than the toilet! You can also pour a weak bleach solution down the drain and garbage disposal to kill bacteria in your drainpipe.

Food Preparation

► **Wash fruits and vegetables well.**

Use water with a drop of dish detergent or with a product designed for washing produce, like Fit Fruit and Vegetable Wash. Thorough washing removes bacteria as well as pesticide residues.

► **Keep raw and cooked foods separate.**

You should also use separate cutting boards and knives for each to prevent transfer of bacteria.

► **Remove skin, head, and inner organs of fish before making soups and stews.**

► **Use a meat thermometer to check the internal temperature of meat, fish, and egg dishes.**

This is the best way to know if food is safely cooked. Minimum internal temperatures:[26]

- Fresh ground beef, ham, veal, lamb, or pork: 160°F or 71°C
- Beef roast or steak: 145°F or 63°C for medium-rare (Cook to higher temperature for medium or medium-well.)
- Whole poultry: 180°F or 82°C
- Ground chicken or turkey: 165°F or 74°C
- Poultry breasts: 170°F or 77°C
- Fish: 145°F or 63°C
- Cooked ham, reheated: 140°F or 60°C
- Eggs: 145°F or 63°C
- Combination dishes, egg dishes, and leftovers: 165°F or 74°C

► **Avoid raw or undercooked animal protein.**

Foods with uncooked or undercooked eggs include homemade Caesar salad dressing, eggnog, ice cream, and cold soufflés.

► **Do not consume marinade used for raw meat unless you boil it first.**

► **Reheat leftovers, deli foods, and ready-to-eat meat and seafood products like hot dogs, lunch meats, and smoked salmon until steaming hot.**

► **Keep hot foods at or above 140°F and cold foods at or below 40°F.**

If you are serving food on a buffet, use a hot plate or Crock-Pot for hot foods and keep cold foods on ice. Foods should not be left at room temperature for more than two hours (one hour on hot days). Refrigerate or freeze leftovers as soon as possible.

Food Storage

▶ **When refrigerating large portions of leftover food, divide the food into smaller containers so it can cool more quickly.**

▶ **Clean your refrigerator regularly and keep its temperature between 35°F and 40°F.**

Listeria can grow in the refrigerator if it gets too dirty or too warm.

▶ **Store fresh fish and meats in the coldest part of the refrigerator and cook them within a day if possible.**

▶ **Don't store fruit juice or acidic foods in ceramic containers (especially imported ones) or crystal containers that may contain lead.**

The acid can cause lead to leach into the food or drink.

▶ **Don't drink hot liquids like coffee or tea from ceramic mugs (especially imported ones) that may contain leaded glaze.**

Hot, acidic beverages can cause small amounts of lead to leach from the glaze.

For more information on food safety or food-borne illnesses, call the USDA Meat and Poultry Hotline at 800-535-4555 (toll-free nationwide), 202-720-3333 (Washington, D.C.), or 800-256-7072 (TDD/TTY). You can also call the FDA's food safety hotline at 888-SAFEFOOD.

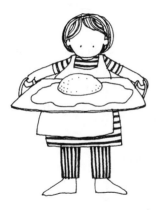

CHAPTER TWELVE

Fast Foods: Eating In and Eating Out

What you will find in this chapter:

- *Tips for Choosing Convenience Foods*
- *Complete, Convenient Meals for One*
- *Convenience Foods for the Whole Family*
- *Healthy Convenience-Food Menus*
- *Last-Minute Meals from the Cupboard*
- *Fifty Quick-and-Easy Meals or Snacks*
- *Choosing Wisely at Restaurants*
- *Choosing Nutritious Fast Foods*
- *Healthy Fast-Food Menus for Pregnancy*

This chapter answers such questions as:

- *What can I add to a frozen entrée to make a quick, complete meal?*
- *Are there any fast foods that are high in iron?*
- *Which fast-food restaurants serve grilled chicken?*
- *Is it possible to eat out and have a low-fat meal?*
- *What can I keep at home to put together a quick meal?*

We live in a fast-paced society and often don't have time to cook. Approximately forty cents of every food dollar is spent on food prepared away from home. You may be wondering whether you can eat out or prepare convenience foods and still have a balanced diet. The answer is yes—with a little planning.

Tips for Choosing Convenience Foods

Convenience foods such as frozen dinners are becoming more and more popular. Some are better than others. Consider these questions when choosing convenience foods:

- Does the product provide a balanced meal (including protein, starch, and vegetable and/or fruit)?
- How much fat does the product contain? Look for no more than 10 grams of fat per 300 calories.
- What is the sodium content? More than 800 milligrams per serving could be excessive. However, since you need more sodium during pregnancy, excess sodium should not be a concern unless you were following a low-sodium diet before pregnancy and your physician has advised you to continue doing so. (See the next page for more on sodium.)
- Is the product a good value? One often pays for convenience. When checking the price of a convenience food, make sure to consider the cost of ingredients that you add, such as chicken or tuna.
- Does the product contain a lot of additives and preservatives?

Watching Your Sodium?

Although your need for sodium increases during pregnancy, you'll get more than enough in your food—especially if you eat any convenience foods. You can balance your daily sodium intake by limiting canned or convenience foods to one serving per day.

If you had hypertension or kidney disease before you became pregnant, your health-care provider may ask you to moderate your salt intake. It will be important for you to read food labels for sodium content.

Most "light" frozen meals and entrées contain 700 milligrams or less of sodium. That's much less than regular frozen dinners, which can contain as much as 1,500 milligrams of sodium per serving! Canned soups and entrées are also known for being high in sodium. Two exceptions are Healthy Choice and Campbell's Select Soups.

Going Meatless?

If you prefer meatless meals, note that the convenience-food menus marked with asterisks on the following pages contain no meat. They may contain cheese and/or eggs. Cascadian Farms and Amy's brands are both meatless and organic.

▼

Complete, Convenient Meals for One

The following frozen dinners offer both convenience and good nutrition. I've also suggested what to add to the different types of convenience foods to create a balanced meal. Thousands of new products enter the market every year. Exclusion of an item from the list below does not imply that it is a bad choice.

Low-Calorie Entrées

> Budget Gourmet
> Healthy Choice Entrées
> Weight Watchers Ultimate 200 Entrées
> Lean Cuisine Entrées

For a complete meal, start with one of the entrées above and add:

- 1 cup milk or yogurt
- 1 serving fruit and/or raw veggies (Consider buying a bag of oranges, apples, or canned individual servings of fruit to keep at work.)
- 1 piece of bread, bagel, bran or corn muffin, or roll

Then maybe add a dessert, and you have a complete meal!

Low-Calorie Dinners

Each of these dinners offers more than an entrée but still contains only about 300 calories. For a complete meal, add milk or yogurt, a roll or piece of bread, and a fruit or vegetable.

> Healthy Choice Dinners
> Budget Gourmet Light and Healthy Dinners
> Budget Gourmet Hearty and Healthy Dinners
> Lean Cuisine

"Light" or lower-calorie meals are good choices because they are low in fat. Too

Doing Your Math

Remember, the average pregnant woman needs about 2,200 calories. (Your calorie needs can range anywhere from a modest 2,000 calories to more than 3,000 calories, depending on your size and activity level.) You can count on about 400 calories for breakfast, 500 calories for lunch and dinner, and two 300-calorie snacks or three 200-calorie snacks. Most low-cal dinners have 300 calories. Adding milk, fruit, and starch makes 550 calories and a well-balanced meal for you and your baby.

much fat could give you heartburn and add too many extra calories. However, entrée-type meals don't always include a fruit or vegetable and can be too low in calories. Additional foods are necessary to make a balanced meal.

Reading nutrition labels can help you pick the healthiest meals. By studying labels, you can pick meals with lower fat, lower sodium, fewer additives, or more vitamin C. Scanning the percentage of vitamins A and C at the bottom of a label can help you determine the amount and quality of fruits and vegetables in a meal.

Meal Starters

These offer yet another choice for a quick, nutritious meal; they can be prepared in the microwave or on the stove top. Some include meat, such as Tyson Fajita Kit. Others, like Green Giant Create-A-Meal and Birds Eye Meal Starter, don't, so you can choose whether to add chicken, shrimp, or beef or leave the meal meatless. One benefit of meal starters is that if you cook them as little as possible, the vegetables will retain more vitamins. These meals are especially nutritious because they include a lot of vegetables. You just need to add a starch, fruit, and milk for a complete, healthy meal.

Pot Pies, Frozen Pizza, Fried Chicken, Chicken Nuggets, Fish Sticks

These foods are usually less expensive than other frozen dinners, but they get 50 percent or more of their calories from fat. However, many "light" versions of these foods are now available. These are better (but more expensive) choices. If you are having a hard time gaining weight or don't have an appetite, you can eat the regular versions in moderation. Just watch out for indigestion due to their high fat content.

Burritos and Pocket Sandwiches

These foods are often less expensive than other convenience foods, but they are missing the vegetables. Some are high in fat, so read the labels. Make sure to add some fruit and vegetables to make a balanced meal.

Shelf-Stable Foods

Don't have access to a refrigerator? Or are you stuck on bed rest? Shelf-stable foods don't need refrigerating until you open them. Good examples are microwaveable boxed meals, stews and soups in microwaveable containers, and Cup-of-Soup-type meals. Many canned soups are also quick, healthy meals. These foods are truly fast; they can be ready to eat in under two minutes! To top off shelf-stable meals, keep dried fruit or individual servings of applesauce, fruit, or pudding on hand.

Read the labels on the shelf-stable products; some of the smaller products are soups or side dishes, not entrées. Make sure to add milk or yogurt, fruit or a vegetable, and a starch to the entrées so that you get adequate calories and nutrients. Products marked with asterisks are meatless.

Chef Boyardee 99% Fat-Free Beef Ravioli
Dennison's 99% Fat-Free Turkey Chili
    with Beans
*Fantastic Foods Bombay Curry Soup
*Fantastic Foods Jumpin' Black Bean Soup
*Healthy Choice Country Vegetable Soup
Healthy Choice Split Pea Soup with Ham
Healthy Choice Zesty Gumbo with
    Chicken and Sausage
Hormel Micro Cup Chili
*Near East Minestrone Soup
*Progresso Lentil Soup
Star Kist Tuna Salad Lunch Kit

Quick Extras to Add to Your Meal

Starches: Bulgur, instant brown rice, whole-wheat English muffin or bagel, bran muffin, bread sticks, canned legumes, corn, or peas.

Fruit: Any fresh fruit, frozen bananas or grapes, frozen melon balls, canned pineapple, instant pudding with bananas, fruit shake, yogurt parfait, fresh fruit, or fruit juice.

Vegetables: Ready-to-make coleslaw or salad, precut vegetable sticks, shelf-stable vegetables, canned or frozen vegetables, or vegetable soup.

▼

Convenience Foods for the Whole Family

Frozen meals are fine for just one person, but how about when you need something quick for the whole family? Any of the products in the following list can be the basis of a family-size meal. Consider stocking some of these items in your freezer for days when you have no time to cook. (See page 242 for "Fifty Quick-and-Easy Meals or Snacks.")

Birds Eye Meal Starter Primavera
Birds Eye Meal Starter Teriyaki Meal Starter
Contessa Classics Shrimp Fajitas
Frozen turkey roasts
Garden Chef Gardenburgers
Gorton's Grilled Italian Herb Fish Fillets
Gorton's Grilled Lemon Pepper Fish Fillets
Gorton's Shrimp and Seafood Stir-Fry
    Teriyaki
Green Giant Create-A-Meal Garlic Herb
Green Giant Create-A-Meal Sweet and
    Sour Stir-Fry
Jennie-O Chicken Breast Fillets in
    Cacciatore Sauce
Morningstar Farms Recipe Crumbles
Morningstar Farms Veggie Burger
Mrs. T's Pierogies
Rosetto Cheese Ravioli or Tortellini
Tuna Helper Au Gratin Creamy Broccoli
Tuna Helper Garden Cheddar
Tyson Chicken Stir-Fry Kit
Tyson Chicken Fried Rice Kit
Van de Kamp's Crisp and Healthy Fish
    Fillets

▼

Healthy Convenience-Food Menus

These menus can help you make complete, balanced meals starting with frozen dinners. Products marked with asterisks are meatless.

Mexican/Southwestern

Dennison's 99% Fat-Free Turkey Chili
2 wheat tortillas
1 ounce reduced-fat cheese
Orange

Healthy Choice Chicken Enchiladas Suiza
Baked tortilla chips (or homemade chips)
Refried black beans
Tomato slices
Strawberries
Milk

Howlin' Coyote Grilled Fajita-Style Chicken
Refried vegetarian beans
Frozen melon balls and bananas
Milk

*Cascadian Farms Vegetarian Enchiladas
3-bean salad with tomato
Yogurt with peaches
Vegetable juice

*Weight Watchers Smart Ones Santa Fe Style Rice and Beans
Raw broccoli and carrots
Bran muffin
Watermelon
Milk

Italian

*Michelina's Rigatoni with Pomodoro Sauce, Broccoli, and Olives
Wheat roll
Green beans in vinaigrette
Yogurt with blueberries

*Cascadian Farms Spinach Lasagna
Bread sticks
Spinach salad with artichoke hearts
Melon
Milk

Lean Cuisine Shrimp with Angel Hair Pasta
Garlic toast
Tossed salad with green peppers
Grapefruit half

Budget Gourmet Italian Style Vegetables with White Chicken
Minestrone soup or Minute Minestrone (See page 300 for recipe.)
Wheat crackers
Fresh peach
Milk

Healthy Choice Supreme French Bread Pizza
Caesar salad
Strawberry sorbet
Milk

*Michelina's Layered Vegetable Lasagna
French bread
Lemon sorbet with peaches
Milk

Michelina's Linguine with Seafood Sauce
Peas and carrots
Canteloupe

*Amy's Tofu Vegetable Lasagna
Wheat toast
Apricots
Gingersnaps
Milk

American

*Lean Cuisine Roasted Potatoes with
  Broccoli and Cheddar Cheese Sauce
Tossed salad with kidney beans
Fresh apple
Vanilla pudding with banana
Milk

Weight Watchers Smart Ones Tuna
  Noodle Casserole
Spinach
Corn muffins
Fresh mango
Milk

Healthy Choice Mesquite Beef with
  Barbecue Sauce
Coleslaw
Lemon yogurt with blueberries

*Amy's Veggie Loaf
Spinach salad with mandarin oranges
Mixed fruit
Sugar cookies
Milk

*Budget Gourmet Cheese Ziti Parmesano
  or Macaroni and Cheese Romano
Carrot-and-raisin salad
Cherries
Milk

Continental

Budget Gourmet Beef Pepper Steak with
  Rice
Cucumber and tomato slices
Dinner rolls
Tangerine
Milk

Budget Gourmet Rigatoni in Cream
  Sauce with Broccoli and White
  Chicken
Wheat rolls
Vegetable soup
Mixed fruit salad
Yogurt

Lean Cuisine Honey Roasted Pork
Carrots
Bran muffin
Fresh strawberries with yogurt

Lean Cuisine Grilled Chicken
Tossed salad with carrot and bell pepper
  strips
Fruit cocktail
Milk

Healthy Choice Garlic Lemon Chicken
  with Rice
Zucchini slices with dip
French bread
Apple slices
Milk

Michelina's Chicken Pesto with Penne
Vegetable soup
Sourdough roll
Tropical fruit salad
Milk

Budget Gourmet Orange Glazed
   Chicken
Caesar salad
French bread
Frozen yogurt with raspberries

*Cascadian Farms Veggie Bowl Cascade
   Veggies au Gratin
Half bagel
Strawberry yogurt with sliced banana

Asian

Yu Sing Sweet and Sour Chicken
Peach halves
Graham crackers
Milk

Yu Sing Chicken Fried Rice
Red peppers and cauliflower with dip
Wheat roll
Cinnamon applesauce
Milk

Uncle Ben's Rice Bowl Teriyaki Stir-Fry
   Vegetables
Roll
Grapes
Milk

Yu Sing Shrimp Lo Mein
Wheat roll
Chocolate frozen yogurt with raspberries

Budget Gourmet Mandarin Chicken
Cabbage with vinaigrette dressing
Honeydew melon
Milk

Yu Sing Garlic Chicken
Raw broccoli
Wheat roll
Yogurt with raisins and sugar cookie

Grab-and-Go Lunches

These sandwich-type meals are great to eat
at your desk while working.

Chicken Broccoli Supreme Lean Pocket
Yogurt
Banana
Milk

*Morningstar Farms Meat-Free Corn Dogs
Baby carrots
Fresh apple
Milk

Chicken Fajita Lean Pocket
Yogurt
V-8 juice

Tina's Pizza Burrito or Chicken Burrito
Tomato slices
Banana
Yogurt

Healthy Choice French Bread Pizza
Baked tortilla chips
Salsa
Grapes
Milk

*Garden Chef Gardenburger on wheat
  bun with lettuce and tomato
Baby carrots
Fresh pear
Milk

---

*Amy's Spinach Feta in a Pocket
  Sandwich
Kiwi
Milk

Economy Frozen Meals

One often pays for the extra convenience of frozen meals, but there are exceptions. Budget Gourmet and Michelina's meals are affordable at less than $1.50 per meal. Other well-known economy frozen meals are generally higher in fat. These can also fit into a healthy diet—just don't make a habit of eating them!

*Bean-and-cheese burrito
Shredded lettuce and tomato
Orange slices
Milk

Fish sticks
Microwave-baked sweet potatoes
Shredded cabbage with Italian dressing
Peach halves
Milk

Totino's Canadian Style Bacon Pizza
Tossed salad
Pineapple slices
Milk

Banquet Turkey Meal
Fresh apple
Milk

Macaroni and cheese
Carrot-and-pineapple salad
Tomato juice
Pudding

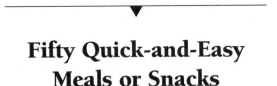

Last-Minute Meals from the Cupboard

The time is ten minutes to famished. You look in the cupboard and see a can of tomato sauce, some olives, and a can of salmon. What do you do? Improvise! If you think creatively, you can make a lot of great meals from the cans in your pantry. And by keeping a supply of staple ingredients on hand, you can avoid spending too much of your food budget on convenience foods or calling out for pizza!

Using the ingredients on the left side of the chart on page 244, you can make all the tasty dishes on the right.

Fifty Quick-and-Easy Meals or Snacks

Some of my best meals are the kind thrown together in a hurry from what's available. On the following pages, you'll find lots of ideas for quick, healthy meals.

Pizzas

Crusts

English muffin
French bread
Pita bread
Corn bread baked in a round pan
Flour or corn tortilla
Boboli crust
Refrigerated pizza dough
Pizza dough mix
Homemade crust
Frozen bread dough

Hot Toppings

Italian: Marinara sauce, cheese, and your choice of meat or veggies.

Mushroom: Cream-of-mushroom soup, mushrooms, onions, and mozzarella and Parmesan cheeses.

Spinach: Marinara sauce, cooked chopped spinach mixed with cream cheese, and mozzarella cheese.

Ratatouille: See page 344 for recipe.

California: Sun-dried tomatoes, cheese, marinara sauce, ham, mushrooms, and chopped fresh basil.

Chile con Queso: Refried beans with sauce of melted Velveeta cheese and salsa over baked corn tortilla or English muffin.

All-White: White sauce, shrimp, crab, mushrooms, and mozzarella cheese. (My version of the sauce is flour, margarine or butter, and milk; another is olive oil and garlic; or you can just skip the sauce altogether.)

Pepper and Olive: Using light creamy Italian or creamy garlic dressing, add a mix of red, yellow, and green peppers and black and green olives. Top with mozzarella cheese.

Hawaiian: Ham and crushed pineapple.

Mexican: For sauce, mix salsa and tomato sauce. For topping, use refried beans, Monterey Jack and Cheddar cheeses, chili or bell peppers, chopped tomatoes, and cilantro or parsley.

Grilled Veggie: Marinara sauce with grilled eggplant, mushrooms, zucchini, and olives. Add grilled chicken pieces if desired.

Cold Toppings

Seafood: Cream cheese, cocktail sauce, and boiled shrimp or crab.

Veggie: For sauce, use cream cheese and ranch dressing mix. Top with chopped broccoli, carrots, green onions, cauliflower, peppers, shredded cheese, and sliced black olives.

Layered Mexican: Start with Boboli crust or other baked crust. Top with refried beans, guacamole, sour cream flavored with taco seasoning, chopped tomatoes, shredded cheese, and sliced black olives. This can be made fat-free or full-fat. Also works well as a dip without crust.

Sandwiches

Tired of the same old peanut butter and jelly on white bread? Try these ideas for a change of pace!

Last-Minute Meals from the Cupboard

Ingredients	Meals
Pasta	Spaghetti with marinara sauce
Marinara sauce	Pizza with artichoke hearts
Boboli pizza crust, canned biscuits,	Chicken with mushrooms and
English muffin, or pita bread	capers over pasta with
Canned chicken	marinara sauce
Canned mushrooms	Quick calzone (using biscuits)
Capers	Chicken tetrazzini
Artichoke hearts	
Mozzarella cheese	Fettuccine Alfredo with
Cottage cheese	tuna or peas
Tuna	Tuna casserole
Salmon	Linguine, salmon, and
Evaporated skim milk	Parmesan cheese toss
Pasta	Macaroni and cheese
Parmesan cheese	
Olives	
Canned peas	
Mushroom soup	
(reduced-salt and reduced-fat)	
Refried beans	Bean tostadas
Taco shells	Chicken tacos
Pineapple tidbits	Chicken salad with pineapple
Tostada shells	Spanish rice with chicken
Instant brown rice	Baked potatoes with chicken topping
Mixed vegetables	Black bean and chicken soup
Canned tomatoes	Black bean tostadas
Canned chicken and vegetables	Black Bean and Corn Salad (page 270)
Potatoes	with tortilla chips
Black beans	
Corn	
Chicken broth	
Fat-free dressing	
Tostadas/corn tortillas	
Black bean soup	
Baked beans	Corn bread and bean bake
Corn bread mix	Hoppin' John (See page 357 for recipe.)
Kidney beans	
Rice or bulgur	

Breads

Rye
Whole-wheat pita
French bread
Flour tortilla
Graham crackers
Saltine crackers
Melba toast
Wheat bread
Sourdough bread
Oat bread
Hamburger bun

Warm Fillings

Leftover stir-fry vegetables (with or without chicken, pork, beef, or tofu) in pita pocket or tortilla.

Light pastrami and sauerkraut with Swiss cheese on rye.

Grilled vegetables and cheese on crusty whole-wheat French bread.

Refried beans and cheese in flour tortilla or on baked corn tortilla. Top with shredded lettuce and tomato.

Vegetarian burger found in frozen food section.

Salmon patties.

Cold popcorn shrimp with melted mozzarella on top of tomato slice on an English muffin.

Grilled fish-fillet burger.

Sloppy joe with lean ground beef, ground turkey, or textured vegetable protein (TVP).

Spiced black beans with reduced-fat cheese and bell peppers in a folded tortilla.

Delightful Spinach (page 266) in a whole-wheat tortilla.

Thinly sliced roast beef and microwave-steamed bell peppers on a French roll with beef broth for dipping on the side.

Cold Fillings

Chef salad stuffed in a pita pocket with light Italian dressing on the side.

Cooked and chilled asparagus spears rolled up with ham and cheese in a whole-wheat tortilla.

Chopped chicken with light mayonnaise, fat-free sour cream, curry powder, green onion, mango, and raisins stuffed in a pita pocket or served as a salad over torn spinach leaves.

Boursin Cheese Spread (page 334) or light cream cheese, chopped parsley, alfalfa sprouts, and thinly sliced cucumbers and tomatoes on thinly sliced bread.

Popcorn shrimp or imitation crab in a sauce of light mayonnaise and ketchup over English muffin topped with chopped tomato and avocado.

Peanut butter with banana on graham crackers.

Light ricotta cheese on raisin English muffin topped with fruit of choice.

Cottage cheese with chopped carrots, broccoli, green onion, and celery on wheat-berry English muffin.

Main-Dish Salads

These are great in the summer when no one feels like having a hot meal. To save time, keep chopped, cooked chicken in the freezer or use canned, chopped white chicken meat.

Tortellini with ham, shredded cheese, tomatoes, artichoke hearts, and vinaigrette.

Rice or bulgur with corn, kidney beans, green beans, chopped red peppers, reduced-fat Cheddar cheese, and vinaigrette dressing.

Linguine with imitation crab, steamed carrots and broccoli, and creamy Italian dressing.

Mixed greens with grilled fish, walnuts, and cucumber dressing.

Black Bean and Corn Salad (See page 270 for recipe.)

Spaghetti with stir-fried chicken, snow peas, and red peppers with peanuts and teriyaki sauce.

Asian Salad with grilled chicken (See page 269 for recipe.)

Leaf lettuce, canned tuna in water, white beans, kidney beans, cherry tomatoes, cucumbers, olives, and green onion with light ranch dressing.

Small shell pasta, popcorn shrimp, chopped avocado, and tomato over bed of shredded romaine lettuce with fat-free vinaigrette dressing.

Chicken-and-Spinach Salad (See page 272 for recipe.)

Chicken and pineapple chunks over shredded cabbage with Catalina dressing.

Mixed fresh fruit salad with fruit-flavored yogurt and bran muffins.

Peas with light mayonnaise and cheese chunks over mixed greens garnished with tomato slices and yellow bell pepper rings.

Fajita salad: Grilled marinated chicken, beef, or shrimp with peppers and onions over torn lettuce. Serve with baked flour tortilla triangles or Baked Tostitos.

Rotini pasta with honey-dijon dressing, ham chunks, and 3-bean salad.

Taco salad with Baked Tostitos topped with shredded romaine lettuce, canned or leftover warmed chili, reduced-fat cheese, chopped tomatoes or salsa, and fat-free sour cream.

▼

Choosing Wisely at Restaurants

Dining out offers many choices; which foods are best for the mom-to-be? If you eat out often, your diet will most likely be higher in fat and lower in nutrients like calcium, folacin, and vitamin C—unless you make your choices wisely! Following are some challenges for the pregnant diner:

- Large servings may tempt you to overeat. Take half your meal home in a doggie bag. Or order a half portion or an appetizer.
- High-fat foods and fried foods may cause heartburn. Foods you might think

of as low-fat, such as Asian food, can sometimes surprise you.

• Servings of vegetables and fruits may be minimal, leaving your meal mostly meats and starches. Consider ordering a side salad, coleslaw, or an appetizer vegetable to round out your meal.

• Milk may not be available; this could be a problem if you dine out regularly.

Need help in eating out more healthfully? Check out *The Restaurant Companion* by Hope Warshaw, M.S., R.D., C.D.E. (Surrey Books).

Salad Bar Savvy

Most people think a trip to the salad bar means a healthy meal. It can be—but beware of the high-fat foods! Here are a few tips for making your trip to the salad bar a healthy one.

▶ **Watch out for hidden fats.**

Sunflower seeds, Chinese noodles, coconut, salad dressing, bacon bits, olives, marinated vegetables, puddings, mousses, and salads made with mayonnaise, such as potato salad, coleslaw, and egg salad, can all be high in fat. Also try to stay away from fried zucchini and potato skins.

▶ **Make sure to eat enough protein foods.**
Ham, turkey, cottage cheese, kidney beans, chickpeas, and Cheddar cheese are all good options.

At the Table

▶ **Try to avoid meals described with these words:** *butter, butter sauce, hollandaise, raw* (**as in seafood**),
au gratin, Alfredo, creamed, cream, sautéed, pan-fried, **or** *fried.*

▶ **Choose wisely from the menu.**

You should be able to order a healthy entrée by looking for these key words: *marinara sauce, vegetarian, grilled, baked, poached, steamed, stir-fried, lean,* and *light.*

▶ **Order a meal that contains one or two servings of vegetables.**

You may need to order à la carte to get what you want. Pasta, potatoes, and brown or wild rice are good side dishes. Avoid fried potatoes.

▶ **Order all salad dressings or sauces on the side.**

▶ **Are you tempted by the chips or bread brought to your table before you order?**

Eat a raw fruit on the way to the restaurant or before you leave home; you'll then be less likely to overindulge in before-dinner snacks. Or ask that chips and bread not be brought to your table and request a salad to snack on.

Common Healthy Entrées

Mexican
Chicken, beef, or shrimp fajitas
Chicken enchiladas
Bean tostadas or burritos

Italian
Pasta with marinara sauce
Pasta primavera
Tortellini or ravioli with marinara sauce
Vegetable lasagna

Bistro

Grilled chicken sandwich
Chef salad
Chicken caesar salad
Grilled shrimp with pasta

Steak House

Filet mignon
Seafood brochette
Grilled salmon

Healthy Menu Items from Chain Restaurants

Au Bon Pain

Minestrone soup
Turkey breast and Swiss cheese on four-grain bread
Vegetarian chili with onion bagel

Boston Market

Chicken soup
Chicken breast
New potatoes
Home-style mashed potatoes
Zucchini marinara
Steamed vegetables
Cinnamon apples
Fruit salad

California Pizza Kitchen

Field greens salad
Moo shoo chicken calzone
Mixed grill vegetarian pizza with honey-wheat crust
Sorbet

Chili's

Chicken fajitas
Southwest salad
Nonfat frozen yogurt

Cracker Barrel

Tossed salad
Grilled farm-raised catfish fillets
Carrots
Country vegetable plate
Corn bread

Houlihan's

Dinner salad
Vegetable lasagna
Chinese chicken salad
Fruit sorbet

Kenny Roger's Roasters

Side salad
BBQ chicken pita
Roasted chicken salad
Cinnamon apples

Olive Garden

Salad with bread sticks
Minestrone soup with bread sticks
Shrimp primavera
Grilled herb chicken with peppers
Raspberry sorbet

Ponderosa

Salad bar
Broiled salmon
Teriyaki steak
Baked potato
Rice pilaf
Carrots
Green beans

Quincy's Family Steakhouse

Dinner salad

Club steak with mushroom sauce

Baked potato

Broccoli spears

Red Lobster

Caesar salad

Shrimp cocktail

Seafood gumbo

Lemon sole

Baked potato

Fresh vegetables

Cheese-garlic biscuit

T.G.I. Friday's

House salad

Gardenburger with house salad

Pacific coast tuna sandwich

Thai chicken salad with dressing on
the side

Sherbet

What's for Dessert?

Fresh fruit, sorbet, sherbet, and low-fat
frozen yogurt are good choices. If you want
to indulge in something heavier, split it with
your dining partner.

▼

Choosing Nutritious Fast Foods

Which fast foods are healthiest? It depends
on what you're looking for: low fat content?
High vitamin C or A content? High fiber

content? Every day the choices available at
the drive-through seem to expand. You can
now eat a healthy, balanced diet even when
you eat fast food regularly. The key is to
make the best choices and to round out your
diet by snacking on fruits and vegetables
that might not be available when you eat in
the fast lane.

Tips for Making a Healthy Fast-Food Meal

▶ **Remember that having a food high in
vitamin C with your meal will
increase the amount of iron your
body absorbs.**

Drink orange juice; eat a salad with high-
vitamin-C veggies such as tomatoes, broccoli, or cauliflower; or choose fresh fruit or
vegetables from the salad bar.

▶ **Cut the fat on sandwiches by asking
for no mayonnaise or sauce.**

You can also ask for sauces on the side.
Skipping the cheese will also cut the fat, but
don't skip it if it's your primary source of
calcium.

▶ **If you eat at the salad bar, balance
your selections.**

Choose raw vegetables, like tomatoes, broccoli, cauliflower, carrot sticks, and fresh
fruits. Have cottage cheese, beans, ham, or
chopped eggs for a protein source. Be sure
to have a source of starch, such as bread sticks
or crackers. Go easy on the puddings, olives,
and mayonnaise-based salads.

▶ **Bring along fresh fruit or vegetables to go with your meal or order a side salad.**

▶ **If you are trying to keep your weight gain down, choose lower-calorie fare such as grilled chicken, fajitas, or bean burritos.**

Skip the additional toppings such as cheese, sour cream, and guacamole. Choose low-calorie or fat-free salad dressings.

▶ **If you have trouble with heartburn, avoid French fries, burgers, fried pies, and other fried foods.**

Fried foods are high in fat and will aggravate your heartburn.

▼

Healthy Fast-Food Menus for Pregnancy

The following menus have been chosen because of their lower fat content as well as higher values for some nutrients. All foods listed have less than 50 percent of their calories from fat. The main dishes marked with asterisks have 30 percent or fewer of their calories from fat. Most meals average 500 calories (according to the manufacturers' nutrient analyses).

Fast Foods Highest in Calcium	
Calcium is very important to your future bone health, and you can jeopardize that health if you don't have enough calcium in your diet while you are pregnant or breast-feeding. But be aware that if you choose a fast food just for its calcium, you're likely to get a lot of extra fat and sugar that you probably don't need. Sometimes it's worth it to splurge. Just don't do it too often!	
Food	**% DRI* of Calcium for Pregnancy**
Carl's Jr. Vanilla shake (13½ ounces)	45
Wendy's Frosty Dairy Dessert (medium)	41
Wendy's Taco Salad	37
Carl's Jr. Breakfast Burrito	35
McDonald's Shake, any flavor (small)	35
McDonald's Quarter Pounder with cheese	35
Taco Bell Cheese Quesadilla	35
Pizza Hut Thin 'n' Crispy Veggie Lovers Pizza (2 medium slices)	26
Arby's Broccoli and Cheddar Baked Potato	25
Taco Bell Mexican Pizza	25
Arby's Light Grilled Chicken Salad	20
McDonald's Ham, Cheese, and Egg Bagel	20
Domino's pizza with ham, mushroom, and green pepper (2 medium slices)	19
TCBY 86% Fat-Free Frozen Yogurt	16
McDonald's Reduced Fat Vanilla Cone	10

*Dietary Reference Intake

Source: Calculated from manufacturers' nutrition information.

Breakfast Fast-Food Menus

With a few exceptions, a fast-food breakfast means a high-fat, low-fiber meal. The closest thing to fresh fruit is orange juice. So, if you do eat fast-food breakfasts regularly, try to supplement the meal with fresh fruit of your own or make healthier choices the rest of the day.

Arby's

*Blueberry muffin
Low-fat milk

Ham biscuit
Orange juice
Low-fat milk

Carl's Jr.

Bran muffin
Low-fat milk

Scrambled eggs
*English muffin with margarine
Low-fat milk

Del Taco

Breakfast burrito
Water or hot chocolate

Dunkin' Donuts

*Bran muffin with raisins
Low-fat milk
Orange juice

Apple and spice muffin
Low-fat milk
Juice

Hardee's

Apple, cinnamon, and raisin biscuit
Orange juice

Fast Foods Highest in Iron

Iron is fairly easy to get from fast foods. Beef, chicken, and beans are good sources. You can increase your absorption of iron by drinking orange juice or having another vitamin-C-rich food with your meal.

Food	% DRI* of Iron for Pregnancy
Wendy's Single with everything	33
Wendy's Broccoli and Cheese Potato	32
McDonald's Quarter Pounder with cheese	32
McDonald's Ham, Egg, and Cheese Bagel	32
Carl's Jr. Famous Star Burger	32
Arby's Regular Roast Beef Sandwich	32
Wendy's Large Chili with cheese	30
Taco Bell 7-Layer Burrito or Mexican Pizza (chicken or beef)	25
Wendy's Garden Veggie Pita	23
Burger King BK Broiler or Whopper Junior with cheese	19
Taco Bell Gordita Santa Fe (steak)	19
Taco Bell Bean Burrito	19

*Dietary Reference Intake
Source: Calculated from manufacturers' nutrition information.

Jack in the Box

Pancakes with bacon
Orange juice
Low-fat milk

Breakfast Jack
Orange juice
Low-fat milk

McDonald's

*Apple bran muffin
Low-fat milk
Orange juice

Egg McMuffin
Low-fat milk
Grapefruit juice

*Hotcakes with margarine and syrup
Low-fat milk

Whataburger

Egg omelet sandwich
Orange juice

Blueberry muffin
Low-fat milk

Lunch and Dinner Fast-Food Menus

Arby's

*Roast beef deluxe sandwich
Low-fat milk

*Roast chicken deluxe sandwich
Orange juice

*Light roast beef deluxe sandwich
*Side salad
Low-fat milk

*Roast chicken salad with light Italian
  dressing
Low-fat milk

Jr. roast beef sandwich
Garden salad with light Italian dressing
Low-fat milk

Burger King

BK Broiler (no mayonnaise)
Orange juice

Captain D's

Broiled fish or broiled shrimp platter
Low-fat milk

Fast Foods Highest in Zinc	
Food	**% DRI* of Zinc for Pregnancy**
Arby's Beef and Cheddar Sandwich	36
Taco Bell Regular Taco	26
Arby's Regular Roast Beef Sandwich	22
KFC fried chicken (drumstick and thigh)	21
Taco Bell Beefy Tostada	21
Taco Bell Bean Burrito	20

*Dietary Reference Intake
Source: *Nutritionist III Analysis Software.*

Carl's, Jr.
*BBQ chicken sandwich
Garden Salad-to-Go
Low-fat milk

Broccoli and cheese baked potato
Orange juice

Charbroiled chicken Salad-to-Go with
   reduced-calorie French dressing
Low-fat milk

Dairy Queen
*Grilled chicken fillet sandwich
Side salad
Low-fat milk
Nonfat vanilla yogurt

Fish fillet sandwich
Low-fat milk

Domino's Pizza
*2 slices 14-inch cheese, bell pepper, and
   mushroom pizza
Tossed salad
Fresh fruit salad (from home)
Low-fat milk

El Pollo Loco
BRC burrito
Cucumber salad
Spiced apples
Low-fat milk

Grilled chicken breast
Honey-glazed carrots
Corn on the cob
Low-fat milk

Chicken fajita soft taco
Orange juice
Flan

Hardee's
*Grilled chicken sandwich
*Mashed potatoes
Orange juice

Roast beef sandwich
Side salad
Low-fat milk

Jack in the Box
*Chicken Teriyaki Bowl
Low-fat milk

Fast Foods Highest in Folate	
Food	**% DRI* of Folate for Pregnancy**
Taco Bell Regular Tostada	12
Taco Bell Bean Burrito	12
Arby's Ham and Swiss Sandwich	12
McDonald's Egg McMuffin	7.5
Taco Bell Burrito Supreme	7.5
Arby's Beef and Cheddar Sandwich	7
McDonald's French Fries (large)	7
Arby's Regular Roast Beef Sandwich	7

*Dietary Reference Intake
Source: *Nutritionist III Analysis Software.*

*Chicken fajita pita
Guacamole
Side salad
Low-fat milk

Garden chicken salad with low-calorie
  Italian dressing
Crackers
Low-fat milk

KFC

Tender Roast sandwich
Garden salad
Corn on the cob
Low-fat milk

Meatless Meal at KFC
*Baked beans
*Corn on the cob
*Coleslaw
Low-fat milk

Long John Silver's

*Flavor-Baked fish with coleslaw and
  green beans
Low-fat milk

*Ocean Chef Salad
Baked potato
Low-fat milk

McDonald's

*Hamburger
Garden salad
Low-fat milk

*Chef Salad Shaker
Crackers
Vanilla reduced-fat ice-cream cone
Low-fat milk

Pizza Hut

The Edge pizza (The Works or veggie),
  2 slices
Salad bar
Water

Cheese Thin 'n' Crispy pizza, 2 slices
Salad bar
Water or low-fat milk

Subway

Following are the best choices; choose the 6-inch sandwich on a wheat roll. In addition to one of the toppings listed, add lettuce, tomato, vinegar, peppers, and so on, but

Fast Foods Highest in Vitamin B$_6$	
Food	**% DRI* of Vitamin B$_6$ for Pregnancy**
KFC fried chicken (breast and wing)	30
Arby's Beef and Cheddar Sandwich	17
KFC fried chicken (leg and thigh)	17
McDonald's French fries (large)	16
Taco Bell Burrito Supreme	14
Arby's Regular Roast Beef Sandwich	14

*Dietary Reference Intake
Source: *Nutritionist III Analysis Software.*

skip the oil. It doesn't add anything but empty calories!

*Chicken Parmesan Ranch Wrap
*Ham
*Roast beef
*Roasted Chicken Breast
*Seafood and crab
*Steak and Cheese Wrap
*Subway Club
 Tuna
*Turkey Breast

Good accompaniments include Veggie Delite salad and Fruizle Smoothies.

Taco Bell

*Bean burrito
 Low-fat milk

*Grilled chicken soft taco
 Pintos 'n' Cheese
 Orange juice

Grilled steak soft taco
Low-fat milk

Gordita Supreme
Low-fat milk

Wendy's

*Grilled chicken sandwich
 Low-fat milk

Hot stuffed chili-cheese baked potato
Side salad
Low-fat milk

Fast Foods Highest in Vitamin C

It's fairly easy to find fast food that contains vitamin C. One of the best sources may be what you least expect: pizza! Of course, the vitamin C content of pizza depends on what you choose for toppings. Baked potatoes and salads are also high on the vitamin C list. Salad bars are a great way to get many vitamins, including vitamin C, depending on your choices. And of course there's always orange juice, which can be found at most fast-food restaurants.

Food	% DRI* of Vitamin C for Pregnancy
Domino's hand-tossed pizza with ham, green pepper, and mushroom (2 medium slices)	175
Orange juice (1 cup)	138
Arby's Light Grilled Chicken Salad	107
Wendy's Broccoli and Cheese Baked Potato	103
Arby's Garden Salad	103
Arby's Broccoli and Cheddar Baked Potato	91
Wendy's Garden Ranch Chicken Pita	77
Wendy's Garden Veggie Pita	77
Wendy's Grilled Chicken Salad	51
Arby's Plain Baked Potato	47
Wendy's Taco Salad	45

*Dietary Reference Intake
Source: Calculated from manufacturers' nutrition information.

*Grilled chicken salad
Bread stick
Low-fat milk
Garden ranch chicken wrap
Low-fat milk

Whataburger

Chicken fajita
Garden salad
Low-fat milk

**Check Out Your Favorite
Fast Foods on the Web!**

www.arbys.com
www.burgerking.com
www.carlsjr.com
www.dominos.com
www.mcdonalds.com
www.pizzahut.com
www.tacobell.com
www.tcby.com

Luscious Snacks and Desserts

When you feel like splurging on dessert, the following are low in fat and delicious.

*Arby's chocolate shake
*Baskin Robbin's nonfat frozen yogurt
*Dairy Queen small strawberry (yogurt) Breeze
*I Can't Believe It's Yogurt's nonfat frozen yogurt
*McDonald's reduced-fat ice cream
*Dairy Queen's nonfat frozen yogurt
*TCBY's nonfat frozen yogurt or sorbet
 Wendy's Frosty dairy dessert

Sugar-free yogurt is also available at TCBY and I Can't Believe It's Yogurt.

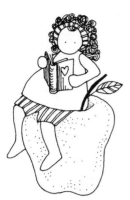

CHAPTER THIRTEEN

Menus and Recipes for the First Trimester

What you will find in this chapter:

• *About the Eating Expectantly Menus*

• *About the Eating Expectantly Recipes*

• *First-Trimester Menus*

— *Don't Feel Like Eating Menus*

— *Don't Feel Like Cooking Menus*

— *Don't Feel Like Cooking or Eating Menu*

— *Feel Like Staying in Bed but Can't Menu*

— *Feel Great Menu*

— *Blender Breakfasts (or Snacks to Go)*

— *Snack Ideas*

— *High-Energy Snack Ideas*

• *First-Trimester Recipes*

About the Eating Expectantly Menus

Many people have trouble planning menus. Menu planning can be even tougher when you're dealing with the food moods of pregnancy. You know—when you're so hungry you could eat a horse, but nothing sounds good. Or when you'd rather stay in bed because you feel queasy, but you've got to get your kids ready for school. Or when you're exhausted, and you'd like to get dinner on the table in fifteen minutes or less. At the beginning of each chapter of recipes, I've tried to take some work out of menu planning by giving you lots of menu ideas. The types of menus in each chapter are listed at the beginning of each recipe chapter and at the ends of Chapters Three, Four, and Five.

Beverages are not included in all the menus. It is assumed that milk will be your choice at least two times per day. Other good choices include vegetable and tomato juice, fruit juice, soymilk, and sparkling water mixed with fruit juice. Of course, you should also try to drink plenty of water throughout the day.

Some menus include recipes found in this book. Page numbers are shown in parentheses following these recipes.

▼

About the Eating Expectantly Recipes

When it comes to food, I have preferences like anyone else, and the recipes in this book reveal my own food biases. For example, you won't find any recipes that contain mustard greens or liver, because I don't care for these foods. You will find some French recipes and southern recipes, because my husband is French, and I am originally from Texas. The Eating Expectantly recipes were developed and chosen primarily for their taste, and then for nutritional value and ease of preparation. (After all, if food doesn't taste good, who would eat it even if it is nutritious?) Most recipes call for ingredients that are readily available. Vegetarian recipes may call for a few ingredients from a large health-food store.

Nutrient Analysis

All recipes were analyzed using Nutritionist III Software Version 7.2 from N-Squared Computing. All numbers are rounded to the nearest whole number. When an alternate ingredient or serving amount is listed, the first listing is the one used for nutrient analysis.

Protein content is listed to help you compare each recipe to your total goal for protein intake. Fat content is listed because most people are interested in fat these days. Women who have heartburn will be especially interested in choosing the lowest-fat recipes. Carbohydrate content is listed to help diabetics and health professionals plan

special diets. The fiber listed is dietary fiber. A recipe that contains less than 1 gram of fiber per serving will list no fiber.

Key Nutrients

I've compared the Eating Expectantly recipes to the Dietary Reference Intakes (DRIs) for pregnancy and listed each key nutrient as a percentage of the DRI. By looking at the key nutrients, you can pick foods high in important nutrients and compare the nutritional values of various dishes.

Diabetic Exchanges

Diabetic exchanges are included to help women who have diabetes or gestational diabetes plan meals. Exchanges are calculated according to the Exchange Lists for Meal Planning developed by the American Diabetes Association and the American Dietetic Association. Exchanges are rounded to the nearest half-exchange. If you have diabetes, consult with a registered dietitian to get an individualized meal plan based on your weight and activity level.

The diabetic exchanges are based on principles of good nutrition, so women who are not diabetic can also use them for keeping track of how many servings from the different food groups they are eating.

Diabetic Variations

A few of the recipes are high in sugar; a sugar-free variation follows each of these recipes. The diabetic variations use Equal. (See page 123 for information about the use of artificial sweeteners during pregnancy.) Use Equal only with your physician's approval. When a diabetic variation is listed, the exchanges that follow it refer to the diabetic variation.

▼

First-Trimester Menus

Keep in mind that during the first trimester, your priority is not to gain weight but to make your diet and health habits as high-quality as possible. Don't worry if you don't eat much for a while because of nausea. Lack of appetite should only become a concern if you begin losing weight.

Don't Feel Like Eating Menus

Many women find that drinking beverages between instead of with meals helps prevent nausea. Remember: Eating what you crave may help you get past nausea, so don't worry if a craving seems a little weird.

Cream-of-mushroom soup
Wheat toast
Peach slices

Chicken-noodle soup
Saltine crackers
Lime sherbet

Jell-O with pears
Cottage cheese
Toast

Low-fat yogurt-and-banana shake
Graham crackers

Egg custard
Graham crackers

Granny Smith apple slices with peanut
butter
Pretzels

Plain pasta
Applesauce

Macaroni and cheese
Frozen grapes

Creamy Asparagus Soup (page 268)
Wheat crackers

Boursin Cheese Spread (page 334) or
cream cheese on bagel
Pears

Don't Feel Like Cooking Menus

See "Vegetarian Convenience-Food Choices" in Chapter Six and "Using Leftovers with Flair" in Chapter Fifteen for more ideas.

Grilled cheese-and-tomato sandwich
Fresh apple

Black Bean and Corn Salad with Baked
Tortilla Chips (page 270)
Strawberry sorbet

Tostadas with Basic Black Beans (page
303), cheese, lettuce, avocado, and
tomato
Low-fat milk
Frozen banana

Quick and Easy Lunches for Friends

Salmon Pâté (page 267) on crusty bread
Shrimp-stuffed avocado with ranch
    dressing
Fresh pineapple slices

Tuna-and-pasta salad with artichoke
    hearts
Rye crackers
Cantaloupe quarters

Cold Sesame Beef (page 361) served
    warm over mixed greens
Marinated vegetables
Tropical Pudding (page 288)

Melted Boursin Cheese Spread (page
    334) on toast rounds over mixed
    greens and vegetables
Wheat roll
Berry Mousse Parfait (page 319)

Black Bean Enchilada Casserole (page
    349)
Carrot-apple salad
Wheat roll
Watermelon

Aspen Black Bean Soup (page 337)
Corn-bread muffin
Grilled grapefruit

Tabouli salad with cheese
French bread
Fresh fruit salad

Pasta with Quick Alfredo Sauce (page 276)
Peas
Tossed salad
Wheat rolls
Frozen yogurt with strawberries

Light Lunch:

Thrive-on-Five Bread (page 281) with
    fat-free cream cheese
Apple Pie à la Mode Shake (page 282)

Don't Feel Like Cooking or Eating Menu

Breakfast

Frozen melon balls
Dry toast
Fruit spread or jam
Milk or juice (later)

Snack

Pretzels or baked chips
Milk or vegetable juice

Lunch

Fresh fruit with cottage cheese
Vanilla wafers

Snack

Lemon-lime float with lime sherbet and
    lemon-lime soda

Dinner

Poached or scrambled eggs
Wheat toast
Milk

Snack

Peach Pops (page 284)
Milk

Feel Like Staying in Bed but Can't Menu

Before-Rising Snack

Saltine crackers or other salty snack
Ginger ale (later)

Breakfast

Jell-O with peaches

Graham crackers

Snack

Lemonade

Lunch

Pasta with mozzarella cheese

Sliced tomatoes

Snack

Frozen fruit juice bars

Snack

Pretzels

Tomato juice

Dinner

Chicken or tuna salad

Vegetables in Vinaigrette (page 346)

Wheat crackers

Apple slices

Bedtime Snack

Raspberry Surprise Shake (page 287)

Feel Great Menu

If you are lucky, you will feel almost normal and will want to eat that way. You may even feel especially hungry! Here's an example of a good day's diet:

Breakfast

Raisin bran

Blueberries

Pumpkin Muffin (page 279)

Milk

Snack

Dried figs or prunes

Lunch

Turkey-and-cheese sandwich

Fresh or canned peaches

Raw broccoli and carrots with dip

Milk

Snack

Vegetable juice

Popcorn

Dinner

Asian Salad (page 269)

Broiled salmon steak

Roasted New Potatoes (page 345)

Carrots Antibes (page 273)

Snack

Tangy Salad (page 302)

Blender Breakfasts (or Snacks to Go)

Banana-Orange Flip (page 283)

Cinnamon graham crackers

___

Piña Colada Frappé (page 286)

Oat bran toast

___

Very Berry Shake (page 289)

½ toasted whole-wheat bagel

___

Raspberry Surprise Shake (page 287)

Bran muffin

___

Apple Pie à la Mode Shake (page 282)

Peanut butter on crackers

___

Peanut-Butter-Chocolate Shake (page 285)

Biscotti

Snack Ideas

Here are dozens of snack ideas for the first, second, and third trimesters to help you avoid between-meals boredom:

First Trimester

Rye crisp and pimiento cheese

Apple with peanut butter

Tangy Salad (page 302)

Cottage cheese and blueberries on ½ English muffin

Melba toast and reduced-fat Laughing Cow cheese

Caramel corn cakes and yogurt

Rice pudding with raisins

Bran flakes and granola with milk

Dried figs and farmer cheese

Apple-Date Bran Muffin (page 278)

Jell-O with peaches

Creamy Asparagus Soup (page 268)

Health Valley Date Bake Bar

Graham crackers and milk

Stewed prunes

Favorite Snack Cake (page 367)

Pumpkin Muffins (page 279)

Pretzels

Second and Third Trimesters

Toasted cheese-and-tomato sandwich

Neufchâtel cheese, raisins, and cinnamon spread on toasted English muffin

Deviled eggs and rye crackers

Pear and cottage cheese

Apple and Colby cheese

Thin-sliced turkey breast rolled up with light cream cheese

Oven-Fried Zucchini (page 274) with marinara sauce

McDonald's low-fat frozen yogurt

Banana and peanut butter

Baked sweet potato

Apple slices with Caramel Dip (page 335)

Berry Mousse Parfait (page 319)

Popcorn cakes with string cheese

½ pita bread stuffed with salad, light Cheddar cheese, and vinaigrette dressing

Popcorn

Tuna salad with apple and crackers

Boiled eggs and saltines

Quick and Healthier Pancakes with fresh fruit (page 298)

Chicken-and-Spinach Salad (page 272)

Refried beans with baked tortilla chips

Quesadilla with mushrooms, tomato, and cheese

Tropical Pudding (page 288)

Leek-and-Potato Soup (page 299) with milk

Rocky Mountain Quesadillas (page 277)

Harvest Crisp wheat crackers with spinach-cottage-cheese dip

Cheerios with peaches and milk

Figs stuffed with light cream cheese

Frozen yogurt with fresh strawberries and blueberries

Toasted wheat-berry English muffin and yogurt

Fiber bar and milk

Leftover pizza and vegetable juice

Guiltless Gourmet nachos

Raw vegetables, ranch dressing, and crackers

Orange juice with club soda and yogurt with Post Grape Nuts and raisins

Strawberry Bread (page 280) and milk

Hot apple cider and Thrive-on-Five Bread (page 281)

Ham and cheese in wheat tortilla

Chicken salad on ½ bagel or bagel crisps (baked)

Corn muffin with Monterey Jack cheese and tomato juice

Orange, pimiento cheese on celery, and carrots and cucumbers

Fruit kebab with strawberries, kiwi, pineapple, and cheese

High-Energy Snack Ideas

Peanut-Butter-Chocolate Shake (page 285)

Fig Newtons

Egg custard and gingersnaps

Oven-baked potato chips with Parmesan cheese and Italian seasoning

Delightful Spinach (page 266) in a flour tortilla and milk

Macho Nachos (Corn tortilla toasted and served with melted Cheddar cheese, refried vegetarian beans, bell pepper strips, lettuce, tomato, light sour cream, and avocado)

Egg-and-olive salad on rye with tomato juice

Mocha Java Cake (page 320) with strawberries and vanilla yogurt

Wendy's Frosty and graham crackers

Tortellini salad with ham

Peanut-butter cookies and vanilla frozen yogurt

English muffin with melted part-skim mozzarella cheese, sun-dried tomatoes, and marinated artichoke hearts

Fruit Pizza for a Crowd (page 369)

Fruit Crisp (page 368) with vanilla frozen yogurt

Fat-free chocolate frozen yogurt with strawberries and granola

Old-fashioned banana pudding with vanilla wafers

Raspberry Surprise Shake (page 287) and granola bar

Refried beans, cheese, and baked tortilla chips with vegetable juice

Low-fat cheesecake with fresh peaches and blueberries

Pound cake topped with peaches and raspberry yogurt and milk

Favorite Snack Cake (page 367) with cream cheese

Avocado-and-shrimp salad with hard rolls

First-Trimester Recipes

Dips and Spreads
Delightful Spinach, 266
Salmon Pâté, 267

Soups
Creamy Asparagus Soup, 268

Salads
Asian Salad, 269
Black Bean and Corn Salad with
   Baked Tortilla Chips and Yogurt
   Sauce, 270
Bridget's Garden Salad, 271
Chicken-and-Spinach Salad, 272

Side Dishes
Carrots Antibes, 273
Oven-Fried Zucchini Sticks, 274
Spring Vegetables in Cream Sauce,
   275

Entrées
Pasta with Quick Alfredo Sauce, 276
Rocky Mountain Quesadillas, 277

Breads and Muffins
Apple-Date Bran Muffins, 278
Pumpkin Muffins, 279
Strawberry Bread, 280
Thrive-on-Five Bread, 281

Sweets
Apple Pie à la Mode Shake, 282
Banana-Orange Flip, 283
Peach Pops, 284
Peanut-Butter-Chocolate Shake, 285
Piña Colada Frappé, 286
Raspberry Surprise Shake, 287
Tropical Pudding, 288
Very Berry Shake, 289

Delightful Spinach

Do you groan at the thought of eating greens? This simple recipe will tempt you to ask for seconds! The creamy sauce boosts calcium and protein content. This delightful dish can be used as a side dish or a dip.

Makes: 3 servings

1 10-ounce package frozen spinach, chopped

4 ounces fat-free or low-fat cream cheese

½ teaspoon mixed herbs

Salt and pepper to taste

2 drops Tabasco sauce (optional)

1. Cook spinach (or thaw completely) and squeeze out all its water; place in small saucepan over low heat.

2. Add remaining ingredients and stir until well blended.

Variations

You can prepare this recipe using Swiss chard, kale, mustard greens, or any greens–even cooked lettuce.

Nutrient Analysis per Serving

44 calories
4 grams carbohydrate
7 grams protein
less than 1 gram fat
1 gram fiber

Key Nutrients

61% vitamin A
15% folate
15% magnesium
8% vitamin B_{12}

Diabetic Exchanges

1 very lean meat
1 vegetable

Salmon Pâté

This creamy spread can be used as a dip or a sandwich filling. It tastes so good you won't believe its low fat content!

Makes: 20 servings

1 15½-ounce can salmon with skin removed

2½ tablespoons grated onion

1½ teaspoons white horseradish

2 tablespoons lemon juice

1 teaspoon dry dill or
1 tablespoon fresh dill

2 teaspoons dry parsley or
2 tablespoons fresh parsley, chopped

1 teaspoon Liquid Smoke

8 ounces fat-free cream cheese or 8 ounces low-fat cottage cheese

1. Place cheese in food processor and blend until smooth.

2. Add remaining ingredients and blend until smooth. When you taste it you shouldn't feel any bones.

Variations

Serve on rye crackers, toasted pita bread, or on a sandwich with thinly sliced cucumbers. For appetizers, stuff cherry tomatoes or mushroom caps, or spread on crackers.

Nutrient Analysis per Serving

50 calories
1 gram carbohydrate
7 grams protein
2 grams fat

Key Nutrients

41% vitamin B_{12}
22% selenium
5% calcium

Diabetic Exchanges

1 very lean meat

Creamy Asparagus Soup

If you like homemade soup but don't have much time to cook, this is the recipe for you. Precooking the asparagus in the microwave preserves its important nutrients.

Makes: 3 servings

1 10-ounce package frozen asparagus

¼ cup each onion and celery, finely chopped, or 1 tablespoon dehydrated onion flakes and a few pinches celery salt

1 to 2 garlic cloves, chopped, or garlic powder to taste

1 chicken bouillon cube or 1 heaping teaspoon broth mix

½ cup hot water

1 12-ounce can skim evaporated milk

1½ tablespoons flour

½ teaspoon seasoned salt or garlic salt

⅛ teaspoon pepper or to taste

1. Place asparagus, onion, celery, and garlic in bottom of microwave-safe dish. Add 1 tablespoon water, cover, and cook on high in microwave for 2 minutes. Rearrange spears and cook 3 minutes more, or until tender. Leave covered several minutes to cool and cut into 1-inch pieces.

2. Meanwhile, dissolve 1 bouillon cube (or enough to make 1 cup broth) in ½ cup hot water. Pour into blender pitcher. Add milk and flour. Blend on low speed; then on high, until well blended.

3. Pour mixture into large saucepan, leaving about ¾ cup in blender. Add asparagus and blend until asparagus is well puréed.

4. Add asparagus mixture to saucepan. Cook over medium-low heat, stirring well until it reaches the desired thickness. Add seasoned salt and pepper.

5. Serve with Bridget's Garden Salad (page 271) and bran muffins.

Variation
Use a 10-ounce package of frozen broccoli instead of asparagus for a creamy broccoli soup.

Nutrient Analysis per Serving

150 calories
23 grams carbohydrate
14 grams protein
1 gram fat
2 grams fiber

Key Nutrients

33% vitamin C
21% folate
36% calcium
26% vitamin A

Diabetic Exchanges

1 skim milk
1 vegetable
½ starch

Asian Salad

Makes: 6 servings

Salad

4 cups romaine lettuce, shredded

1 celery stalk, finely chopped

1 or 2 green onions, sliced

½ cup sliced water chestnuts, rinsed

1 10-ounce package frozen snow peas, thawed or steamed; then cooled

1 teaspoon toasted sesame seeds

½ cup mung bean sprouts

1 11-ounce can mandarin oranges (optional)

Dressing

¾ cup white wine vinegar

¼ cup sugar

½ teaspoon sesame oil

1 teaspoon soy sauce

¼ teaspoon pepper

1. Toss salad ingredients in large salad bowl.

2. Combine dressing ingredients and toss with salad.
(If you are accustomed to having more oil in your salad dressing, add a few extra teaspoons of vegetable oil.)

Nutrient Analysis per Serving

76 calories

12 grams carbohydrate

1 gram protein

3 grams fat

Key Nutrients

16% vitamin C

11% folate

14% vitamin A

Diabetic Exchanges

1 vegetable

½ fat

½ starch

Black Bean and Corn Salad with Baked Tortilla Chips and Yogurt Sauce

This easy-to-make dish is chock-full of important nutrients for you and your baby! You can prepare it for a light meal or eat a smaller portion as a snack.

Makes: 4 servings

Salad

1 16-ounce can black beans, drained

1 cup corn, drained

½ cup fat-free Italian dressing

4 cups romaine or leaf lettuce leaves, torn

4 ounces reduced-fat Cheddar or Monterey Jack cheese

2 tomatoes

Yogurt Sauce

½ cup plain nonfat yogurt

½ teaspoon cumin

⅛ teaspoon garlic powder

Tortilla Chips

6 corn tortillas

Cooking spray

1. Mix corn, beans, and dressing. Marinate in refrigerator at least 30 minutes.

2. Spoon corn and bean mixture over lettuce. Sprinkle 1 ounce of cheese on each serving. Garnish with 2 tomato quarters.

3. Mix yogurt with cumin and garlic powder.

4. Serve with homemade tortilla chips, Baked Tostitos, or Guiltless Gourmet chips and yogurt sauce.

Baked Tortilla Chips

1. Preheat oven to 350°F. Cut each tortilla into 6 pieces, spray with cooking spray, and sprinkle with salt and/or spices.

2. Bake on cookie sheet for 20 to 30 minutes, turning once.

Nutrient Analysis per Serving

350 calories
52 grams carbohydrate
21 grams protein
8 grams fat
12 grams fiber

Key Nutrients

32% vitamin C
24% chromium
13% folate

Diabetic Exchanges

3 starches
1½ medium-fat meats
1 vegetable

Bridget's Garden Salad

I often create meals from my refrigerator leftovers or from my garden. Many of my creations work—and my family lets me know when they don't. I created this salad one summer when it seemed as though our garden was producing only green beans.

Makes: 4 servings

4 cups leaf or romaine lettuce, torn

2 cups green beans or a mixture of green and wax beans, cooked

½ cup purple cabbage, shredded

4 large mushrooms, sliced

2 tomatoes, coarsely chopped

4 ounces smoked turkey, cubed

½ cup kidney beans, drained

2 ounces reduced-fat cheese, grated

½ cup fat-free Italian dressing

2 tablespoons low-fat sour cream

Sesame seeds, sunflower seeds, or pine nuts (optional)

1. Toss all ingredients except cheese, dressing, and sour cream.

2. Mix sour cream and dressing in small bowl.

3. Toss salad with dressing. Sprinkle cheese on top. Garnish with toasted sesame seeds or sunflower seeds, if desired.

Variation

Substitute 4 cups of pasta (rotini or shells) for lettuce. Increase fiber content by using whole-wheat pasta.

Nutrient Analysis per Serving

177 calories

16 grams carbohydrate

17 grams protein

6 grams fat

5 grams fiber

Key Nutrients

50% vitamin C

26% vitamin A

22% vitamin B_6

10% zinc

Diabetic Exchanges

2 lean meats

2 vegetables

½ starch

Chicken-and-Spinach Salad

This dish makes a wonderful summertime lunch. Substitute other fruit if fresh strawberries are not available. Try using leftover grilled chicken and prewashed spinach for an especially quick meal.

Makes: 7 servings

Salad

6 ounces fresh spinach

2 oranges, peeled and cut into chunks

2 cups chicken, cooked and cubed

2 cups sliced strawberries

Dressing

3 tablespoons red wine vinegar

3 tablespoons orange juice

1½ tablespoons canola oil

¼ teaspoon dry mustard

⅓ teaspoon poppy seeds

1. Mix dressing ingredients in a bowl and refrigerate.

2. Wash spinach and tear into bite-size pieces into a large bowl.

3. Add oranges, chicken, and strawberries.

4. Serve with dressing.

Source: Reprinted with permission from *Quick and Healthy Recipes and Ideas* by Brenda J. Ponichtera, R.D. (ScaleDown Publishing, Inc.).

Nutrient Analysis per Serving

152 calories

9 grams carbohydrate

14 grams protein

7 grams fat

Key Nutrients

88% vitamin C

39% niacin

27% vitamin A

23% selenium

13% folate

Diabetic Exchanges

1½ lean meats

1 fruit

1 vegetable (free)

Carrots Antibes

While visiting my husband's family in France, I ate this dish in a restaurant on the Mediterranean coast. Europeans love puréed vegetables, and once you try Carrots Antibes, you'll know why! This is my version of the dish, which even kids will love!

Makes: 4 servings

*8 carrots (about 1 pound),
   peeled and sliced*

½ cup water

1 egg

½ teaspoon sugar

¼ teaspoon nutmeg

1. Place carrots and water in microwave-safe dish. Cover and cook 10 minutes in microwave on high, turning halfway once during cooking. Drain liquid.

2. Place carrots in blender or food processor with egg and spices. Blend until well puréed.

3. Return mixture to microwave dish and cook 4 minutes, rotating once.

4. Serve as a side dish or as a snack with crackers.

**Nutrient Analysis
per Serving**

82 calories

15 grams carbohydrate

3 grams protein

2 grams fat

5 grams fiber

Key Nutrients

509% vitamin A

24% potassium

19% vitamin C

Diabetic Exchanges

3 vegetables

Oven-Fried Zucchini Sticks

What a great way to eat vegetables; they taste almost too good to be healthy!

Makes: 4 servings

½ cup Italian bread crumbs

2 tablespoons Parmesan cheese, freshly grated or canned

¼ teaspoon garlic powder

3 medium zucchini

Water or milk

1 cup fat-free or low-fat spaghetti sauce

Cooking spray

1. Preheat oven to 450°F. Spray baking sheet with cooking spray.

2. Place bread crumbs, cheese, and garlic powder in a Ziploc bag and shake well to combine all ingredients. Set aside.

3. Cut each zucchini in half horizontally. Then cut each half lengthwise into 8 pieces. Fill a pie plate with water or milk. Dip each zucchini stick in water or milk, then drop into crumb mixture. Shake until zucchini stick is coated on all sides. Place on cookie sheet. Repeat with rest of sticks.

4. Bake on cookie sheet for 10 to 15 minutes or until brown and tender. Serve with warm spaghetti sauce.

Variation

Use 1 medium peeled eggplant, sliced into thin rounds, instead of zucchini.

Nutrient Analysis per Serving

107 calories
17 grams carbohydrate
5 grams protein
2 grams fat

Key Nutrients

Small amounts of all nutrients

Diabetic Exchanges

2 vegetables
½ starch
½ fat

Spring Vegetables in Cream Sauce

This recipe is very versatile; it can be a side dish, a light meal over angel hair pasta, or a filling for crepes. You can also add cooked chicken breast, shrimp, crab, or white beans for a complete meal.

Makes: 4 servings

Sauce

1½ cups fat-free chicken broth

1 cup skim milk

1 package Butter Buds

3 tablespoons cornstarch

½ teaspoon tarragon

¼ teaspoon each dill and basil

½ teaspoon onion powder

½ teaspoon garlic salt

1 teaspoon lemon pepper

1 teaspoon lemon juice

Vegetables

1 1-pound package Green Giant California Style Vegetables (cauliflower, carrots, asparagus) or other frozen mixed vegetables

1 7- or 14-ounce can artichoke hearts, quartered

½ red bell pepper, sliced thinly

1. Put chicken broth, milk, cornstarch, and Butter Buds in blender. Blend on high until well mixed.

2. Pour mixture into large saucepan and add rest of sauce ingredients.

3. Cook over medium heat, stirring often until thickened.

4. Meanwhile, steam vegetables or cook in microwave.

5. Add steamed vegetables to thickened sauce and serve.

Nutrient Analysis per Serving

103 calories

22 grams carbohydrate

6 grams protein

0 grams fat

4 grams fiber

Key Nutrients

124% vitamin A

56% vitamin C

13% folate

Diabetic Exchanges

1 starch

2 vegetables

Pasta with Quick Alfredo Sauce

Do you love alfredo sauce, but hate its rich ingredients? Try this delicious, healthier version.

Makes: 4 servings

1 cup low-fat cottage cheese

¼ cup Parmesan cheese, preferably freshly grated

¼ teaspoon garlic salt

¼ to ⅓ cup skim evaporated milk or fresh milk

2 dashes nutmeg

1 cup frozen peas, thawed or lightly cooked

4 cups cooked pasta

1. Purée all ingredients except peas and pasta in food processor or blender.

2. Pour into microwave-safe container and cook on medium-high for 2 minutes. Or place in saucepan and cook on a low flame until warm.

3. Toss pasta with peas.

4. Pour sauce over pasta. Garnish with more Parmesan cheese.

Variation

Use canned mushroom pieces instead of peas. Add several ounces of chopped lean ham.

Nutrient Analysis per Serving

313 calories
46 grams carbohydrate
20 grams protein
5 grams fat

Key Nutrients

20% vitamin B_{12}
19% calcium
7% folate

Diabetic Exchanges

3 starches
1½ lean meats

Rocky Mountain Quesadillas

These can be served as a snack, an appetizer, or a light meal. The figs give this dish a real nutritional boost!

Makes: 1 serving

1 small whole-wheat flour
  tortilla

1 ounce farmer cheese,
  grated or sliced

4 figs

1. Cut figs in half. Arrange them on one half of flour tortilla.

2. Top with cheese.

3. Broil until cheese is just melting; then fold over.
OR
Fold over tortilla and cook in microwave on medium-high for 45 seconds to 1 minute.

**Nutrient Analysis
per Serving**

268 calories
44 grams carbohydrate
10 grams protein
7 grams fat
4 grams fiber

Key Nutrients

28% calcium
15% potassium
10% magnesium

Diabetic Exchanges

2 fruits
1 lean meat
1 starch

Apple-Date Bran Muffins

This recipe was developed by Deborah Compton, who loves to cook. Muffins can be baked and served fresh or kept as ready-to-bake dough in the refrigerator for up to one week.

Makes: 24 muffins

1 cup oat flake cereal

2 cups 100% bran cereal

1 cup low-fat buttermilk, scalded, or 1 cup plain nonfat yogurt, heated

2 large eggs or ½ cup egg substitute

½ cup margarine, at room temperature

1½ cups brown sugar, packed

1 cup low-fat buttermilk or 1 cup plain nonfat yogurt

1 cup unsweetened applesauce (Choose one with vitamin C.)

2 cups all-purpose flour

½ cup whole-wheat flour

2½ teaspoons baking soda

¼ teaspoon salt

1 cup chopped dates

Cooking spray, margarine, or muffin liners

1. Preheat oven to 400°F. In a large bowl, combine oat and bran cereals; pour scalding buttermilk over the cereal mixture and stir.

2. Add eggs, margarine, sugar, the second cup of buttermilk, and applesauce; mix to blend.

3. Mix flour, soda, and salt in a separate bowl and then stir into cereal mixture until moistened.

4. Fold in dates.

5. Grease muffin tins, spray with cooking spray, or line with paper liners. Fill muffin tins ⅔ full. Bake 20 to 25 minutes.

Diabetic Variation

Reduce brown sugar to ½ cup and substitute ½ cup thawed apple juice concentrate.

Nutrient Analysis per Serving

147 calories
27 grams carbohydrate
3 grams protein
4 grams fat
2 grams fiber

Key Nutrients

Small amounts of all nutrients

Nutrient Analysis per Serving
(Diabetic Variation)

134 calories
24 grams carbohydrate
3 grams protein
4 grams fat
2 grams fiber

Diabetic Exchanges

1½ starches
1 fat

Pumpkin Muffins

Makes: 12 muffins

2 egg whites or 1 egg

1 tablespoon light margarine or 1½ teaspoons margarine + 1½ teaspoons water

¾ cup + 2 tablespoons canned unsweetened pumpkin

⅔ cup brown sugar

¾ cup skim milk

2 cups all-purpose flour

2 teaspoons baking powder

½ teaspoon baking soda

½ teaspoon salt

¼ teaspoon ground ginger

½ teaspoon each ground cinnamon and nutmeg

½ cup raisins (optional)

Cooking spray

1. Preheat oven to 400°F. In large bowl, combine egg whites, margarine, pumpkin, sugar, and milk.

2. In small bowl, combine remaining ingredients.

3. Fold the wet ingredients into the dry ingredients until blended. Fold in raisins, if desired.

4. Spray muffin pan with cooking spray. Pour batter into pan and bake for 20 to 25 minutes.

5. Remove from pan and cool on wire rack.

Serving Suggestion

Serve with creamy orange spread: Mix fat-free cream cheese, orange marmalade, and powdered sugar to taste.

Nutrient Analysis per Serving

169 calories
36 grams carbohydrate
4 grams protein
1 gram fat

Key Nutrients

50% vitamin A
17% thiamin
12% iron

Diabetic Exchanges

2½ starches

Strawberry Bread

My friend, Peggy Conner, made and served this bread at a baby shower for me.
Serve with fat-free cream cheese that's been whipped with strawberry fruit spread.

Makes: 16 pieces

1½ cups sifted flour

½ cup whole-wheat flour

½ cup old-fashioned rolled oats

2 tablespoons wheat germ

½ teaspoon baking soda

2 teaspoons baking powder

½ teaspoon salt

2½ teaspoons cinnamon

¼ cup sugar

2 tablespoons vegetable oil

2 10-ounce packages frozen, sliced, sweetened strawberries, thawed and drained to make 1¾ cups

½ cup unsweetened applesauce

2 eggs

½ cup chopped pecans (optional)

Cooking spray or margarine

1. Preheat oven to 325°F.

2. Combine first 8 ingredients. Mix well.

3. Add remaining ingredients and mix until moistened. Gently fold in nuts, if desired.

4. Pour into 8-by-8-inch pan that has been sprayed with cooking spray or lightly greased and bake for 45 to 55 minutes.

Quick Tip

No applesauce in the house? Peel a medium-size apple, place in a microwave-safe dish, cover, and cook in microwave 5 minutes. When cool, remove core and mash with fork. One cooked apple makes about ½ cup applesauce.

Nutrient Analysis per Serving

131 calories

24 grams carbohydrate

3 grams protein

3 grams fat

3 grams fiber

Key Nutrients

17% manganese

16% vitamin C

Small amounts of many other nutrients

Diabetic Exchanges

1½ starches

½ fat

Thrive-on-Five Bread

Experimenting with a basic zucchini bread recipe, I added ingredients until I came up with a bread that contained five different fruits and vegetables.

Makes: 1 15-slice loaf

½ cup each whole-wheat flour, white flour, and wheat germ

2 teaspoons baking soda

1 teaspoon baking powder

½ teaspoon cinnamon

¼ teaspoon cloves

¼ teaspoon ginger

¼ cup vegetable oil

1 egg

¼ cup brown sugar

⅓ cup molasses

½ cup crushed pineapple in juice, drained well

½ cup applesauce

1 cup each grated carrot and grated zucchini

½ cup raisins

Cooking spray or margarine

1. Preheat oven to 350°F.

2. Mix together in a bowl all dry ingredients except sugar and set aside. In a separate bowl, mix together oil, egg, brown sugar, and molasses. Add vegetables and fruits.

3. Gradually add dry ingredients to sugar mixture. Mix until moistened.

4. Pour mixture into 9-by-5-inch loaf pan that is lightly greased or sprayed with cooking spray. Bake 50 to 60 minutes.

Nutrient Analysis per Serving

136 calories
23 grams carbohydrate
3 grams protein
5 grams fat
2 grams fiber

Key Nutrients

24% manganese
17% vitamin A
7% iron

Diabetic Exchanges

1½ starches
1 fat
A tiny portion each of fruit and vegetable

Apple Pie à la Mode Shake

All the shakes in this chapter can be made with either plain yogurt or milk. Yogurt adds a little tanginess and makes the shake very thick.

Makes: 2 servings

½ cup applesauce, frozen

2 tablespoons brown sugar

1 cup skim milk or plain nonfat yogurt

½ teaspoon cinnamon or apple pie spice

½ teaspoon vanilla extract

Ice as needed

1. Blend all ingredients in blender and serve.

2. Add ice if needed.

Diabetic Variation

Instead of brown sugar, use Equal to taste.

Nutrient Analysis per Serving

120 calories
26 grams carbohydrate
4 grams protein
0 grams fat
1 gram fiber

Key Nutrients

18% vitamin B$_{12}$
15% potassium
16% calcium

Nutrient Analysis per Serving
(Diabetic Variation)

86 calories
17 grams carbohydrate
4 grams protein
0 grams fat
1 gram fiber

Diabetic Exchanges

⅔ fruit
½ skim milk

Banana-Orange Flip

Makes: 2 servings

½ *cup skim milk or plain nonfat yogurt*

½ *cup orange juice*

1 frozen banana

1. Blend all ingredients in a blender and serve in tall glasses.

2. Add ice if needed.

Nutrient Analysis per Serving

100 calories
22 grams carbohydrate
3 grams protein
0 grams fat

Key Nutrients

38% vitamin C
21% potassium
11% riboflavin

Diabetic Exchanges

1¼ fruits
¼ skim milk

Peach Pops

This recipe may be just the trick for morning sickness. It also makes a great warm-weather snack. If you like chunky treats, experiment with adding a few fresh blueberries, grape halves, or other small pieces of fruit to fruit purée before pouring into freezer-pop molds.

Makes: 8 servings

1 16-ounce can sliced peaches with juice

2 tablespoons sugar

1. In a blender, mix all ingredients until smooth.

2. Pour into freezer-pop molds and freeze about 3 to 5 hours until firm.

Diabetic Variation

Omit sugar or use Equal.

Source: Reprinted with permission from *Quick and Healthy, Volume II* by Brenda J. Ponichtera, R.D. (ScaleDown Publishing, Inc.).

Nutrient Analysis per Serving

36 calories
10 grams carbohydrate
0 grams protein
0 grams fat

Key Nutrients

Small amounts of many nutrients

Diabetic Exchanges

⅔ fruit

Peanut-Butter-Chocolate Shake

This shake is filling. Drink it when you're really hungry, trying to gain weight, or don't feel like preparing or eating an entire meal.

Makes: 1 serving

*1 cup plain nonfat yogurt
or skim milk*

*1 package chocolate
instant breakfast mix*

*2 tablespoons smooth peanut
butter*

Ice as needed

1. Blend all ingredients in blender and serve in tall glasses.

Variations

Chocolate-Mint: Omit peanut butter and substitute ½ teaspoon peppermint flavoring.

Vanilla-Fruit: Use vanilla instant breakfast mix and substitute frozen unsweetened berries, frozen pineapple and banana, or peaches for peanut butter.

Mocha: Dissolve 1 teaspoon of instant decaffeinated coffee mix in milk before blending.

Note: This recipe is high in sugar. If you are watching your sugar intake, use sugar-free hot cocoa mix or sugar-free instant breakfast mix instead of regular.

**Nutrient Analysis
per Serving**

351 calories
43 grams carbohydrate
24 grams protein
9 grams fat

Key Nutrients

66% vitamin A
55% calcium
42% magnesium
41% vitamin C
37% zinc

This recipe's high nutrient content is due to the instant breakfast mix, which is vitamin-fortified. If you eat more than one fortified food in a day, such as instant breakfast and a fortified cereal, plus your prenatal vitamin, you will be getting more than your daily requirements of some vitamins and minerals.

Piña Colada Frappé

Makes: 2 servings

½ *cup frozen pineapple*

½ *frozen banana*

1 *cup plain nonfat yogurt*

½ *teaspoon coconut extract*

2 *teaspoons of sugar or 1 packet of Equal (optional)*

1. Blend all ingredients in a blender and serve in tall glasses.

Nutrient Analysis per Serving

127 calories

25 grams carbohydrate

7 grams protein

0 grams fat

1 gram fiber

Key Nutrients

24% calcium

23% potassium

14% vitamin C

Diabetic Exchanges

1 fruit

¾ skim milk

Raspberry Surprise Shake

Makes: 2 servings

*1 cup plain nonfat yogurt
or 1 cup skim milk*

*2 fresh peaches or nectarines,
peeled, sliced, and frozen*

*½ of 1 10-ounce package frozen
sweetened raspberries*

1. Blend all ingredients in a blender and serve in tall glasses.

Variation

Use frozen strawberries instead of raspberries.

Diabetic Variation

Use unsweetened fruit and add Equal to taste.

Nutrient Analysis per Serving

174 calories

36 grams carbohydrate

8 grams protein

0 grams fat

3 grams fiber

Key Nutrients

27% potassium

26% vitamin B₁₂

26% vitamin C

Nutrient Analysis per Serving
(Diabetic Variation)

135 calories

26 grams carbohydrate

8 grams protein

3 grams fiber

0 grams fat

Diabetic Exchanges

1½ fruits

½ milk

Tropical Pudding

Women who are lactose intolerant will enjoy this dessert.

Makes: 4 servings

*1 package vanilla instant
    pudding*
½ cup orange juice
1 cup plain nonfat yogurt
*½ cup crushed pineapple,
    well drained*
½ teaspoon coconut extract

1. Mix juice into pudding mix using wire whisk.

2. Stir in yogurt and coconut extract. Follow package directions.

3. Stir in pineapple.

4. Chill at least 30 minutes.

5. Garnish with pineapple slice.

Diabetic Variation

Substitute sugar-free instant pudding for regular pudding.

**Nutrient Analysis
per Serving**

*157 calories
36 grams carbohydrate
4 grams protein
0 grams fat*

**Key Nutrients for
Regular and
Diabetic
Variations**

*30% vitamin B$_{12}$
22% vitamin C
12% calcium*

**Nutrient Analysis
per Serving**
(Diabetic Variation)

*86 calories
18 grams carbohydrate
4 grams protein
0 grams fat*

**Diabetic
Exchanges**

*½ fruit
½ starch*

Very Berry Shake

This is my favorite shake. If you have children at home, they will love its pretty purple color.

Makes: 2 servings

1 cup unsweetened frozen
strawberries and blueberries,
or any combination of berries

1 cup vanilla nonfat yogurt or
skim milk plus 1 teaspoon
vanilla and sugar to taste

1. Blend all ingredients in a blender and serve in tall glasses.

Diabetic Variation

Use vanilla sugar-free nonfat yogurt.

**Nutrient Analysis
per Serving**

112 calories
23 grams carbohydrate
6 grams protein
0 grams fat
2 grams fiber

Key Nutrients

60% vitamin C
20% calcium
18% potassium

Diabetic Exchanges

1 fruit
½ skim milk

CHAPTER FOURTEEN

Menus and Recipes for the Second Trimester

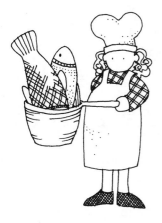

What you will find in this chapter:

• *Second-Trimester Menus*

   – A Month of Breakfast Ideas

   – Menus for a Hungry Appetite

   – I Could Cook All Day Menus

   – Company's Coming! Menus

• *Second-Trimester Recipes*

Second-Trimester Menus

A Month of Breakfast Ideas

Do you get tired of eating the same breakfast day in and day out? Here is a whole month's worth of meal ideas to help relieve your breakfast boredom:

• Peanut butter on toast with banana
• Frozen Nutri-Grain waffles topped with blueberries
• Vanilla yogurt with Health Valley Granola and bran muffin
• Oat bran cereal with strawberries
• Country Brunch Casserole (page 355), oat toast, and milk
• Apple-Date Bran Muffin (page 278), mixed fresh fruit salad, and milk
• Orange slices and wheat-berry English muffin with farmer cheese
• Strawberry Bread (page 280) with light or fat-free cream cheese, mango slices, and milk
• French French Toast (page 296), broiled grapefruit, and milk
• Microwaved scrambled eggs with low-fat cheese, mushrooms, and tomato slices, toast, and milk
• Krusteaz Oat Bran Belgium Waffles with peaches
• Cantaloupe and cottage cheese with blueberry bagel
• Bran cereal with mixed dried fruit and milk
• Oatmeal with raisins, peanut butter on graham crackers, and milk

- Poached egg and ham on English muffin, tangerine, and milk
- Mixed fresh fruit salad, Quick and Healthier Pancakes (page 298), and yogurt
- Bran muffin, honeydew melon, and milk
- Thrive-on-Five Bread (page 281) with fat-free cream cheese and hot cocoa
- Breakfast Pancakes with Raspberry Sauce (page 297) and milk
- Hot wheat cereal with chopped dried figs and milk
- Berry Mousse Parfait (page 319), cinnamon toast triangles, and milk
- Melted Swiss cheese on rye bread, apple pieces, and milk
- Cantaloupe, wheat toast with peanut butter, and milk
- Vegetable juice, boiled eggs, wheat bagel, and milk
- Cheerios, banana, and milk
- Corn muffins, refried beans with cheese, fresh pear, and milk
- Vegetarian Breakfast Tacos (page 366), kiwi, and milk
- Peanut butter and honey on whole-wheat bread, kiwi, peaches, and milk
- Banana-Orange Flip (page 283) and oat bran toast
- Leftover Broccoli Quiche (page 350), watermelon cubes, and milk
- Cinnamon bread with Caramel Dip (page 335)
- Raspberry Surprise Shake (page 287) and poppy-seed muffin
- Very Berry Shake (page 289) and bran muffin

Menus for a Hungry Appetite

Mixed green salad
Stuffed Eggplant Creole (page 316)
Wheat baguette
Frozen yogurt with berries

Vegetable juice
French French Toast (page 296)
Mixed fruit salad

Leek-and-Potato Soup (page 299)
Chicken Roll-Ups (page 307)
Carrots Antibes (page 273)
Wheat rolls
Fruit Crisp (page 368)

Salad with grated carrot, red cabbage, chickpeas, and corn
Pasta with Quick Alfredo Sauce (page 276)
Garlic bread
Tropical Pudding (page 288)

Raw veggies with Boursin Cheese Spread (page 334)
Tortellini with Creamy Pesto Sauce (page 309)
Wheat rolls
Mocha Java Cake (page 320) with strawberries

Caesar salad
Spinach-Stuffed Shells (page 362)
Carrots, zucchini, and yellow squash
Hard rolls
Frozen melon balls

Coleslaw with pineapple
Vegetarian Chili (page 340)
Baked Tortilla Chips (page 270)
Frozen yogurt with blueberries
Sugar cookies

Chicken and Shrimp with Fruit Salsa
(page 352)
Broccoli-and-carrot stir-fry
Roasted New Potatoes (page 345)
Strawberry Bread (page 280)

Piña Colada Frappé (page 286)
Breakfast Pancakes with Raspberry Sauce
(page 297)
Turkey sausage slices
Milk

Creamy Broccoli Soup (page 268)
Greek Island Pita Pockets (page 312)
Banana pudding

I Could Cook All Day Menus

Sesame Beef (page 361)
Asian noodles
Stir-fried vegetables
Tangy Salad (page 302)

Vegetables in Vinaigrette (page 346)
Turkey Pot Pie (page 317)
Mocha Java Cake (page 320)

Mushroom-and-Barley Soup (page 301)
Grilled pork loin chops
Ratatouille (page 344) over rice or bulgur
Frozen yogurt with fresh fruit

Orange-glazed Cornish hens
Thanksgiving Sweet Potatoes (page 306)
Green beans with almonds
Pumpkin Roll (page 321)

3-bean salad
Crab Marinara over angel hair pasta
(page 356)
Herbed dinner rolls
Sunshine Sorbet (page 370)

Homemade cream-of-tomato soup
Hoppin' John (page 357)
Cheese corn bread rolls
Lime sorbet with blueberries

Company's Coming! Menus

Brunch

Watermelon and cantaloupe balls
Country Brunch Casserole (page 355)
Apple-Date Bran Muffins (page 278)
Steamed milk with amaretto flavoring

Asian Salad (page 269)
Broccoli Quiche (page 350)
Strawberry Bread (page 280)

Very Berry Shake (page 289)
Breakfast Pancakes with Raspberry Sauce
(page 297)
Vegetarian breakfast sausage

Creamy Broccoli Soup (page 268)
Chicken-and-Spinach Salad (page 272)
French bread
Apple slices with Caramel Dip (page
335)

Pineapple-orange juice spritzers
Crepes with various fillings (pages
310–311)
Grilled Canadian bacon

Berry Mousse Parfait (page 319)
Strawberry Bread (page 280) and
Pumpkin Muffins (page 279)
Lite or fat-free cream cheese whipped
with orange marmalade and powdered
sugar
Cinnamon-orange herb tea

Lunch or Dinner

Boursin Cheese Spread (page 334) with
  fresh vegetables and French bread
Cranberry juice and sparkling water
  spritzers
Company Fondue (page 308)
Fruit Pizza for a Crowd (page 369)

Spinach-Stuffed Shells (page 362)
Garlic bread sticks
Tossed salad
Frozen blueberry yogurt with raspberries

Mushroom-and-Barley Soup (page 301)
Chicken with Dijon Sauce (page 336)
Bulgur-and-Veggie Mix (page 341)
Wheat rolls
Blueberry Cobbler (page 322)

Apricot-Glazed Chicken (page 347)
Steamed asparagus with lemon
Rice wheat-berry pilaf
Mixed fruit salad
Apple-Date Bran Muffin (page 278)

Mixed green salad
Corn muffins
Spanish Steak Roll with Sautéed
  Vegetables (page 315)
Potatoes Marie Louise (page 305)
Raspberry sorbet

Salmon en Papillote with julienne vegetables (page 314)
Spaghetti squash with warm tarragon
  vinaigrette
Country sourdough bread
Peaches and blueberries topped with
  lemon yogurt

Sliced tomatoes and cucumbers in vinaigrette dressing
Spring Vegetables in Cream Sauce (page
  275) over linguine
Peach Cobbler (page 322)

Coleslaw
Quick Grilled Fish (page 360)
Carrots Antibes (page 273)
Wild rice pilaf
Mocha Java Cake (page 320) with
  strawberries and Lite Cool Whip

Minute Minestrone (page 300)
Crepes (pages 310–311)

Oven-Fried Zucchini (page 274) with
  ranch dip
Crab Marinara (page 356)
Sunshine Sorbet (page 370)

Vegetables in Vinaigrette (page 346)
Veal Piccata with Roasted Red Pepper
  and Cream Sauce (page 275)
Spinach pasta with vegetables
Apple tart

Tossed salad
Cheese-Topped Orange Roughy (page
  351)
French-style green beans and corn
Roasted New Potatoes (page 345)
Fresh melon

Mexican Kale-and-Pork Soup (page 339)
Stuffed Eggplant Creole (page 316)
Low-fat cheesecake with raspberries

Second-Trimester Recipes

These recipes were developed for your second-trimester eating moods. Most women feel their best during these months, so the recipes are hearty and require a bit more preparation time than recipes for the other trimesters.

Breakfast Foods
French French Toast, 296
Pancakes with Raspberry Sauce, 297
Quick and Healthier Pancakes, 298

Soups
Leek-and-Potato Soup, 299
Minute Minestrone, 300
Mushroom-and-Barley Soup, 301

Salad
Tangy Salad, 302

Side Dishes
Basic Black Beans, 303
Beans 101, 304
Potatoes Marie Louise, 305
Thanksgiving Sweet Potatoes, 306

Entrées
Chicken Roll-Ups, 307
Company Fondue, 308
Creamy Pesto Pasta, 309
Crepe Dinner, 310–311
Greek Island Pita Pockets with
    Cucumber Yogurt Sauce, 312
Leg of Lamb, 313
Salmon en Papillote, 314
Spanish Steak Roll with Sautéed
    Vegetables, 315
Stuffed Eggplant Creole, 316
Turkey Pot Pie, 317
Turkey with Hoisin Sauce, 318

Sweets
Berry Mousse Parfait, 319
Mocha Java Cake, 320
Pumpkin Roll, 321
Quick and Easy Blueberry Cobbler,
    322

French French Toast

When you're married to someone from another country, you find out which ethnic foods are authentic. The American version of French toast doesn't exist in France, but my mother-in-law remembers eating French French Toast as a child. This dish is great for those with a hearty appetite or those who need to gain more weight.

Makes: 2 servings

2 large eggs or 4 egg whites

3 tablespoons skim or low-fat milk

Salt and pepper to taste

6 slices stale French bread or 4 slices regular bread

Cooking spray

2 ounces ham

1½ ounces Swiss cheese

1. Mix eggs, milk, salt, and pepper. Soak bread slices in egg mixture. Spray pan with cooking spray.

2. Place bread in pan and cook over medium heat for several minutes.

3. Turn bread slices over and add ham and cheese to each piece. Cook several more minutes, and remove when cheese is melted.

Nutrient Analysis per Serving

347 calories
29 grams carbohydrate
24 grams protein
14 grams fat
1 gram fiber

Key Nutrients

80% selenium
30% calcium
23% chromium

Diabetic Exchanges

2½ medium-fat meats
2 starches
½ fat

Pancakes with Raspberry Sauce

With this dish, Margo Marrow won first place in the bread category of the Delicious and Nutritious Recipe Contest. Margo has a special interest in nutrition because she works for the Women, Infants, and Children (WIC) nutrition program. Her recipe shows her love of good food and nutrition. The variety of grains boosts the recipe's nutrient and fiber content, and the raspberry sauce is high in vitamin C.

Makes: 3 servings

Pancakes

¾ cup soy-wheat pancake flour (or use ¼ cup soy flour and ½ cup wheat flour)

¼ cup each cornmeal, oatmeal, and white flour

3 egg whites

¾ cup skim evaporated milk or skim milk

½ cup orange juice

Margarine, canola oil, or cooking spray

Raspberry Sauce

1 10-ounce package frozen raspberries (unsweetened) or 1¼ cups fresh berries

3 tablespoons sugar

1 tablespoon cornstarch

1 teaspoon vanilla

⅓ cup any juice (orange, apple, or cranberry)

Pancakes

1. Lightly beat egg whites. Add milk, flours, and orange juice. Spray pan with cooking spray or using paper towel, lightly grease pan with oil.

2. Pour 3-inch pancakes using 1 full tablespoon for each.

3. Serve on plates kept hot in the oven.

Raspberry Sauce

1. Strain thawed berries, reserving juice. Heat raspberry juice in saucepan until it simmers.

2. Dissolve cornstarch in cold juice. Add with sugar to simmering raspberry juice. Stir occasionally to prevent sticking.

3. Cook until slightly thick and clear. Add vanilla and berries.

4. Serve warm over pancakes.

Diabetic Variation

Omit sugar and use ⅓ cup diluted frozen juice concentrate instead of regular juice in sauce.

Diabetic Exchanges

2 starches
1 fruit
½ skim milk
½ fat

Nutrient Analysis per Serving

298 calories
58 grams carbohydrate
12 grams protein
2 grams fat
5 grams fiber

Key Nutrients

32% vitamin C
20% magnesium
13% calcium

Nutrient Analysis (Diabetic Variation)

292 calories
55 grams carbohydrate
13 grams protein
2 grams fat
5 grams fiber

Key Nutrients (Diabetic Variation)

90% vitamin C
31% potassium
20% folate

Quick and Healthier Pancakes

I developed this recipe for those who aren't quite ready for 100-percent whole-grain pancakes but want something healthier than "all-white" pancakes.

Makes: 4 servings

1 cup reduced-fat Bisquick mix

½ cup old-fashioned oatmeal

½ cup wheat germ

4 tablespoons molasses

½ cup skim or 1% milk (or low-fat yogurt)

1 teaspoon cinnamon

1 egg or 2 egg whites

Cooking spray or oil

1. Mix all ingredients together until blended.

2. Spray pan with cooking spray or grease it with a small amount of oil. Pour about ⅛ cup of batter for each pancake.

3. Cook over medium heat until bubbles form on top and batter looks set.

4. Flip pancakes and cook briefly until golden brown.

Variation

After pouring batter, add raisins and/or thinly sliced bananas on top of batter. Gently push into batter. Cook as usual. Fruit makes the pancakes sweet, so you can reduce or omit the syrup. The leftovers also make a good snack.

Nutrient Analysis per Serving

279 calories

47 grams carbohydrate

10 grams protein

5 grams fat

2 grams fiber

Key Nutrients

38% selenium

19% zinc

19% calcium

17% iron

Diabetic Exchanges

3 starches

1 fat

Leek-and-Potato Soup

When you taste this soup, you may swear it has ham in it. It doesn't! This soup is great on a fall or winter day with cheese toast and fresh fruit. Spinach, leftover green vegetables, or mixed vegetables can be substituted for the carrots and leeks.

Makes: 16 servings

2 pounds leeks

4 medium carrots

8 potatoes

2 cups evaporated skim milk

Salt and pepper to taste

1. Peel potatoes and carrots. Trim ends off leeks, then cut lengthwise and rinse thoroughly. Cut all vegetables into 1-to-2-inch pieces.

2. Place all vegetables in large pot of hot water. Bring to boil and simmer, covered, for 45 minutes, or until potatoes and carrots are tender. (Since carrots take longer to cook, you may want to give them a head start in the pot.)

3. Drain 90 percent of water. Purée in batches in blender, adding small amount of milk to each batch.

4. Place all puréed batches in large bowl. Stir well, adding additional milk if needed. Add salt and pepper to taste.

Nutrient Analysis per Serving

141 calories

30 grams carbohydrate

6 grams protein

0 grams fat

3 grams fiber

Key Nutrients

74% vitamin A

28% vitamin B$_6$

17% vitamin C

11% folate

Diabetic Exchanges

2 vegetables

1 starch

½ skim milk

Minute Minestrone

This hearty vegetable soup can't be beat for a quick, nutritious meal on a cold night.

Makes: 4 servings

5 ounces frozen spinach, thawed or cooked and not drained

1 8-ounce can tomato sauce

1 14½-ounce can diced tomatoes

1 cup green beans

1 cup chickpeas or kidney beans

¾ to 1 cup pasta, cooked

1 cup water

½ teaspoon onion powder

½ teaspoon garlic powder

1 teaspoon Italian spices

½ teaspoon basil, dried

Parsley, 1 teaspoon dried or 2 teaspoons fresh

1. Combine all ingredients in 1½-quart saucepan.

2. Simmer 10 to 15 minutes, until heated. Add more water for thinner soup.

Variation

Omit green beans and spinach and add 1 10-ounce package frozen mixed vegetables to soup. Cook until vegetables are done.

Nutrient Analysis per Serving

182 calories

36 grams carbohydrate

9 grams protein

2 grams fat

Key Nutrients

51% vitamin A

46% vitamin C

41% potassium

15% iron

Diabetic Exchanges

3 vegetables

1½ starches

½ fat

Mushroom-and-Barley Soup

You can make this a main dish by adding 2 cups cooked chicken or white beans.

Makes: 6 servings

½ cup pearl barley, uncooked

4½ cups water

1 medium onion, chopped

2 medium cloves garlic, minced

1 pound mushrooms, sliced

1 to 2 tablespoons dry sherry

3 cups fat-free chicken broth

Freshly ground black pepper

1. Place barley and 1½ cups water in large saucepan. Bring to boil, cover, and simmer until barley is tender (20 to 30 minutes).

2. Meanwhile, heat 1 to 2 tablespoons water in a skillet. Add onions and sauté for about 5 minutes over medium heat; add garlic and mushrooms. Cover and cook, stirring occasionally, until everything is very tender (about 10 to 12 minutes).

3. Add sauté with all its liquid to cooked barley, along with remaining 2 cups water, sherry, and broth. Grind in generous amount of black pepper and simmer, partially covered, another 20 minutes over very low heat. Season to taste and serve.

Nutrient Analysis per Serving

87 calories

17 grams carbohydrate

3 grams protein

0 grams fat

3 grams fiber

Key Nutrients

14% selenium

13% niacin

10% potassium

Diabetic Exchanges

1 starch

½ vegetable

Tangy Salad

Gwen Shaw often serves this to her family. Even picky children should enjoy this salad. It tastes like a Waldorf salad, but yummier!

Makes: 4 servings

Salad

1 green apple, peeled and chopped

1 large carrot, peeled and thinly sliced

1 celery stalk, chopped

1 medium orange, peeled, seeded, and sectioned (or use 1 11-ounce can mandarin oranges, drained)

4 tablespoons raisins

2 tablespoons walnuts, chopped

4 large leaves lettuce

Dressing

¾ cup plain nonfat or low-fat yogurt

1½ tablespoons honey

1 tablespoon lemon juice

¼ teaspoon each cinnamon and nutmeg

Fresh mint or orange twists for garnish

1. Combine ingredients for dressing in small bowl. Set aside.

2. Wash and drain lettuce. Line each plate with 1 whole lettuce leaf.

3. Combine fruits and vegetables and toss with dressing. Divide into equal portions on plates. Garnish each with orange slice and/or mint sprig.

Diabetic Variation

Substitute 2 packets of Equal for honey.

Nutrient Analysis per Serving

170 calories
30 grams carbohydrate
5 grams protein
3 grams fat
3 grams fiber

Nutrient Analysis (Diabetic Variation)

145 calories
23 grams carbohydrate
5 grams protein
3 grams fat
3 grams fiber

Key Nutrients

67% vitamin A
37% vitamin C
19% potassium

Diabetic Exchanges

1 fruit
1 vegetable
½ fat

Basic Black Beans

Black beans often satisfy my craving for something creamy and rich that sticks to my ribs. I often eat them for lunch topped with fresh tomatoes and melted cheese. Or I make a soft taco or tostado. If you don't have time to cook beans from scratch, keep a stock of canned beans on hand. This recipe can easily be turned into soup or a dip.

Makes: 10 servings

*1 pound dry black beans
  or any dry bean*

4 cloves garlic

*3 medium shallots or 1 onion,
  chopped*

*1 teaspoon each cumin and
  chili powder*

½ teaspoon pepper

*2 to 3 pieces turkey bacon or
  ham (optional)*

1. Soak beans overnight or use the quick-soak method. (See next page.) Discard soaking water.

2. Combine all ingredients in large pot. Add enough water to cover (about 6 cups).

3. Cook 4 to 6 hours, or until beans are tender.

Variations

"Refried" Black Beans: To 2 cups cooked beans, add 1 to 2 cloves minced garlic or garlic powder, cumin, and salt to taste. Mash by hand or in food processor or blender.

Quick Soup: Blend cooked beans and chicken broth in blender to desired consistency. Add onion and garlic powder, cumin, and chili powder to taste. (See Aspen Black Bean Soup, page 337.)

Dip: Place 1½ cups cooked beans in food processor. Add 1 tablespoon vinegar, 1 to 2 cloves mashed garlic, and ½ teaspoon salt (or use garlic salt to taste in place of garlic and salt). Process until smooth. Serve with baked tortilla chips or pita crisps.

Nutrient Analysis per ⅔-Cup Serving

*201 calories
34 grams carbohydrate
14 grams protein
1 gram fat
6 grams fiber*

Key Nutrients

*43% folate
34% magnesium
12% zinc and iron*

Diabetic Exchanges

*2½ starches
1 very lean meat*

Beans 101

Soaking

Quick Soak

Add 6 to 8 cups hot water to 1 pound beans. Bring to boil and boil for 2 minutes; set aside and cover. Let soak 1 hour. Drain and rinse before cooking.

Overnight Soak

Add 6 cups cold water to 1 pound dry beans. Let soak overnight or at least 6 hours in cool place; do not refrigerate. Drain and rinse before cooking.

Cooking

Standard Method

Place beans in large pot with 6 cups hot water. Boil gently, with lid tilted, to desired tenderness.

Savory Method

Place beans in large pot with 3 cups hot water. Add:

    2 teaspoons onion salt
    ¼ teaspoon garlic salt
    ¼ teaspoon white pepper
    1 tablespoon chicken-broth base or 3 bouillon cubes.

Boil gently, with lid tilted, to desired tenderness. Add water as needed to keep beans covered.

Helpful Hints

- Simmer beans slowly; cooking too fast and stirring frequently breaks skins.
- Add 1 to 2 tablespoons oil to prevent foaming.
- Acid slows down cooking. Add tomatoes, vinegar, and other acidic foods last.
- At high altitudes, beans take longer to cook.
- When cooking in hard water, add ⅛ to ¼ teaspoon baking soda (no more) per pound of beans to shorten cooking time.
- When cooking beans for casseroles and stews, avoid overcooking. (Beans should not be falling apart.) To purée or mash, cook until very soft.
- Some old recipes call for cooking unsoaked beans with meats, vegetables, and so on. This is acceptable. However, soaking, draining, and rinsing beans improves their flavor and digestibility and shortens their cooking time. Nutrient loss from soaking is minimal.
- Long, slow cooking in water is essential for rehydration and digestibility of dry beans.
- Microwave ovens can be used for reheating cooked or canned beans.

Source: *Favorite Recipes of Four Generations, Featuring California's Large Lima Beans,* by the Large Lima Council of the California Dry Bean Advisory Board.

Bean Math

1-pound package
    = 2 cups dry beans
    = 5 cups soaked beans
1 15½-ounce can
    = 1⅔ cups beans

Potatoes Marie Louise

This is a favorite dish in our home. It's a great way to sneak more vegetables into your diet, and picky children will gobble it up! Vary the amount of carrots for a different flavor and color.

Makes: 18 servings

**10 medium potatoes
(about 7 ounces each),
peeled and cubed**

**5 medium carrots, peeled and
sliced**

**1 to 1½ cups evaporated
skim milk**

2 tablespoons soft margarine

Salt and pepper to taste

1. Place potatoes and carrots in large pot; cover with water. Cook 45 minutes to 1 hour, or until both are tender.

2. Drain; place vegetables in large bowl. Whip with electric beater, adding milk, margarine, and seasoning. Add more milk until desired consistency is reached.

Variation

Add 3 ounces Light Velveeta cheese while beating for a richer, creamier dish.

Nutrient Analysis
per Serving

127 calories
26 grams carbohydrate
3 grams protein
1 gram fat
2 grams fiber

Key Nutrients

70% vitamin A
23% potassium
12% vitamin C

Diabetic Exchanges

1½ starches
1 vegetable

Thanksgiving Sweet Potatoes

Have Thanksgiving anytime with this variation of a classic French dish!

Makes: 6 servings

*3 medium sweet potatoes,
  peeled and thinly sliced*

2 tablespoons margarine, melted

2 tablespoons brown sugar

*1 teaspoon ginger root, minced
  or in a jar (prepared)*

Cooking spray

1. Preheat oven to 400°F.

2. Spray a 9-inch glass pie plate with cooking spray.

3. Toss potatoes with 1 tablespoon melted margarine, sugar, and ginger.

4. Line bottom and sides of pie plate with a layer of overlapping potato slices.

5. Brush the remaining melted margarine on the potatoes. Cover with foil and place another pie plate upside down on top.

6. Bake on the bottom rack for 30 minutes. Remove foil and top pie plate and bake another 30 minutes or until potatoes are brown and caramelized.

Nutrient Analysis per Serving

126 calories
18 grams carbohydrate
1 gram protein
2 grams fiber

Key Nutrients

158% vitamin A
20% vitamin C

Diabetic Exchanges

1 starch
1 fat

Chicken Roll-Ups

This can be an elegant meal for company or just a casual meal for family.

Makes: 4 servings

4 skinless, boneless chicken breast halves

3 tablespoons light or fat-free cream cheese

2 teaspoons fresh parsley, minced

2 ounces lean ham, thinly sliced

⅓ cup Italian-style bread crumbs

1 teaspoon lemon pepper

½ teaspoon garlic salt

½ teaspoon basil

1 tablespoon grated Parmesan cheese, fresh or canned

1 egg plus 1 tablespoon milk, beaten

Fresh parsley and lemon wedges for garnish

Cooking spray

1. Preheat oven to 350°F. Place all chicken breast halves between wax paper or plastic wrap and pound flat until they're almost ¼-inch thick.

2. In a small bowl, combine cream cheese with parsley. In a shallow dish, mix bread crumbs, spices, and Parmesan cheese.

3. Lay out 1 chicken breast half on a clean surface. Place 1 slice ham (½ ounce) on top. Spread ½ tablespoon cream cheese mixture evenly over ham.

4. Roll up chicken breast, starting with small end. Secure with toothpicks, if necessary.

5. Beat 1 egg and 1 tablespoon milk in a shallow bowl. Dip rolled chicken breast in egg mixture and roll in crumb mixture. Place in small baking dish coated with cooking spray.

6. Repeat steps 3 to 5 with remaining chicken halves.

7. Bake uncovered for 30 minutes or until tender. Increase oven heat to broil last 2 to 3 minutes of cooking. Remove toothpicks before serving.

8. Serve with fresh chopped parsley and lemon wedges.

Nutrient Analysis per Serving

270 calories
38 grams protein
8 grams carbohydrate
8 grams fat

Key Nutrients

79% niacin
60% selenium
35% vitamin B_6
21% chromium

Diabetic Exchanges

4½ very lean meats
½ starch

Company Fondue

The first time I ate this dish was at a gathering of coworkers. It was great fun because everyone brought a small portion of the meal, so the host didn't have much to prepare. For a last-minute company meal, I can't think of a faster meal to cook and serve.

Makes: 8 servings

Fondue

6 cups chicken or beef broth

4 pounds any combination of beef, chicken, shellfish, or tofu

1 pound fresh spinach, washed and trimmed

2 pounds fresh mushrooms, washed and trimmed

Dipping Sauces

Teriyaki sauce

Dijon cream sauce:
Mix ½ cup plain nonfat yogurt with ½ cup low-fat sour cream and 1 or 2 tablespoons Dijon mustard to taste.

Sweet and sour sauce:
Heat ½ cup fruit spread (apricot or plum) with 1 tablespoon soy sauce and 1 or 2 teaspoons vinegar to taste.

Horseradish mayonnaise:
Mix 1 tablespoon white horseradish with ½ cup low-fat or fat-free mayonnaise.

Honey-mustard sauce

Steak sauce

Barbecue sauce

1. Cut meat and chicken into 1-inch pieces.

2. Heat broth to boiling. Pour into fondue pot or Crock-Pot.

3. Arrange meats and vegetables on separate platters.

4. Using fondue forks, guests cook meat and vegetables to desired doneness and dip in sauces.

5. When everyone is finished eating, add dash of sherry or sherry vinegar into broth, divide it among guests, and pass out soup spoons.

Variation

Serve fondue with noodles or brown rice and tossed green salad.

Nutrient Analysis per Serving
(not including broth or sauces)

259 calories
3 grams carbohydrate
41 grams protein
9 grams fat

Key Nutrients

23% vitamin B_6
20% zinc
17% iron
11% folate

Diabetic Exchanges

5½ lean meats
½ vegetable

Creamy Pesto Pasta

If you like a lot of flavor without a lot of fat, you'll love this recipe. Try the sauce over fettuccine or small shells.

Makes: 4 servings

1 cup low-fat cottage cheese

¼ cup Parmesan cheese (preferably freshly grated)

1 cup plain nonfat yogurt

¼ cup prepared pesto sauce (can usually be purchased in produce department)

2 teaspoons tarragon vinegar

Freshly ground pepper

Salt

1. Combine all ingredients except yogurt in food processor or blender.

2. Blend until smooth, adding yogurt to desired consistency.

3. Pour into microwave-safe bowl and heat 2 minutes on medium-high. Or cook slowly, stirring frequently, on stove until hot.

Nutrient Analysis per Serving

179 calories
8 grams carbohydrate
15 grams protein
9 grams fat

Key Nutrients

30% vitamin B_{12}
24% calcium
14% potassium

Diabetic Exchanges

1½ lean meats
1 fat
½ skim milk

Crepe Dinner

Crepes are another family favorite. They're so versatile; you can have them for breakfast, lunch, dinner, dessert, or a leftover snack. Consider hosting a make-your-own-crepes party!

Makes: 10 to 12 servings

Batter

1 whole egg or 2 egg whites

2 teaspoons canola oil

¼ teaspoon salt

2 cups flour

2 cups skim or evaporated skim milk

1 cup plus 2 tablespoons water

Cooking spray

For dessert crepes add:
  1 teaspoon vanilla
  2 tablespoons sugar

1. In large bowl, beat eggs, oil, and salt. Gradually stir in flour, milk, and water. Add vanilla and sugar for dessert crepes. Beat until smooth. Let stand several minutes.

2. Using ladle, pour 2 to 3 tablespoons of batter into heated 10-inch nonstick skillet sprayed with cooking spray. It is essential to use a pan with no nicks or scratches. After pouring batter into pan, quickly rotate pan so that batter completely covers bottom of pan.

3. Cook over medium to medium-high heat until 1 side starts browning. Turn crepe over and cook briefly on other side.

4. Fill immediately with one of the fillings listed below (or use your own filling) or place between pieces of wax paper or foil to refrigerate or freeze.

5. Unused batter may be kept several days in refrigerator. Before using, let batter sit at room temperature a few minutes; then beat well.

Fillings

Breakfast

Peanut butter and banana

Berries and strawberry fruit spread or powdered sugar

Ham and cheese

Margarine and sugar or honey

Applesauce and cinnamon

Fresh fruit and yogurt

(continued on next page)

Crepe Dinner
(continued)

Lunch or Dinner

Spinach filling from Spinach-Stuffed Shells (page 362)

Ham and Swiss cheese, topped with Dijon Sauce (page 336)

Chicken and mushrooms topped with thick cream-of-mushroom soup

Ratatouille (page 344) and mozzarella cheese

Salmon Pâté (page 267) with Cucumber Yogurt Sauce (page 312)

Sautéed or steamed shrimp and scallops with white sauce

Boursin Cheese Spread (page 334)

Dessert

Peaches with Caramel Dip (page 335)

Fresh fruit with vanilla yogurt

Chocolate frozen yogurt topped with raspberries

Margarine and sugar or honey

Vanilla frozen yogurt and blueberries with heated strawberry all-fruit spread

Vanilla frozen yogurt with bananas cooked in orange juice and brown sugar

Nutrient Analysis per Serving
(2 unfilled crepes)

120 calories
22 grams carbohydrate
5 grams protein
1 gram fat

Key Nutrients

Small amounts of all nutrients. Depending upon the fillings you choose, your crepes can be chock-full of nutrients.

Diabetic Exchanges

1 starch
½ fat

Greek Island Pita Pockets
with Cucumber Yogurt Sauce

This dish mimics the flavor of a gyro sandwich, but contains less fat.

Makes: 4 servings

Pita Stuffing

**1 pound boneless pork loin
or loin chops**

1 clove garlic, minced

½ cup lemon juice

1 teaspoon dry oregano

1 tablespoon Dijon mustard

Cooking spray

4 pieces whole-wheat pita bread

1 tomato, chopped

**Leaf or romaine lettuce,
shredded**

Cucumber Yogurt Sauce

½ cup plain low-fat yogurt

**½ small clove garlic (Use less if
you can't tolerate garlic. You
may want to use only a few
dashes of garlic powder.)**

¼ teaspoon oregano

1 teaspoon lemon juice

½ cucumber, peeled and chopped

⅛ teaspoon salt

1. Cut pork into ¼-inch strips.

2. Mix together garlic, lemon juice, and spices in Ziploc bag or glass container. Add pork and marinate in refrigerator at least 1 hour.

3. Spray pan with cooking spray. Over medium-high heat, stir-fry pork 6 to 8 minutes until it is no longer pink and is thoroughly cooked. Stuff meat, lettuce, and tomato inside pita bread.

4. To make sauce, place all sauce ingredients in food processor or blender and blend until cucumbers are finely chopped but not puréed. Or chop cucumber finely by hand and mix with all other ingredients.

5. Top stuffed pita with Cucumber Yogurt Sauce.

**Nutrient Analysis
per Serving**

417 calories

26 grams carbohydrate

38 grams protein

15 grams fat

2 grams fiber

Key Nutrients

88% thiamin

43% niacin

28% vitamin B₆

19% zinc

**Diabetic
Exchanges**

4½ lean meats

1½ starches

½ vegetable

Leg of Lamb

If not for my husband, I may never have had the joy of discovering leg of lamb. The French usually eat it with *flagolet* (a legume similar to a northern bean), green beans, and some type of potato. The leftovers are good served cold with Dijon mustard or as a sandwich on an onion roll. *Bon appétit!*

1 leg of lamb, with or without bone

4 to 6 garlic cloves, peeled and sliced into 2 or 3 pieces

1½ teaspoons each rosemary, oregano, thyme, and marjoram

OR

3 to 4 teaspoons Herbes de Provence (found in gourmet shops)

1. Preheat oven to 450°F.

2. Cut small slits in leg. Insert garlic clove pieces as deep as possible into slits.

3. Sprinkle outside of leg with spices.

4. Reduce oven heat to 325°F.

5. Bake 30 minutes per pound. If you prefer pink or rare meat, reduce cooking time to 15 or 20 minutes per pound. Internal temperature of meat should be 175°F to 180°F for well-done and 160°F to 165°F for medium-rare.

6. Serve with pan juices or mint jelly.

Nutrient Analysis per 4-Ounce Serving

217 calories
0 grams carbohydrate
32 grams protein
9 grams fat

Key Nutrients

46% zinc
16% iron
9% folate

Diabetic Exchanges

4 lean meats

Salmon en Papillote

The beauty of fish is that it cooks so quickly. This recipe is based on the "dash of this and a dash of that" principle—so use your imagination! This dish is traditionally cooked in parchment paper; I use aluminum foil. Some people like to add a teaspoon of dry white wine or tarragon vinegar for flavor. Salmon is a good source of omega-3 fatty acid, which is important for the development of your baby's nervous system and brain.

Makes: 4 servings

*4 pieces salmon steak
(about 1 pound)*

Lemon pepper

Dill, preferably fresh

Green onion and garlic, chopped

Basil, fresh

Lemon juice (fresh or bottled)

Wine, soy sauce, or vinegar

Tomatoes, chopped

Garlic powder

*Zucchini and carrots,
cut julienne-style (optional)*

Lemon slices

1. Preheat oven to 400°F. Place each piece of fish on top of piece of foil or parchment paper big enough to wrap the fish in.

2. Top each piece of fish with spices, lemon juice, and dash of wine, soy sauce, or vinegar. Add or delete any spices according to your tastes. Add herbs and vegetables. Top with several very thin lemon slices.

3. Bring together edges of paper above fish and crimp sides and ends of paper so that fish is enclosed in an almost airtight package.

4. Place on baking sheet and bake for 10 minutes per each inch of thickness of fish. Or cook on medium-hot grill for 15 to 20 minutes.

5. Serve fish still wrapped in its baking package, so your guests can open their packages and enjoy the aroma.

Nutrient Analysis per Serving

210 calories
0 grams carbohydrate
31 grams protein
9 grams fat

Key Nutrients

53% niacin
53% selenium
12% magnesium

Diabetic Exchanges

4 lean meats

Spanish Steak Roll with Sautéed Vegetables

Sandy Collins won first place with this recipe in a National Beef Cookoff. I'm sure you'll agree that this dish is delicious! Omit the chilies if you can't tolerate spicy foods.

Makes: 6 servings

1½ pounds boneless 1-inch-thick beef top sirloin steak

1 teaspoon garlic powder

¼ teaspoon black pepper, freshly ground

2 teaspoons vegetable oil

1 teaspoon butter

¾ teaspoon salt

1 red and 1 green bell pepper, cut lengthwise into strips

1 small white onion, thinly sliced

1 cup fresh mushrooms, sliced

⅓ cup walnuts, chopped

¼ teaspoon chili powder

1 tablespoon sour cream or low-fat yogurt

1 4-ounce can green chilies, chopped

Lemon slices

Cilantro sprigs

1. Pound boneless beef top sirloin steak to about ¼-inch thickness. Sprinkle with pepper and ½ teaspoon garlic powder.

2. Heat butter and 1 teaspoon oil in 12-inch heavy frying pan over medium-high heat until hot.

3. Pan-fry steak 5 to 7 minutes for medium-rare, turning once.

4. Remove steak to heated platter and sprinkle with ½ teaspoon salt. Keep warm.

5. Add remaining 1 teaspoon oil to frying pan. Add red and green peppers, onion, mushrooms, and walnuts. Cook 2 minutes, stirring frequently.

6. Add remaining ½ teaspoon garlic powder, ¼ teaspoon salt, and chili powder; continue cooking 2 minutes, stirring frequently.

7. Spread steak with sour cream and top with chilies.

8. Starting at long side of steak, roll up jelly-roll fashion; secure with 6 wooden picks. Place vegetables around steak roll; garnish with lemon slices and cilantro sprigs. To serve, slice steak roll between wooden picks, then remove and discard picks.

Reprinted with permission, 1991 National Beef Cookoff.

Nutrient Analysis per Serving

320 calories
7 grams carbohydrate
37 grams protein
16 grams fat
2 grams fiber

Key Nutrients

58% vitamin C
52% zinc
16% magnesium
15% iron

Diabetic Exchanges

5 lean meats
1 vegetable

Stuffed Eggplant Creole

This recipe is pretty mild, so most pregnant women should be able to tolerate it. Add more Tabasco sauce if you like it hot!

Makes: 4 servings

*2 small eggplants
(1 pound each)*

1 tablespoon vegetable oil

*1 pound shrimp, crawfish, ground beef, or tofu
(or a combination)*

1 clove garlic, crushed

¼ cup each finely chopped onion, green pepper, and celery

1 14½-ounce can tomatoes, undrained

¼ teaspoon dried thyme

½ teaspoon salt

Dash of Tabasco sauce or cayenne pepper (optional)

1 cup seasoned or unseasoned dry bread crumbs

½ cup low-fat sour cream

1. Preheat oven to 375°F.

2. Wash eggplant; cut in half lengthwise. Place in large pan and cover with water. Bring to boil, cover, and simmer 15 minutes. Drain and cool.

3. Scoop out pulp from eggplant, taking care to leave shell ¼-inch thick.

4. In skillet, heat vegetable oil. Sauté garlic with either beef, seafood, or tofu.

5. Add raw vegetables and cook 5 minutes over low flame, stirring occasionally.

6. Stir in tomatoes, thyme, salt, and dash of Tabasco or cayenne pepper, if desired.

7. Add ½ cup bread crumbs. Add eggplant pulp and sour cream. Stir.

8. Stuff mixture back into 4 eggplant shells and top with remaining bread crumbs.

9. Place in baking dish and bake 30 minutes.

Nutrient Analysis per Serving

*347 calories
37 grams carbohydrate
29 grams protein
9 grams fat
6 grams fiber*

Key Nutrients

*35% vitamin C
23% magnesium
19% iron
15% zinc*

Diabetic Exchanges

*3 lean meats
3 vegetables
1½ starches*

Turkey Pot Pie

This recipe is a great way to use holiday leftovers. Divide leftovers into individual microwave/freezer containers for pot pies to go.

Makes: 4 servings

Filling

4 medium carrots, peeled and sliced

1 teaspoon oil

¼ cup hot water

2 green onions, thinly sliced

1 clove garlic, minced

2 tablespoons cornstarch

¾ cup chicken broth

2 cups white turkey meat, skin removed, diced

½ cup frozen peas, thawed

½ cup evaporated skim milk

2 tablespoons parsley, chopped

¼ teaspoon each thyme, salt, and pepper

Topping

1 can (8 biscuits) prepared biscuit dough

1. Preheat oven to 375°F.

2. Place carrots, green onions, garlic, and oil in microwave-safe dish; add ¼ cup hot water and cover. Cook 5 to 8 minutes on high. Drain (reserving liquid) and set aside.

3. Mix cornstarch with ¼ cup broth. Stir in rest of broth, cooking liquid from carrots, and evaporated skim milk. Cook, stirring constantly, until thickened (about 5 minutes).

4. Stir in remaining ingredients. Pour into pie pan or baking dish.

5. Arrange 8 pieces of biscuit dough over mixture. Bake 15 to 20 minutes or until biscuits are browned.

Nutrient Analysis per Serving

326 calories
39 grams carbohydrate
29 grams protein
6 grams fat

Key Nutrients

247% vitamin A
32% vitamin B₆
15% zinc
10% iron

Diabetic Exchanges

3 lean meats
2 starches
1½ vegetables

Turkey with Hoisin Sauce

I've discovered that turkey breast is even more versatile than chicken breast. It's larger, so you can cook it as a "roast," slice it into "fillets" or "scallopini" (as in veal), or slice it thin for stir-fry dishes. Also, turkey is often less expensive than boneless chicken breast!

Makes: 4 servings

2 teaspoons canola oil

1 clove garlic, minced

**1 pound turkey cutlets
or turkey tenderloin,
sliced into ½-inch slices**

2 green onions, chopped

1 teaspoon cornstarch

½ cup water

**2 tablespoons frozen orange
juice concentrate, thawed**

2 tablespoons soy sauce

**1 tablespoon hoisin sauce
(found in the Asian section of
your grocery)**

1. Heat oil in nonstick pan over medium-high heat.

2. Add garlic. Sauté for 1 to 2 minutes.

3. Add turkey and sauté for 2 to 3 minutes on each side. Remove and keep warm.

4. Add green onions to pan and sauté briefly.

5. In small bowl, mix cornstarch with ½ cup water. Add mixture to pan along with orange juice, soy sauce, and hoisin sauce. Bring to boil and cook until slightly thickened.

6. Pour sauce over turkey and serve.

Serving Suggestions

Serve with brown rice and stir-fried vegetables.

Nutrient Analysis
per Serving

197 calories

3 grams carbohydrate

34 grams protein

4 grams fat

Key Nutrients

47% niacin

34% vitamin B$_6$

17% vitamin B$_{12}$

Diabetic Exchanges

5 very lean meats

Berry Mousse Parfait

This delicious dish can be a dessert or a snack. You can vary the types of yogurt and fruit.

Makes: 4 servings

*2 8-ounce containers fat-free or
low-fat blueberry yogurt*

1 cup Lite Cool Whip

*2 cups strawberries and
blueberries, sliced*

Sprig of mint

1. Gently stir Cool Whip into blueberry yogurt.

2. In 4 parfait or wineglasses, layer yogurt mixture, then berries, then yogurt mixture.

3. Garnish with additional Cool Whip, a few berries, and a sprig of mint.

Diabetic Variation

Use sugar-free yogurt instead of regular yogurt.

**Nutrient Analysis
per Serving**

152 calories
31 grams carbohydrate
5 grams protein
2 grams fat
2 grams fiber

Key Nutrients

52% vitamin C
19% potassium
18% calcium

**Nutrient Analysis
per Serving**
(Diabetic Variation)

106 calories
19 grams carbohydrate
5 grams protein
2 grams fat
2 grams fiber

Diabetic Exchanges

1 fruit
½ skim milk

Mocha Java Cake

Just because you're pregnant doesn't mean you need to give up chocolate—just make it a little healthier! This cake is so moist, it reminds me of chocolate cheesecake; just a small piece should be enough to satisfy your craving.

Makes: 15 servings

1¾ cups flour
½ cup brown sugar, packed
¼ cup canola oil
¾ cup evaporated skim milk
¼ cup cocoa powder
½ cup applesauce
1 cup strong decaffeinated coffee
1 teaspoon baking powder
1 teaspoon baking soda
1 teaspoon vanilla
Margarine and flour

1. Preheat oven to 375°F.

2. Mix all ingredients until well blended, about 1 to 2 minutes with electric mixer.

3. Pour into 8-by-8-inch or 9-inch round cake pan that has been lightly greased and floured.

4. Bake 35 to 40 minutes.

5. Sprinkle cake with powdered sugar and serve with low-fat frozen yogurt and strawberries for a special treat!

Nutrient Analysis per Serving

155 calories
26 grams carbohydrate
3 grams protein
4 grams fat

Key Nutrients

11% potassium
11% thiamin
7% calcium

Diabetic Exchanges

2 starches
1 fat

Pumpkin Roll

Although this recipe may look complicated, it's actually easy to prepare. It makes an elegant (and healthy) dessert for company or a potluck.

Makes: 12 servings

Cake

**3 eggs (or 2 eggs and
    2 egg whites)**

⅔ cup unsweetened pumpkin

¾ cup sugar

¾ cup whole-wheat or white flour

1 teaspoon baking soda

1½ teaspoons cinnamon

Powdered sugar

Filling

**1 8-ounce package
    any type cream cheese
    (fat-free, light, or regular)**

½ cup powdered sugar

1 teaspoon vanilla

1. Preheat oven to 375°F. In bowl, beat together eggs, pumpkin, and sugar.

2. In separate bowl, mix together flour, baking soda, and cinnamon; then add to pumpkin mixture. Spread on jelly roll pan (15-by-10-by-1-inch) that has been covered with wax paper, well coated with cooking spray, or greased. Bake 15 minutes.

3. Sift generous amount of powdered sugar onto clean tea towel.

4. Turn hot cake onto towel and roll up towel with cake jelly-roll fashion. Refrigerate at least 1 hour.

5. In bowl, beat together cream cheese, sugar, and vanilla.

6. Unroll cake. Spread filling onto cake, roll up cake without towel, wrap in foil, and keep chilled until ready to serve. Freezes well.

7. When you're ready to serve, sprinkle again with powdered sugar.

Nutrient Analysis per Serving

141 calories
28 grams carbohydrate
5 grams protein
1 gram fat

Key Nutrients

40% vitamin A
9% manganese
9% selenium

Diabetic Exchanges

2 starches

Quick and Easy Blueberry Cobbler

If you like cobbler, you'll find this one worth the small effort.

Makes: 6 servings

1 cup flour

⅔ cup sugar

1½ teaspoons baking powder

½ teaspoon salt

1 package dry Butter Buds

1 teaspoon almond extract

*¾ cup canned evaporated
skim milk*

*1 21-ounce can "more fruit"
blueberry pie filling*

Slivered almonds (optional)

Cooking spray

1. Preheat oven to 350°F.

2. Spray 2-quart casserole with cooking spray.

3. Mix together flour, sugar, baking powder, salt, Butter Buds, almond extract, and milk. Pour into casserole.

4. Spoon pie filling on top.

5. Bake for 35 to 40 minutes or until golden brown. If desired, sprinkle almonds on top of cobbler during last 10 minutes of baking.

Variation

Use peach pie filling instead of blueberry to make a Peach Cobbler.

Note: This recipe is high in simple sugar. Diabetic moms should eat only a small amount or none at all.

Nutrient Analysis per Serving

275 calories
64 grams carbohydrate
5 grams protein
0 grams fat

Key Nutrients

15% riboflavin
12% calcium

Diabetic Exchanges

3½ starches
½ fruit

CHAPTER FIFTEEN

Menus and Recipes for the Third Trimester

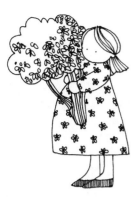

Third-Trimester Menus

Using Leftovers with Flair

What you will find in this chapter:

- Third-Trimester Menus
  - Using Leftovers with Flair
  - Meals in Minutes
  - Feel Full Meals
  - Best Bite Snacks
  - Vegetarian Budget Menus
- The Bean Routine
- Third-Trimester Recipes

Day 1
> Tossed salad
> Grilled chicken
> Rotini pasta
> Steamed zucchini and yellow squash

Day 2
> Colorado Stuffed Peppers (page 354)
> (Cook black beans in Crock-Pot during the day.)
> Corn bread
> Fresh fruit salad

Day 3
> Grilled chicken (from Day 1) in pita pocket with lettuce, tomatoes, and vinaigrette dressing
> OR
> Chicken-and-Spinach Salad (page 272)

Day 4
> Bridget's Garden Salad (page 271)
> (Use rotini pasta and leftover veggies from Day 1.)
> Strawberries and vanilla yogurt

Day 5

Black bean soup with cheese (Use beans
from Day 2.)
Corn bread
Tomato and avocado slices with fat-free
Italian dressing

Day 6

Fajitas with chicken, beef, or shrimp
Guacamole dip (Use tomato and avocado
from Day 5.)
Lettuce, tomato, and reduced-fat cheese

Day 7

Salmon en Papillote (page 314)
Steamed asparagus
Easy Microwave Potatoes (page 342)
Sorbet

Day 8

Tossed salad with leftover fajita strips
(from Day 6), canned kidney beans,
tomatoes, carrots, and cheese
Aspen Black Bean Soup (Use black beans
from Day 5.)
Baked Tortilla Chips (page 270)

Day 9

Linguine with salmon, canned artichoke
hearts, and Parmesan cheese (Use fish
from Day 7.)
Delightful Spinach (page 266)
Crusty whole-wheat French bread
Coleslaw
Fruit salad

Day 10

Creamy Asparagus Soup (page 268)
(Use asparagus from Day 7.)
Baked chicken
Potatoes Marie Louise (page 305)
Green beans
Tangerine

Day 11

Spinach, mushroom, and cheese que-
sadillas with tomatoes (Use spinach
from Day 9.)
OR
Curried chicken salad and romaine let-
tuce in pita pocket (Use chicken from
Day 10.)
Fresh melon

Day 12

Grilled fish with grilled pineapple
Grilled vegetable shish kebabs: zucchini,
mushrooms, eggplant, tomatoes
Bulgur or brown rice pilaf

Day 13

Fish on a Kaiser roll
Tossed salad with vinaigrette dressing
Black Bean and Corn Salad (page 270)
Apple slices with Caramel Dip (page
335)

Day 14

Tangy Salad (page 302)
Vegetable tacos with zucchini, mush-
rooms, eggplant, tomatoes, and cheese
(Use vegetables from Day 12.)
Roasted New Potatoes/Home Fries (page
345)

Day 15

    Ratatouille (page 344)

    Brown rice (from Day 12) with poached egg

    Kiwi and peaches over angel food cake

Day 16

    Chicken with Dijon Sauce (page 336)

    Pasta with steamed vegetables

    Fruit Crisp (page 368)

Day 17

    Ratatouille (from Day 15) and cheese on Boboli bread

    Tossed salad

    Frozen melon balls

Day 18

    Crepes (pages 310–311) with chicken and Dijon Sauce (from Day 16)

    Black Bean and Corn Salad (from Day 13)

    Frozen vanilla yogurt with Fruit Crisp (from Day 16) as topping

Day 19

    Vegetarian Chili (page 340)

    Coleslaw

    Sunshine Sorbet (page 370)

Day 20

    Vegetarian tacos or taco salad (Use chili from Day 19.)

    Tossed salad

    Berry Mousse Parfait (page 319)

Meals in Minutes

Cup of won ton soup
Turkey with Hoisin Sauce (page 318)
Instant brown rice with snow peas
Frozen banana

Healthy Choice split-pea soup
Microwaved grilled cheese sandwich
Tomato slices
Fresh fruit

Bean tostadas with lettuce and tomato
Frozen yogurt with strawberries
Scallop-and-shrimp stir-fry with frozen veggie mix
Angel hair pasta
Fresh peach

Salad with smoked turkey, cherry tomatoes, and romaine lettuce
Bread sticks
Fresh orange

Hoppin' John (page 357)
Steamed broccoli
Strawberries and banana slices

Minute steak on wheat bun
Spinach salad (in a bag)
Banana pudding

Minute Minestrone (page 300)
Turkey breast and cheese quesadilla in whole-wheat tortilla
Apple

Turkey with Hoisin Sauce (page 318)
Kids' Carrots (page 343)
Spinach pasta twists

Tomato soup
Cheese-Topped Orange Roughy (page 351)
Bulgur-and-Veggie Mix (page 341)
Mixed fruit salad

Raw vegetables with ranch dip
Hoppin' John (page 357)
Very Berry Shake (page 289)

Apricot-Glazed Chicken (page 347)
Easy Microwave Potatoes with Italian seasoning (page 342)
Delightful Spinach (page 266)

Quick Grilled Fish (page 360) with grilled vegetables
Angel hair pasta, fresh
Tropical Pudding (page 288)

Caesar salad (in a bag)
Shrimp cocktail
Garlic French bread with melted low-fat cheese
Frozen grapes
Sugar cookies

European-style salad (in a bag)
Aspen Black Bean Soup (page 337)
Baked Tortilla Chips (page 270) with salsa
Fresh pineapple rings

Salad with leftover grilled chicken, romaine lettuce, corn, and tomato
Bread sticks
Cantaloupe chunks
Strawberry ice milk

Bean tostada
Sliced tomatoes and cucumbers
Frozen fruit salad (peaches, raspberries, grapes)

Tossed salad
Crab Marinara (page 356) over linguini
Lemon sorbet with fresh raspberries

Feel Full Meals

These menus give you the very most nutrition per bite when you can't eat much!

Crab Marinara (page 356)
Tossed romaine salad
Cantaloupe slices

Spanish Steak Roll (page 315)
Delightful Spinach (page 266)
Bulgur pilaf

Leg of Lamb (page 313)
Green beans and northern beans
Potatoes Marie Louise (page 305)
Raspberries

Sesame Beef (page 361)
Stir-fried bell peppers and tomatoes
Brown rice or bulgur pilaf
Berry Mousse Parfait (page 319)

Black Bean and Corn Salad (page 270)
Baked Tortilla Chips (page 270)
Fresh orange

Asian Salad (page 269)
Cheese-Topped Orange Roughy (page 351)
Steamed broccoli
Mango slices

Stuffed Eggplant Creole (page 316)

Brown rice or quinoa

Sunshine Sorbet (page 370)

Country Brunch Casserole (page 355)

Very Berry Shake (page 289)

Raw veggies with Boursin Cheese Spread (page 334)

Spinach-Stuffed Shells (page 362)

Bread sticks

Watermelon balls

Chicken and Shrimp with Fruit Salsa (page 352)

Carrots Antibes (page 273)

Barley pilaf

Veal Piccata with Roasted Red Pepper Sauce (page 364)

Whole-wheat pasta

Strawberry and banana slices

Broccoli Quiche (page 350)

Tomato slices

Wheat baguette

Fruit Crisp (page 368)

Spanish Steak Roll with Sautéed Vegetables (page 315)

Roasted New Potatoes (page 345)

Cantaloupe

Apricot-Glazed Chicken (page 347)

Romaine lettuce salad

Piña Colada Frappé (page 286)

Vegetables in Vinaigrette (page 346)

Black Bean Enchilada Casserole (page 349)

Tangy Salad (page 302)

Best Bite Snacks

These snacks have the most nutrients per calorie:

Boursin Cheese Spread (page 334)

Favorite Snack Cake (page 367)

Spiced refried beans with Baked Tortilla Chips (page 270)

Very Berry Shake (page 289)

Raspberry Surprise Shake (page 287)

Stuffed Figs (page 53)

Berry Mousse Parfait (page 319)

Pumpkin Muffins (page 279)

Thrive-on-Five Bread (page 281)

Layered Mexican Dip (page 243)

Tropical Pudding (page 288)

Tangy Salad (page 302)

Oven-Fried Zucchini or Eggplant (page 274)

Aspen Black Bean Soup (page 337)

Peach Pops (page 284)

Vegetarian Budget Menus

The following two weeks' worth of sample menus can help if you are becoming vegetarian or are just looking for ways to cut food costs. Meatless meals can be very affordable and very healthy! The Week 1 menus require ingredients found in most kitchens and little preparation. Week 2 introduces meals using some common recipes. These menus do include milk and eggs. If you are vegan, you can use egg substitute, soymilk, or soy cheese instead.

These menus use 2-percent milk and may contain fats like margarine, butter, or oil added while cooking. The menus average 2,200 calories and assume serving sizes such as 1½ cups cereal or soup, ½ to 1 cup fruit, ½ to 1 cup vegetables, 2 tablespoons peanut butter, 1 cup milk, and so on. Unlike other menus in this book, these vegetarian menus include beverages because beverages have been used to calculate calories and nutrients.

A recommended vegetarian cookbook for busy people is *Meatless Meals for Working People: Quick and Easy Vegetarian Recipes,* available from the Vegetarian Resource Group at www.vrg.org.

Week 1

Monday

Breakfast
  Quick and Healthier Pancakes (page 298) with sliced peaches
  Low-fat milk

Lunch
  Tomato soup
  Grilled cheese sandwich with whole-wheat bread
  Apple

Dinner
  Vegetarian Chili (page 340)
  Corn bread muffins
  Coleslaw
  Watermelon
  Low-fat milk

Snacks
  Crackers with peanut butter and low-fat milk
  Tortilla chips with bean dip and tomato juice

Tuesday

Breakfast
  Total Raisin Bran
  Banana
  Low-fat milk

Lunch
  Sloppy joes made with textured vegetable protein (TVP)
  Carrot-and-raisin salad
  Low-fat milk

Dinner
  Broccoli Quiche (page 350) (a good way to use leftovers)
  Wheat toast
  Broiled tomato halves
  Roasted New Potatoes/Home Fries (page 345)

Snacks
  Graham crackers with low-fat milk
  Canned pineapple with cottage cheese and fruit juice

Wednesday

Breakfast
  Oatmeal with raisins and molasses
  Banana bread
  Low-fat milk

Lunch
  Black Bean and Corn Salad (page 270)
  Baked corn tortillas with cheese
  Fruit Crisp (page 368)

Dinner
  Hoppin' John (without ham—page 357)
  Corn bread
  Collard greens or spinach
  Carrot sticks
  Grapes

Snacks

Popcorn and low-fat milk

Piña Colada Frappé (page 286) and
gingersnaps

Thursday

Breakfast

Poached eggs on wheat toast
Grapefruit
Low-fat milk

Lunch

Macaroni and cheese
Tossed salad with kidney beans and
tomato slices
Kiwi

Dinner

Vegetables in Vinaigrette (page 346)
Colorado Stuffed Peppers (page 354)
Fresh cantaloupe slices
Low-fat milk

Snacks

Cheese and crackers
Pumpkin Muffins (page 279) and low-fat
milk

Friday

Breakfast

Hot wheat cereal
Peanut butter and banana on toast
Low-fat milk

Lunch

Bean and brown rice burritos
Spinach salad with orange pieces
Apple

Dinner

Tossed salad with chickpeas
Whole-wheat pasta with marinara sauce
and cheese
Wheat rolls
Cinnamon grilled peach halves

Snacks

Oatmeal cookies and low-fat milk
Brown rice pudding with raisins

Saturday

Breakfast

Cheese toast
Apple-and-pear salad
Low-fat milk

Lunch

Lentil Soup (page 338)
Celery and carrot sticks
Strawberries with yogurt
Low-fat milk

Dinner

Whole-wheat couscous with mushrooms,
zucchini, tomato sauce, and Parmesan
cheese
Kids' Carrots (page 343)
Garlic bread
Fruit salad
Low-fat milk

Snacks

Hot cocoa
Fig bars
Very Berry Shake (page 289)
Favorite Snack Cake (page 367)

Sunday

Breakfast

Vegetarian Breakfast Tacos (page 366)
Mango slices
Low-fat milk

Lunch
  Grilled vegetable-and-cheese sandwich
    on rye toast
  Banana
  Low-fat milk

Dinner
  Cabbage salad
  Tofu Loaf (page 363)
  Steamed zucchini
  Strawberry Bread (page 280) with light
    cream cheese
  Fresh orange

Snacks
  Frozen yogurt sundae
  Granola bar and low-fat milk

Week 2

Monday

Breakfast
  French toast with strawberries
  Low-fat milk

Lunch
  Leek-and-Potato Soup (page 299)
  Whole-wheat English muffins
  Celery with low-fat cream cheese
  Frozen grapes
  Low-fat milk

Dinner
  Ratatouille (page 344) over brown rice
    or bulgur
  Macaroni, black beans, and corn
  Kiwi slices

Snacks
  Graham crackers with peanut butter
  Low-fat milk
  Thrive-on-Five Bread (page 281)

Tuesday

Breakfast
  Oatmeal with raisins
  Fresh orange
  Apple-Date Bran Muffin (page 278)
  Low-fat milk

Lunch
  Grilled Swiss cheese and sauerkraut on
    rye bread
  Potato salad
  Fresh apple

Dinner
  Oat-Nut Burgers (page 359)
  Thanksgiving Sweet Potatoes (page 306)
  Wheat rolls
  Fruit cocktail
  Low-fat milk

Snacks
  Bran muffin and low-fat milk
  Fat-free cream cheese dip, cauliflower
    and carrot sticks, and wheat crackers

Wednesday

Breakfast
  Cheese grits
  Cantaloupe
  Wheat toast

Lunch
  Boursin Cheese Spread (page 334) on
    wheat roll with lettuce, cucumber,
    tomato, and sprouts
  Carrot-and-pineapple salad
  Sugar cookies

Dinner
Tomatoes in vinaigrette
Black Bean Enchilada Casserole (page 349)
Wheat garlic toast
Fresh fruit salad
Low-fat milk

Snacks
Tangerine and string cheese
Leftover veggies, beans, and cheese in
    wheat tortilla with low-fat milk

Thursday

Breakfast
Whole-grain cereal
Sliced banana
Low-fat milk

Lunch
Sliced avocado, cheese, tomato, and
    lettuce on wheat bread
Salad
Plums
Low-fat milk

Dinner
Bean and Corn Bread Bake (page 348)
Coleslaw
Strawberries over angel food cake
Low-fat milk

Snacks
Yogurt with fruit
Refried vegetarian beans and homemade
    tortilla chips or toasted pita bread tri-
    angles

Friday

Breakfast
Poached eggs
Cinnamon-raisin bagels
Apple juice
Low-fat milk

Lunch
Minute Minestrone (page 300)
Cottage cheese with raw vegetables
Corn bread
Grapes

Dinner
Asian Salad (page 269)
Vegetable-and-Tofu Stir-Fry (page 365)
Chinese noodles or brown rice
Pineapple slices

Snacks
Crackers and peanut butter with low-fat
    milk
Granola bar and low-fat milk

Saturday

Breakfast
Country Brunch Casserole (page 355)
Raisins or prunes
Toast
Low-fat milk

Lunch
Oven-Fried Eggplant Slices (page 274)
    with marinara sauce and cheese
Crusty French bread
Watermelon
Low-fat milk

Dinner
Spring Vegetables in Cream Sauce (page
    275)
Spinach salad
Garlic bread
Low-fat milk

Snacks
Berry Mousse Parfait (page 319)
Vegetarian nachos made with Baked
    Tortilla Chips (page 270) and V-8 juice

Sunday

Breakfast
Frozen waffles
Frozen strawberries
Low-fat milk

Lunch
Aspen Black Bean Soup (page 337)
Crackers
Carrot and celery sticks
Apple slices with Caramel Dip (page 335)
Low-fat milk

Dinner
Spinach-Stuffed Shells (page 362)
3-bean salad with cherry tomatoes
Melon

Snacks
Popcorn and tomato juice
Banana, peanut butter, and low-fat milk

▼

The Bean Routine

Dry beans are a nutritional gold mine for today's mom-to-be! They are high in protein, complex carbohydrate, and fiber; low in fat; and full of important nutrients. They make a great main dish when you can't tolerate meat. Beans will save you money on your food budget, and you can save time by using canned beans.

One cup of cooked dried beans provides 27 percent of a pregnant woman's daily need for protein, 25 percent of her requirement for manganese, 18 percent of her requirement for iron, and 31 percent of her requirement for folacin. Plus, beans provide about 9 grams of fiber. Pregnant women should eat 20 to 35 grams of fiber per day.

Beating Bean Bloat

One common concern about beans is that they can cause gas. A University of California-Berkeley study reported greater intestinal tolerance after three weeks of eating beans regularly. Here are some tips for adjusting to the bean routine.[1]

1. Build up your body's tolerance. Eat small servings at first; then increase your intake slowly over a period of weeks.

2. Soak beans overnight, cook your beans properly, and always pour off the soaking water and add fresh water for cooking. Proper cooking can break down starches, making the beans more digestible.

3. Chew well and slowly. This assists in digestion and can minimize your bloating problem.

4. Drink enough fluids. Sufficient fluid intake helps your digestive system handle the increased dietary fiber.

Third-Trimester Recipes

Dips, Sauces, and Spreads
Boursin Cheese Spread, 334
Caramel Dip, 335
Dijon Sauce, 336

Soups
Aspen Black Bean Soup, 337
Lentil Soup, 338
Mexican Kale-and-Pork Soup, 339
Vegetarian Chili, 340

Side Dishes
Bulgur-and-Veggie Mix, 341
Easy Microwave Potatoes, 342
Kids' Carrots, 343
Ratatouille, 344
Roasted New Potatoes/Home Fries, 345
Vegetables in Vinaigrette, 346

Entrées
Apricot-Glazed Chicken, 347
Bean and Corn Bread Bake, 348
Black Bean Enchilada Casserole, 349
Broccoli Quiche, 350

Cheese-Topped Orange Roughy, 351
Chicken and Shrimp with Fruit Salsa, 352–353
Colorado Stuffed Peppers, 354
Country Brunch Casserole, 355
Crab Marinara, 356
Hoppin' John, 357
Mock Egg Foo Yung, 358
Oat-Nut Burgers, 359
Quick Grilled Fish, 360
Sesame Beef, 361
Spinach-Stuffed Shells, 362
Tofu Loaf, 363
Veal Piccata with Roasted Red Pepper Sauce, 364
Vegetable-and-Tofu Stir-Fry, 365
Vegetarian Breakfast Tacos, 366

Sweets
Favorite Snack Cake, 367
Fruit Crisp, 368
Fruit Pizza for a Crowd, 369
Sunshine Sorbet, 370

Boursin Cheese Spread

This recipe is from *More Low-Fat Favorites* by Ceacy Thatcher. Try it with pita bread crisps, crackers, raw vegetables, or in crepes with veggies. Or thin it with a little skim milk to make a sauce for pasta or vegetables or to use as salad dressing.

Makes: 12 servings

8 ounces fat-free margarine

16 ounces fat-free cream cheese

2 cloves fresh garlic, minced, or 1 teaspoon chopped garlic from jar

½ teaspoon dried oregano

¼ teaspoon dried marjoram

¼ teaspoon dried thyme

¼ teaspoon dried basil

¼ teaspoon dried dill weed

¼ teaspoon white pepper

1. Using a hand mixer or spoon, mix all ingredients until well blended.

2. Chill 1 hour before serving.

Nutrient Analysis per Serving

40 calories
3 grams carbohydrate
5 grams protein
1 gram fat
373 milligrams sodium

Key Nutrients

Small amounts of all nutrients

Diabetic Exchanges

½ very lean meat
¼ milk

Caramel Dip

This is Cindy McKee's recipe, and you won't believe it's fat-free! Serve it with apple slices or graham crackers.

8 ounces fat-free cream cheese, softened

⅓ cup brown sugar, packed

1 teaspoon Watkin's Caramel Flavor

1 teaspoon vanilla

1. Beat all ingredients with mixer.

Variation

Caramel Sauce: Over very low heat, thin mixture with small amount of milk until desired consistency is reached. Serve over crepes, fruit, or frozen yogurt.

Diabetic Variation

Instead of brown sugar, use Equal to taste.

Nutrient Analysis per Serving

57 calories
11 grams carbohydrate
4 grams protein
0 grams fat

Key Nutrients

Small amounts of many nutrients

Nutrient Analysis per Serving
(Diabetic Variation)

23 calories
2 grams carbohydrate
4 grams protein
0 fat

Diabetic Exchanges

1 very lean meat

Dijon Sauce

In France, this sauce is made with crème fraîche and makes any meat taste divine! This healthy version goes well with chicken breast, pork tenderloin chops, or new potatoes.

Makes: 4 servings

½ *cup low-fat or fat-free sour cream*

½ *cup plain nonfat yogurt*

1 to 2 tablespoons Dijon mustard

Salt, pepper, and garlic powder to taste

1. Mix all ingredients in saucepan.

2. If you are serving with meat, blend sauce with pan juices. Heat until very warm.

Nutrient Analysis per Serving

52 calories
6 grams carbohydrate
3 grams protein
2 grams fat

Key Nutrients

Small amounts of all nutrients

Diabetic Exchanges

½ skim milk

Aspen Black Bean Soup

Serve this hearty, delicious soup after your morning walk.

Makes: 6 servings

Soup

1 medium onion, chopped

3 cloves garlic or 3 teaspoons chopped garlic in jar

1 teaspoon dried whole oregano

½ teaspoon dried whole thyme

½ teaspoon cumin

¼ teaspoon cayenne pepper (optional)

2 15-ounce cans (3 cups) black beans, drained and rinsed

3 cups fat-free chicken broth

Cooking spray

Garnish

½ cup part-skim mozzarella cheese

2 tomatoes, chopped

1 onion, finely minced (optional)

1. Spray skillet with cooking spray. Cook onion and garlic until tender (about 5 minutes); add water if needed.

2. Stir in spices; cook 2 to 3 minutes.

3. Place ½ of beans in blender and purée until smooth, adding broth as needed to help make it smooth.

4. Add puréed beans, remaining broth, and remaining beans to onion mixture. Bring to boil and then lower to medium heat and simmer 20 to 30 minutes.

5. Serve garnished with chopped tomatoes, onions, and cheese.

Serving Suggestion

For a complete meal, add a salad, fruit, and corn bread, or a grilled vegetable sandwich.

Nutritional Analysis per Serving

240 calories
37 grams carbohydrate
15 grams protein
4 grams fat
8 grams fiber

Key Nutrients

25% folate
21% magnesium
18% zinc
15% chromium

Diabetic Exchanges

2 starches
1 lean meat
1 vegetable

Lentil Soup

Lentils cook quickly and don't need to be soaked before cooking. They are also delicious!

Makes: 6 servings

2 medium onions, chopped

6 large garlic cloves, crushed

2 stalks celery, chopped

1 pound dry lentils

7 cups water

1 cup chicken broth

½ teaspoon basil

1½ teaspoons each thyme
 and oregano

1 bay leaf

1 to 2 teaspoons salt

2 to 3 medium carrots, sliced

Freshly ground black pepper
 to taste

Cooking spray

Garnish

Red wine vinegar

Tomatoes, chopped

1. Brown onions, garlic, and celery in pan sprayed with cooking spray, adding 1 tablespoon water as needed.

2. Place lentils, water, chicken broth, spices, and salt in kettle. Bring to boil, lower heat to very slow simmer, and cook covered for 20 to 30 minutes.

3. Add carrots and black pepper. Cover and let simmer another 30 to 45 minutes, stirring occasionally. Remove bay leaf.

4. Serve hot, with sprinkle of red wine vinegar and chopped tomatoes on top of each bowl.

Nutrient Analysis per Serving

182 calories

33 grams carbohydrate

13 grams protein

1 gram fat

9 grams fiber

Key Nutrients

41% folate

38% vitamin A

16% magnesium

Diabetic Exchanges

2 starches

1 very lean meat

Mexican Kale-and-Pork Soup

This recipe offers an interesting combination of flavors and textures.

Makes: 8 servings

1 teaspoon canola oil

1 medium onion, chopped

1 clove garlic, minced

16 ounces pork loin or loin chops, trimmed of all fat and cut into 1-inch cubes

5 cups water

1 bunch fresh kale, trimmed and cut into 1-inch pieces

1 16-ounce can whole peeled tomatoes

5 Roma tomatoes, halved and sliced, or 3 medium tomatoes, chopped

1½ teaspoons ground cumin

¾ teaspoon chili powder

1 15-ounce can hominy

½ can tomato paste

Salt, pepper, and hot pepper sauce to taste

1. In saucepan, heat oil over medium heat. Add onion, garlic, and pork. Cook about 10 minutes, stirring occasionally.

2. Place pork in large microwave-safe dish. Add water. Cook 5 minutes on high.

3. Add kale. Cook 5 minutes on high.

4. Add canned and fresh tomatoes, spices, hominy, and tomato paste. Cook 15 minutes on high, or until kale reaches desired tenderness. Add more tomato paste for thicker soup.

Serving Suggestion

Serve with homemade corn chips and guacamole.

Vegetarian Variation

Substitute tofu or pinto beans for pork.

Nutrient Analysis per Serving

229 calories

19 grams carbohydrate

19 grams protein

9 grams fat

4 grams fiber

Key Nutrients

49% vitamin C

43% thiamin

40% vitamin A

21% vitamin B_6

Diabetic Exchanges

2 medium-fat meats

2 vegetables

½ starch

Vegetarian Chili

This hearty chili is chock full of nutrients and makes a great potluck dish or casual dinner.

Makes: 6 servings

1 medium onion, chopped

2 large cloves garlic, minced

1 medium zucchini or 1 medium bell pepper, chopped

1 28-ounce can crushed tomatoes in purée

1 15-ounce can tomato sauce

2 15-ounce cans kidney beans, drained

2 to 4 teaspoons chili powder

2 teaspoons cumin

½ teaspoon oregano

¼ cup uncooked bulgur

Cayenne or black pepper to taste

Garnish

Parsley

Tomato, fresh, chopped

Onion, finely minced

1. Heat small amount of water in nonstick pot. Add onion and garlic. Sauté over medium heat about 5 to 10 minutes.

2. Add zucchini or bell pepper and sauté until all vegetables are tender.

3. Add tomatoes, tomato sauce, beans, spices, and bulgur. Simmer over lowest heat, stirring occasionally, for 15 minutes.

4. Season to taste and serve hot, topped with parsley, chopped fresh tomato, and onion.

Variations

- Spooned over baked tortilla chips and topped with fat-free Cheddar cheese.
- Rolled up in a flour tortilla.
- Stuffed in a bell pepper.

Nutrient Analysis per Serving

220 calories

44 grams carbohydrate

12 grams protein

1 gram fat

11 grams fiber

Key Nutrients

53% vitamin B_6

28% vitamin C

22% iron

12% folate

Diabetic Exchanges

2½ starches

1½ vegetables

1 very lean meat

Bulgur-and-Veggie Mix

Bulgur is a quick and healthy alternative to rice. It is also very versatile.

Makes: 5 servings

*2 cups fat-free chicken broth
  or water*

¼ teaspoon salt (optional)

*2½ cups broccoli, chopped,
  or other vegetable in season*

1 cup dry bulgur

½ teaspoon thyme

1. In saucepan, bring broth or water to boil. Add salt and broccoli. Simmer 5 minutes.

2. Place bulgur in heatproof serving bowl. Pour water and broccoli over bulgur.

3. Cover and let sit until most of water is absorbed.

4. Pour off excess water and fluff with fork.

Variation

Substitute any vegetable, or vegetable combinations, fresh or frozen, for broccoli.

**Nutritional Analysis
per Serving**

103 calories

22 grams carbohydrate

6 grams protein

0 grams fat

6 grams fiber

Key Nutrients

103% vitamin C

16% vitamin A

15% magnesium

14% chromium

Diabetic Exchanges

1 starch

1 vegetable

Easy Microwave Potatoes

With the help of a microwave, the potato can be a quick and nutritious side dish.

Potatoes, any amount, peeled or unpeeled, cut into 1-inch pieces
2 to 3 tablespoons water
Salt and pepper to taste

1. Cook potatoes in water and spices in covered microwave-safe dish on high for 5 minutes.

2. Rotate dish. Cook 5 more minutes on high. Continue cooking until fork can easily pierce potatoes.

Variations

Italian: Add Italian spices before cooking and top potatoes with Parmesan cheese the last few minutes of cooking.

German: Add sautéed onions and bacon bits or ham to potatoes the last few minutes of cooking. Sprinkle with vinegar and toss.

**Nutrient Analysis
per Serving**
(1 medium potato)

178 calories
41 grams carbohydrate
4 grams protein
0 grams fat
2 grams fiber

Key Nutrients

38% potassium
36% vitamin C
30% vitamin B$_6$

Diabetic Exchanges
(per ½-cup serving)

1 starch

Kids' Carrots

You're never too young to be in the kitchen! That philosophy paid off for twelve-year-old Andy Hawk, who placed third in the vegetable category of the Delicious and Nutritious Recipe Contest.

Makes: 5 servings

1 1-pound package frozen baby carrots

2 tablespoons honey

Mint, 1 tablespoon minced fresh or 1½ teaspoons dried

1. Cook carrots according to package directions. Drain.

2. Stir in honey to coat carrots. Stir in mint. Serve.

Nutrient Analysis per Serving

48 calories
19 grams carbohydrate
1 gram protein
0 grams fat
3 grams fiber

Key Nutrients

167% vitamin A

Diabetic Exchanges

1 vegetable
¼ starch

Ratatouille

My husband introduced me to this wonderful and versatile dish. You can serve it over rice with cheese as a main dish, as a side dish, or as a topping on your pizza or potato. In Europe, ratatouille is often served topped with a fried egg.

Makes: 8 servings

1 eggplant, peeled and cut into 1-inch cubes

1 teaspoon olive oil

4 garlic cloves, crushed

8 tomatoes, cut into quarters

3 zucchini, sliced

1 cup mushrooms, sliced

1 teaspoon oregano

1 teaspoon basil

1 teaspoon salt

¼ teaspoon pepper

1. Brown eggplant in oil in nonstick pan. Add garlic and cook until tender.

2. Add remaining ingredients. Cook over medium heat until vegetables are tender, stirring frequently.

3. Reduce heat, cover, and simmer 10 to 15 minutes.

4. Remove cover and continue cooking until most of liquid has evaporated.

Variations

Add chopped red and green bell peppers and sliced black olives.

Quick Method: Use 16-ounce can of tomatoes and ¼ cup tomato paste instead of fresh tomatoes.

Nutrient Analysis per Serving

58 calories
12 grams carbohydrate
2 grams protein
1 gram fat
4 grams fiber

Key Nutrients

40% vitamin C
29% potassium
6% folate

Diabetic Exchanges

2 vegetables

Roasted New Potatoes/Home Fries

Do you like fried foods, but not the fat in them? Try these crispy roasted potatoes. Their secret is a high oven temperature.

Makes: 4 servings

1 pound new potatoes or baking potatoes, well scrubbed

1 tablespoon olive oil

1 to 2 cloves garlic, crushed

½ teaspoon salt

Rosemary, 1 teaspoon dried or 2 teaspoons fresh, chopped

1. Preheat oven to 450°F.

2. Cut potatoes into 1-inch pieces. Toss in bowl with oil, garlic, salt, and rosemary.

3. Spread potatoes on baking sheet. Roast about 30 minutes until potatoes are tender and brown, turning once halfway through cooking.

Variations

All should cook in about 20 minutes.

Oven Home Fries: Slice white potatoes, sweet potatoes, or yams into ¼-inch slices to make home fries, or slice thinner for home-made potato chips.

Sweet Chips: Thinly sliced sweet potatoes dusted with cinnamon or pumpkin spice makes a sweet snack chip.

French Fries: Cut into thin, long strips for French fries.

Nutrient Analysis per Serving

144 calories
26 grams carbohydrate
2 grams protein
4 grams fat
3 grams fiber

Key Nutrients

24% vitamin C
19% vitamin B₆
11% riboflavin

Diabetic Exchanges

2 starches
1 fat

Vegetables in Vinaigrette

A starting course of raw vegetables in vinaigrette dressing is a French tradition.

Makes: 4 servings

Use one or more of the following vegetables:

7 carrots, finely grated

½ celery root, finely grated (also called celeriac)

2 cucumbers, thinly sliced

⅓ head red cabbage, finely grated

Add

½ cup fat-free or low-fat vinaigrette dressing (Strong-flavored is best.)

¼ cup parsley, finely chopped

Salt and pepper to taste

1. Combine all ingredients. Marinate at least 30 minutes.

Variation

Add 1 to 2 tablespoons fat-free or light sour cream to vinaigrette dressing.

Nutrient Analysis per Serving

30 calories
7 grams carbohydrate
1 gram protein
0 grams fat

Key Nutrients
(for carrots)

194% vitamin A
Small amounts of other nutrients

Diabetic Exchanges

1 vegetable

Apricot-Glazed Chicken

You can cook this chicken in a flash and serve it to family or friends.

Makes: 4 servings

4 chicken breast halves,
   skinned and boned

2 teaspoons margarine

Salt and pepper to taste

⅓ cup apricot or peach all-fruit
   spread

1½ tablespoons tarragon wine
   vinegar or other flavored
   vinegar

2 teaspoons ginger

¼ cup cashews, chopped

1. Rinse chicken and pat dry with paper towels.

2. Melt margarine in nonstick pan.

3. Sauté chicken over medium heat for 8 to 10 minutes. Remove chicken and keep warm. Sprinkle with salt and pepper. Set aside pan juices.

4. Stir preserves, vinegar, and ginger into pan juices. Cook over medium heat until hot.

5. Spoon glaze over chicken breasts. Sprinkle with cashews.

Nutrient Analysis per Serving

240 calories

11 grams carbohydrate

28 grams protein

9 grams fat

Key Nutrients

66% niacin

28% vitamin B₆

13% magnesium

Diabetic Exchanges

4 lean meats

1 fruit

Bean and Corn Bread Bake

This one-dish meal is easy to make, and it's high in fiber, too!

Makes: 6 servings

Beans

1 16-ounce can pinto beans, drained

1 16-ounce can kidney beans, black beans, or black-eyed peas, drained (Any combination will work!)

¼ cup each chopped green pepper, onion, and celery

2 tablespoons ketchup

1 8-ounce can tomato sauce

1 teaspoon dry mustard

Oil or cooking spray

Corn Bread Topping

1 small package (7 to 8½ ounces) corn bread mix

¼ cup reduced-fat or fat-free Cheddar cheese, grated

¼ cup green chilies (optional)

1. Preheat oven to 375°F.

2. Mix together beans and vegetables. Pour into baking dish that has been lightly oiled or sprayed with cooking spray.

3. Prepare corn bread according to package directions, adding cheese and chilies if desired. Pour over beans.

4. Bake for 30 to 35 minutes or until corn bread is golden brown.

5. Serve with spinach salad and fresh fruit.

Nutrient Analysis per Serving

360 calories
53 grams carbohydrate
16 grams protein
10 grams fat
7 grams fiber

Key Nutrients

29% potassium
25% folate
21% magnesium
11% iron

Diabetic Exchanges

3½ starches
1½ fats
1 lean meat

Black Bean Enchilada Casserole

This quick and easy casserole was modified from Janet Boyd's recipe.

Makes: 4 servings

1 15-ounce can Southwestern style black beans (with spices), undrained

1 15-ounce can Del Monte Chili Style Tomatoes

¼ cup picante sauce

3 corn tortillas

4 to 6 ounces fat-free or low-fat cheese

Cooking spray

1. Preheat oven to 350°F.

2. In bowl, mix beans, tomatoes, and sauce. Spray 2-quart round casserole dish with cooking spray.

3. Place 1 corn tortilla in bottom of dish. Add ⅓ of bean mixture, ⅓ of cheese, another tortilla, ⅓ of bean mixture, another tortilla, and rest of bean mixture.

4. Bake 20 minutes. Sprinkle remaining 2 tablespoons cheese on top during last 5 minutes of cooking.

5. To make this recipe in 9-by-13-inch pan, use 3 cans black beans, 3 cans tomatoes, and 12 tortillas, overlapping 6 tortillas for each layer.

Low-Sodium Variation

Cook 1 sliced onion, 1 teaspoon chopped garlic, and 1 sliced bell pepper until tender. Add 15-ounce can stewed tomatoes and ¾ cup picante sauce. Use 1½ cups cooked black beans with 1½ teaspoons cumin and 1 teaspoon chili powder.

Nutritional Analysis per Serving

269 calories
35 grams carbohydrate
20 grams protein
8 grams fat
10 grams fiber

Key Nutrients

28% folate
28% magnesium
26% vitamin C
18% copper

Diabetic Exchanges

2 starches
1½ lean meats
1 vegetable
½ fat

Broccoli Quiche

This recipe, from the book *Quick and Healthy Volume II* by Brenda Ponichtera, is great for a luncheon or brunch. Serve with a fruit cup or orange wedges.

Makes: 6 servings

*3 flour tortillas
(7½-inch diameter)*

*2 cups broccoli, cooked, drained,
and chopped into bite-size
pieces*

½ cup green onion, sliced

*4 ounces reduced-fat Cheddar
cheese, grated*

8 eggs or 2 cups egg substitute

¼ cup skim milk

¼ teaspoon paprika

Salt and pepper (optional)

6 tomato slices

Cooking spray

1. Preheat oven to 350°F.

2. Spray 9-inch pie pan with cooking spray.

3. Cut 2 tortillas in half and place each half in pan so that rounded edge is ¼ inch above rim. Place remaining tortilla in center of pan. Add broccoli, onion, and cheese.

4. In separate bowl, mix eggs with milk and add salt and pepper (if desired). Pour into pan; sprinkle with paprika.

5. Bake 45 minutes or until knife inserted in center comes out clean. Let sit 10 minutes before cutting into 6 wedges.

6. Top each piece with tomato slice.

Source: Adapted with permission from *Quick and Healthy Volume II* by Brenda Ponichtera, R.D. (ScaleDown Publishing, Inc.).

Nutrient Analysis per Serving

*213 calories
14 grams carbohydrate
16 grams protein
11 grams fat*

Key Nutrients

*33% vitamin A
31% riboflavin
28% vitamin C
20% calcium*

Diabetic Exchanges

*2 medium-fat meats
½ starch
½ vegetable*

Cheese-Topped Orange Roughy

This recipe is from *Simply Colorado,* a cookbook by the Colorado Dietetic Association. Using this recipe, you can serve dinner in 15 to 20 minutes!

Makes: 6 servings

*2 pounds orange roughy
(or sole, cod, or red snapper)*

Cooking spray

Topping

⅓ cup light mayonnaise

⅓ cup Parmesan cheese, grated

¼ cup green onion, sliced

½ teaspoon lemon juice

¼ to ½ teaspoon garlic powder

Hot sauce to taste (optional)

1. Preheat oven to 350°F.

2. Place fish in shallow glass casserole coated with cooking spray; bake 8 minutes or until fish flakes easily when tested with fork.

3. Meanwhile, mix topping ingredients. Spread topping evenly over cooked fish fillets. Broil 6 inches from heat for 5 minutes or until topping is lightly browned.

Source: Reprinted with permission from Simply Colorado, Inc.

**Nutrient Analysis
per Serving**

164 calories

2 grams carbohydrate

27 grams protein

5 grams fat

Key Nutrients

102% vitamin B$_{12}$

18% potassium

17% magnesium

12% niacin

Diabetic Exchanges

3 very lean meats

½ fat

Chicken and Shrimp with Fruit Salsa

My friend Debbie Russell is a wizard in the kitchen. She has won several regional and national cooking contests, and this recipe is one of her winners.

Makes: 6 servings

1 pound large shrimp, shelled and deveined

1 pound boneless, skinless chicken breasts, cut into pieces

Marinade

¼ cup mild picante sauce

1 tablespoon lime or lemon juice

1 tablespoon soy sauce

½ teaspoon coriander, ground

½ teaspoon fresh ginger root, grated

1 clove garlic, crushed

Fruit Salsa

½ cup peaches, diced

½ cup pineapple, diced

½ cup green apple, diced

½ cup red bell pepper, diced

2 tablespoons green onion, chopped

1 teaspoon lime or lemon juice

1 teaspoon sugar

Garnish

12 thin slices pineapple or peaches

Cilantro or parsley sprigs

1. In dish or plastic bag, combine marinade ingredients.

2. Add shrimp and chicken, turning to coat pieces well. Cover dish or close bag and marinate at least 30 minutes in refrigerator.

3. In small bowl, combine salsa ingredients. Cover and set aside.

4. Drain shrimp and chicken, reserving marinade for basting. Thread shrimp and chicken alternately on skewers.

5. Broil chicken and shrimp over medium-hot coals or broil at 400°F until shrimp turns pink and chicken is well cooked (7 to 10 minutes), basting often with marinade.

6. Serve with fruit salsa on the side. Garnish with pineapple or peach slices and cilantro or parsley.

(continued on next page)

Chicken and Shrimp with Fruit Salsa
(continued)

Variations

• Stir-fry the chicken and shrimp instead of broiling.

• Serve with Peanut-Butter Sauce instead of Fruit Salsa:

½ cup plain nonfat yogurt

2 teaspoons peanut butter

½ teaspoon Dijon mustard

⅛ teaspoon Worcestershire sauce

**Nutrient Analysis
per Serving**
(with Fruit Salsa)

256 calories
18 grams carbohydrate
37 grams protein
4 grams fat
1 gram fiber

Key Nutrients

90% selenium
64% niacin
30% vitamin C
30% vitamin B_6

Diabetic Exchanges

5 very lean meats
1 fruit
½ vegetable

**Nutrient Analysis
per Serving**
(with Peanut-Butter
Sauce)

223 calories
4 grams carbohydrate
38 grams protein
5 grams fat

Key Nutrients

92% selenium
64% niacin
28% vitamin B_6
15% magnesium

Diabetic Exchanges

5 very lean meats

Colorado Stuffed Peppers

Makes: 4 servings

3 *Roma tomatoes or 2 medium tomatoes, chopped coarsely*

2 *green onions, chopped*

¼ *medium red onion, finely chopped*

1 *clove garlic, minced*

½ *sweet red pepper, chopped*

2 *teaspoons olive or canola oil*

1 *cup cooked brown rice or bulgur*

1½ *cups cooked black beans*

½ *cup plus 2 teaspoons reduced-fat Cheddar cheese, grated*

4 *bell peppers, cored and seeded*

1. Sauté tomatoes, both onions, garlic, and red pepper in oil until cooked to desired tenderness. (The less the tomato and pepper are cooked, the more vitamin C they retain.)

2. Add brown rice, black beans, and ½ cup cheese to pan and gently stir until warm and cheese is melted.

3. Meanwhile, steam whole peppers in microwave until tender-crisp; then fill with bean mixture.

4. Sprinkle remaining 2 teaspoons of cheese on top before serving. (To increase protein content, add some lean meat, chicken, tofu, or more cheese to the filling.)

Nutrient Analysis per Serving

237 calories

37 grams carbohydrate

12 grams protein

6 grams fat

5 grams fiber

Key Nutrients

106% vitamin C

32% selenium

25% magnesium

20% folate

Diabetic Exchanges

2 starches

1½ vegetables

1 lean meat

½ fat

Country Brunch Casserole

This recipe is from *Simply Colorado,* a cookbook by the Colorado Dietetic Association. It's perfect to serve to house guests; just prepare the dish the night before, and enjoy a leisurely brunch.

Makes: 8 servings

½ cup onion, chopped

2 tablespoons water

3 cups bread stuffing cubes

⅓ pound Canadian bacon, thinly sliced and cut into bite-size pieces (you can also use very lean ham)

1 cup (4 ounces) reduced-fat Cheddar cheese, shredded

3 eggs

2 egg whites

2 cups skim milk

½ teaspoon dry mustard

½ teaspoon onion salt

Cooking spray

1. Microwave onion and water on high for 2 minutes, stirring occasionally.

2. Place stuffing cubes in bottom of 12-by-8-by-2-inch baking dish that has been coated with cooking spray.

3. Sprinkle pan with microwaved onion, sliced ham, and shredded cheese.

4. In separate bowl, mix eggs, egg whites, milk, and seasonings; pour over stuffing mixture. Cover and refrigerate overnight.

5. Bake uncovered at 325°F for 1 hour. Let stand 10 minutes before serving.

Source: Reprinted with permission from Simply Colorado, Inc.

Nutrient Analysis per Serving

202 calories

13 grams carbohydrate

18 grams protein

9 grams fat

Key Nutrients

19% vitamin B₁₂

19% calcium

17% riboflavin

12% vitamin A

Diabetic Exchanges

1½ medium-fat meats

1 starch

Crab Marinara

This is a quick, delicious meal. If tomato sauce gives you heartburn, you may be able to tolerate this dish because the sour cream reduces the acidity of the sauce. You can keep the sauce on hand in the freezer for those times when you have no time to cook. Freeze leftovers for lunch.

Makes: 6 servings

12 ounces spaghetti, uncooked

4 cups prepared marinara sauce

¾ cup fat-free sour cream

¼ cup olives, sliced

1 7-ounce or 14-ounce can artichoke hearts (depending on how well you like artichokes)

½ teaspoon tarragon

¼ teaspoon dill

12 ounces imitation crab or other shellfish, cooked

1. Cook spaghetti according to package directions.

2. Meanwhile, drain artichokes and chop into ½-inch pieces.

3. In saucepan, combine marinara sauce with sour cream, olives, artichokes, and spices.

4. Break crab into bite-size pieces, add to sauce, and stir until thoroughly combined. Heat over medium heat until warm.

5. Serve sauce over pasta with salad and whole-wheat garlic bread.

Nutrient Analysis per Serving

351 calories
64 grams carbohydrate
17 grams protein
3 grams fat

Key Nutrients

50% thiamin
30% vitamin C
23% magnesium

Diabetic Exchanges

3½ starches
1½ vegetables
1 very lean meat
½ fat

Hoppin' John

This southern classic dish can be prepared in a flash with canned beans and quick-cooking brown rice or bulgur.

Makes: 4 servings

2 16-ounce cans red kidney beans or black-eyed peas, undrained

2 cups cooked brown rice or bulgur

6 ounces lean ham, chopped

¼ teaspoon onion powder

Pepper and salt to taste

Garnish

Fresh parsley and red onion, chopped (optional)

1. Combine undrained beans with rice, ham and spices. Cook over medium heat, stirring frequently.

2. Serve topped with parsley and chopped onion, if desired. If you can't tolerate raw onion, cook onion with beans.

Nutrient Analysis per Serving

262 calories
39 grams carbohydrate
17 grams protein
4 grams fat
2 grams fiber

Key Nutrients

89% selenium
19% vitamin B$_6$
17% zinc

Diabetic Exchanges

2½ starches
1½ lean meats

Mock Egg Foo Yung

This recipe provides a good way to incorporate soy into your diet.

Makes: 4 servings

16 ounces firm, low-fat tofu

2 eggs, beaten

4 green onions, finely chopped

1 cup mung bean sprouts,
    cut into 1-inch pieces

1 garlic clove, minced,
    or ¼ teaspoon garlic powder

1 tablespoon soy sauce

1 teaspoon salt

2 tablespoons old-fashioned
    oatmeal

1 carrot, finely grated

½ teaspoon sesame oil

1. Stir all ingredients together until well blended.

2. Form into 3-inch patties and cook in small amount of oil until lightly browned.

Nutrient Analysis per Serving

119 calories

7 grams carbohydrate

13 grams protein

5 grams fat

4 grams fiber

Key Nutrients

73% vitamin A

42% iron

35% magnesium

25% calcium

Diabetic Exchanges

2 lean meats

1 vegetable

Oat-Nut Burgers

This recipe is modified from a recipe in *Meatless Meals for Working People*. When my picky friends ate these, they wanted seconds! If you have hamburger lovers at your house, you can put just about any type of burgers between the buns, and they'll be happy.

Makes: 3 to 4 servings

⅔ *cup rolled oats*

⅔ *cup cashews (or other nuts), chopped*

1 onion, chopped

3 stalks celery, chopped

2 carrots, grated (or use 1 carrot and ½ small zucchini, grated)

¼ *cup whole-wheat flour*

¼ *cup water*

1 teaspoon soy sauce (optional)

Salt and pepper to taste

Oil or cooking spray

1. Mix all ingredients. Season to taste with salt, pepper, or soy sauce.

2. Shape into 6 burgers.

3. Cook in lightly oiled pan (or pan sprayed with cooking spray) until brown on both sides; or broil burgers in oven.

4. Serve on toasted buns with lettuce, tomato, and so on. Oven-fried potatoes (page 345) go great with these burgers.

Nutrient Analysis per Serving

189 calories

25 grams carbohydrate

7 grams protein

8 grams fat

4 grams fiber

Key Nutrients

49% vitamin A

23% magnesium

11% zinc

Diabetic Exchanges

1½ fats

1½ starches

1 vegetable

Quick Grilled Fish

I never enjoyed thick cuts of fish until I started marinating them. Marinating adds flavor and keeps fish moist. We enjoy fish cooked this way at least twice a month!

1 pound halibut, salmon, or other fish steaks

½ cup vinaigrette or fat-free Italian dressing (Experiment with different dressings.)

1. Pour fish and dressing into Ziploc bag. Marinate in refrigerator at least 1 hour; the longer the better.

2. Grill approximately 10 minutes per inch of thickness at thickest part; or broil at 450°F for same amount of time. Fish is cooked when opaque and flakes easily with fork.

Nutrient Analysis per Serving
(4 ounces)

158 calories
less than 1 gram carbohydrate
23 grams protein
6 grams fat

Key Nutrients

81% selenium
47% vitamin B$_{12}$
27% magnesium

Diabetic Exchanges

3 lean meats

Sesame Beef

This recipe was modified from a recipe in the 1991 National Beef Cookoff.

Makes: 6 servings

2 pounds boneless top sirloin

Marinade

¼ cup rice wine or white wine vinegar

¼ cup soy sauce

2 tablespoons dark sesame oil

1 tablespoon granulated sugar

1 teaspoon fresh ginger, minced

1 teaspoon baking soda

2 teaspoons cornstarch

Sauce

8 ounces beef broth

2 tablespoons cornstarch

½ cup light brown sugar, packed

¼ cup hoisin sauce

1½ tablespoons sesame seeds

1 tablespoon teriyaki sauce

½ tablespoon molasses

1 clove garlic, minced

1 tablespoon dark sesame oil

Garnish

1 large head romaine lettuce, shredded

Sesame seeds

Crushed red-pepper pods or hot chili paste (optional)

1. Slice beef into 1-inch strips; remove all fat.

2. Mix together marinade ingredients. Toss with beef and store in plastic bag, turning occasionally. Marinate in refrigerator at least 30 minutes, preferably overnight.

3. Drain marinade. Cook beef quickly in nonstick pan, adding small amount of oil if needed. Keep warm.

4. Mix 2 tablespoons broth with cornstarch; set aside. Mix remaining broth with next 5 sauce ingredients.

5. Add garlic and ½ teaspoon oil to same pan in which you cooked beef. Sauté 1 minute.

6. Add sauce mixture; bring to boil. Add broth-cornstarch mixture. Cook over medium heat until thickened, stirring occasionally.

7. Arrange lettuce on platter. Top with meat and drizzle with sauce or serve sauce on side. Sprinkle with sesame seeds and optional crushed red pepper.

Diabetic Variation

Follow directions for sauce, omitting brown sugar and molasses.

Diabetic Exchanges

6 lean meats

1 vegetable

Nutrient Analysis per Serving

451 calories

30 grams carbohydrate

42 grams protein

17 grams fat

Key Nutrients

65% zinc

36% vitamin B₆

22% iron

11% folate

Nutrient Analysis (meat and lettuce)

357 calories

6 grams carbohydrate

42 grams protein

17 grams fat

Spinach-Stuffed Shells

I recently discovered large pasta shells. Shells can be the busy cook's elegant meal!
They freeze well, so try doubling the recipe and freezing half.

Makes: 4 servings

*1 10-ounce package frozen
    spinach, cooked or thawed
    and well drained*

*1 cup low-fat or fat-free cottage
    cheese*

*⅓ cup Parmesan cheese,
    preferably freshly grated*

½ cup mozzarella cheese, grated

*¼ teaspoon garlic powder
    or to taste*

*½ pound large pasta shells,
    cooked until still slightly firm
    (al dente) and drained*

*2½ cups prepared low-fat
    marinara sauce*

Garnish

*Mozzarella and Parmesan
    cheese, grated*

1. Preheat oven to 350°F.

2. Mix all ingredients except shells until well blended.

3. Stuff shells with spinach mixture. Cover with marinara sauce. Bake 30 minutes.

4. Sprinkle with a bit of extra cheese just before serving.

Variation

Double the amounts of pasta and spinach. Drain 1 pound of firm tofu and squeeze out excess water. In food processor, blend tofu, 2 cloves fresh garlic, and a bunch of fresh basil leaves until smooth. Add cottage cheese and blend until smooth. Remove from processor and stir in spinach. Stuff and cook shells as directed above.

Nutrient Analysis per Serving

388 calories
58 grams carbohydrate
25 grams protein
7 grams fat

Key Nutrients

78% vitamin A
54% calcium
42% vitamin C
34% folate

Diabetic Exchanges

3 starches
2 lean meats
2 vegetables

Tofu Loaf

This recipe is from Norma Robinson. The pecans give it an interesting texture and flavor.

Makes: 8 servings

16 ounces low-fat tofu, firm

¼ cup pecans, chopped

½ cup canned tomatoes, chopped

2 egg whites

¼ cup skim milk

½ cup dry seasoned bread crumbs or old-fashioned oatmeal

½ teaspoon salt

½ teaspoon each onion and garlic powder

1 teaspoon thyme, cumin, oregano, or Italian seasoning

Optional seasonings: finely chopped parsley, green onion, or celery

Cooking spray

1. Preheat oven to 350°F.

2. Squeeze out excess liquid from tofu and crumble. With spoon, mix with rest of ingredients until well blended.

3. Pour into loaf pan that has been sprayed with cooking spray. Bake 50 to 60 minutes.

4. Serve like meat loaf with ketchup, salsa, or pasta sauce, or on a bun like a burger. Leftovers are great as sandwiches.

Nutrient Analysis per Serving

86 calories

5 grams carbohydrate

8 grams protein

4 grams fat

Key Nutrients

26% iron

20% magnesium

14% calcium

Diabetic Exchanges

1 lean meat

1 vegetable

1 fat

Veal Piccata with Roasted Red Pepper Sauce

The sauce makes this dish tasty and colorful.

Makes: 4 servings

16 ounces veal loin

3 tablespoons lemon juice

½ to 1 clove garlic, crushed

Sauce

½ green onion, chopped (If you can't tolerate onions, just use green tops.)

1 heaping cup roasted red bell peppers (can be bought in jar)

2 tablespoons white wine vinegar (can be flavored)

⅓ cup parsley (or 2 fresh spinach or lettuce leaves)

⅓ cup nonfat yogurt or reduced-fat sour cream

Dash cayenne pepper (optional)

1. Marinate veal in lemon juice and garlic in refrigerator for at least 1 hour.

2. Cook over medium-high heat or grill to desired doneness.

3. Purée all sauce ingredients except yogurt in food processor or blender. Place in microwave-safe dish and heat on medium-high 2 minutes.

4. Fold in yogurt or sour cream. Return to microwave for 30 seconds on high. Stir and serve over meat. (The sauce can be made ahead of time and refrigerated.)

Variation

Turkey tenderloin or chicken breast can also be used.

Nutrient Analysis per Serving

301 calories
5 grams carbohydrate
39 grams protein
12 grams fat

Key Nutrients

44% vitamin C
32% zinc
22% vitamin B_6

Diabetic Exchanges

5½ lean meats
1 vegetable

Vegetable-and-Tofu Stir-Fry

You won't even miss the meat!

Makes: 4 servings

2 tablespoons vinegar

½ teaspoon sesame oil

2 tablespoons hoisin sauce

4 tablespoons light soy sauce

¼ cup water

1 pound low-fat, firm tofu, cubed

2 tablespoons chicken broth

1 to 2 teaspoons ginger

2 cloves garlic, minced

3 green onions, chopped

4 cups mixed vegetables
(carrots, bell peppers, bean
sprouts, cabbage, broccoli,
snow peas) or 1 pound
frozen vegetable mixture

1. Mix together vinegar, sesame oil, hoisin sauce, soy sauce, and water. Add tofu and marinate 10 to 20 minutes.

2. Heat chicken broth in nonstick pan. Add ginger, garlic, and green onions. Sauté 2 minutes.

3. Add vegetables (except broccoli) and stir-fry until tender-crisp. Add more chicken broth or water to pan if necessary.

4. Add tofu and cook, turning until brown on all sides. Remove from pan and set aside.

5. Add broccoli to pan along with remaining marinade and stir-fry until broccoli is tender-crisp.

6. Add tofu and continue cooking until warm.

Serving Suggestion

This dish is great served over brown rice, bulgur, or noodles.

Nutrient Analysis per Serving

117 calories

11 grams carbohydrate

15 grams protein

3 grams fat

3 grams fiber

Key Nutrients

133% vitamin C

29% vitamin A

19% potassium

Diabetic Exchanges

2 very lean meats

2 vegetables

Vegetarian Breakfast Tacos

Linda Hood developed this recipe, which won first place for entrées in a local recipe contest. The term *Mexican food* often brings to mind high fat content, but this recipe is low in fat and full of flavor. It is not spicy, and you may make it even milder by reducing garlic and onion and using mild salsa (or chopped tomatoes with lemon juice and onion powder). You can also use parsley instead of cilantro.

Makes: 4 servings

2 teaspoons olive or canola oil

1 small clove garlic

½ cup onion, chopped

½ cup green pepper, chopped

1 medium potato, chopped

1 small zucchini, chopped

*1 egg, plus 2 egg whites
(or 3 whole eggs)*

1 medium tomato, chopped

1 tablespoon cilantro or parsley, chopped

Salt and pepper to taste

*4 whole-wheat flour
or corn tortillas*

1 cup Mexican salsa

*4 ounces part-skim mozzarella
cheese, shredded*

1. In oil, sauté garlic, onion, and green pepper.

2. Add potato and zucchini. Stir until tender.

3. Push veggies aside and scramble eggs in middle of skillet; gradually stir in vegetables.

4. Add tomato and heat thoroughly.

5. Season with cilantro, salt and pepper.

6. Steam tortillas on top of mixture in covered skillet. Fill tortillas with vegetable-egg mixture. Fold over.

7. Spoon salsa over folded tortilla and sprinkle cheese on top.

Nutrient Analysis per Serving

255 calories

27 grams carbohydrate

16 grams protein

10 grams fat

3 grams fiber

Key Nutrients

51% vitamin C

20% calcium

14% vitamin B_{12}

Diabetic Exchanges

1½ lean meats

1½ starches

1 fat

1 vegetable

Favorite Snack Cake

This is one of my son's favorite snacks. Unfortunately, it's also our dog's favorite–
the first time I made this cake, he climbed on the counter and finished it off!

Makes: 12 servings

1¼ cups whole-wheat flour

½ cup rolled oats

¼ cup cornstarch

1 teaspoon baking soda

*1 teaspoon each ground ginger
and cinnamon*

½ teaspoon ground cloves

½ teaspoon salt

1 large egg

2 tablespoons canola oil

½ cup blackstrap molasses

*1¾ cups applesauce
(Use the kind that's fortified
with vitamin C.)*

Margarine and flour

1. Preheat oven to 325°F.

2. Mix together all dry ingredients and spices.

3. In separate bowl, combine egg, oil, molasses, and applesauce.

4. Gradually add egg mixture to dry ingredients.

5. Pour batter into greased and floured 9-by-9-inch pan. (In a pinch you can also use a 9-inch pie plate.)

6. Bake 45 minutes, or until knife inserted in middle comes out clean. Let cool on wire rack.

Nutrient Analysis per Serving

129 calories
25 grams carbohydrate
2 grams protein
3 grams fat
2 grams fiber

Key Nutrients

23% potassium
10% calcium
9% iron

Diabetic Exchanges

1½ starches
½ fat

Fruit Crisp

This recipe from the National Heart, Lung, and Blood Institute is full of fiber and vitamins. Try the summer and winter variations, or come up with your own.

Makes: 6 servings

Winter Variation

Filling

½ *cup sugar*

3 tablespoons all-purpose flour

1 teaspoon lemon peel, grated

¼ *teaspoon lemon juice*

5 cups apples, unpeeled, sliced

1 cup fresh cranberries
  or ½ cup raisins

Topping

⅔ *cup rolled oats*

⅓ *cup brown sugar, packed*

¼ *cup whole-wheat flour*

2 teaspoons ground cinnamon

1 tablespoon soft margarine,
  melted

1. To prepare filling, in medium bowl, combine sugar, flour, and lemon peel; mix well. Add lemon juice, apples, and cranberries and stir to mix.

2. To prepare topping, in small bowl, combine oats, brown sugar, flour, and cinnamon. Add melted margarine and stir to mix.

3. Pour apple mixture into baking pan and sprinkle oat mixture on top.

4. Bake in 375°F oven for approximately 40 to 50 minutes. Serve warm or at room temperature. It's delicious with low-fat yogurt!

Summer Variation

Instead of apples and cranberries, substitute 4 cups fresh or unsweetened frozen (thawed) peaches and 3 cups fresh or frozen (unthawed) blueberries. If frozen, thaw peaches completely (do not drain). Do not thaw blueberries before mixing or they will be crushed.

Note: This dish contains a significant amount of carbohydrate, and women with diabetes should eat it only in very small amounts.

Nutrient Analysis per Serving
(winter variation)

283 calories
62 grams carbohydrate
4 grams protein
4 grams fat
5 grams fiber

Key Nutrients

13% magnesium
10% vitamin C
8% chromium

Nutrient Analysis per Serving
(summer variation)

309 calories
68 grams carbohydrate
5 grams protein
4 grams fat
7 grams fiber

Key Nutrients

37% manganese
24% vitamin C
21% potassium
11% vitamin A

Diabetic Exchanges

Winter	*2 fruits*	
	2 starches	
Summer	*2½ fruits*	
	2 starches	

Fruit Pizza for a Crowd

This recipe is adapted from the book *Quick and Healthy Recipes and Ideas* by Brenda Ponichtera. The secret to this impressive dessert is to arrange the fruit in attractive patterns—try combinations of strawberries, raspberries, blueberries, and kiwi fruit. You can also add light whipped topping. (See notation below for using different-size pans.) This dessert is considered a "somewhat healthy" splurge, so go easy on portion sizes!

Makes: 18 servings

*1 package (20 ounces)
Pillsbury Sugar Cookie Dough*

*1 quart strawberries
(or other fresh fruit),
washed and hulled*

*1 large box (5.1 ounces) vanilla
instant pudding*

3 cups skim milk

*6 ounces fat-free cream cheese,
room temperature*

Cooking spray

Source: Reprinted with permission from *Quick and Healthy Recipes and Ideas* by Brenda J. Ponichtera, R.D. (ScaleDown Publishing, Inc.).

1. Preheat oven to 350°F.

2. Spray pizza pan with cooking spray.

3. Slice cookie dough into ¼-inch slices.

4. Arrange slices on pizza pan so that they are ½ to 1 inch apart. Bake 18 to 20 minutes or until golden and set. Cool.

5. In small mixing bowl, combine pudding mix and milk. Beat on low to mix. Add cream cheese and beat until smooth and thickened.

6. Pour over cooled cookie crust. Arrange fruit on top.

Note: This amount will also make four 8-inch pizzas or one 11-by-14-inch and one 8-inch pizza. Eight-inch cake pans work fine.

Diabetic Variation

Use sugar-free pudding instead of regular pudding. This diabetic variation still contains significant amounts of sugar. Women with diabetes should either skip this recipe or eat only in limited amounts.

Nutrient Analysis per Serving

*191 calories
31 grams carbohydrate
5 grams fat
4 grams protein*

Key Nutrients

*27% vitamin C
Small amounts of
many other nutrients*

Nutrient Analysis per Serving
(Diabetic Variation)

*167 calories
25 grams carbohydrate
5 grams fat
4 grams protein*

Diabetic Exchanges

*1½ starches
1 fat
½ very lean meat*

Sunshine Sorbet

The beauty of this dessert is that it's made entirely of fruit, with no added sugar or thickener!

Makes: 5 servings

1 20-ounce can crushed
  pineapple, in its own juice

1 ripe banana, sliced

3 nectarines, peeled and sliced,
  or 1 cup canned peaches,
  in their own juice

1 cup strawberries, fresh or
  frozen, unsweetened

2 teaspoons orange or lemon
  rind, freshly grated

Garnish

Fresh mint

1. Freeze fruit before preparing. Thaw pineapple enough to slice into chunks.

2. Place all fruit in food processor, and process until smooth. Scrape down sides occasionally.

3. Serve immediately; garnish with mint sprigs or place in 8-by-8-inch pan and freeze.

4. To serve after freezing: Thaw enough to break into chunks. Process again in food processor and store in airtight freezer container.

Nutrient Analysis per Serving

112 calories
1 gram protein
less than 1 gram fat
2 grams fiber

Key Nutrients

36% vitamin C
19% potassium
12% vitamin B_6

Diabetic Exchanges

2 fruits

References

Chapter 1

1. "Knowledge and Use of Folic Acid by Women of Childbearing Age–United States, 1995 and 1998." *Morbidity and Mortality Weekly Report,* 1999 Apr. 30; 48(16): 325–7.

2. Willett, W. C. "Folic Acid and Neural Tube Defects: Can't We Come to Closure." *American Journal of Public Health,* 82, 5, May 1992: 666.

3. Fall, C., et al. "Fetal and Infant Growth and Cardiovascular Risk Factors in Women." *British Medical Journal,* 310, 1995: 428–432.

4. Godfrey, K. M., et al. "Maternal Nutritional Status in Pregnancy and Blood Pressure in Childhood." *British Journal of Obstetrics and Gynæcology,* 101, 5, May 1994: 398.

5. Kitzmiller, J., et al. "Pre-Conception Care of Diabetes. Glycemic Control Prevents Congenital Anomalies." *Journal of the American Medical Association,* 265, 6, 1991: 731.

6. Achadi, E. L., et al. "Women's Nutritional Status, Iron Consumption and Weight Gain during Pregnancy in Relation to Neonatal Weight and Length in West Java, Indonesia." *International Journal of Gynæcology and Obstetrics,* 48, suppl., June 1995: S103.

7. Crawford, M. "The Role of Essential Fatty Acids in Neural Development: Implications for Perinatal Nutrition." *American Journal of Clinical Nutrition,* 57, suppl., 1993: S703.

8. Buchanan, T. A., and S. L. Kjos. "Gestational Diabetes: Risk or Myth." *Journal of Clinical Endocrinology and Metabolism,* 1999 Jun; 84(6): 1854–7.

9. Olds, D. "Intellectual Impairment in Children of Women Who Smoke Cigarettes during Pregnancy." *Pediatrics,* 93, 2, 1994: 221.

10. Sasco, A. J., and H. Vainio. "From in Utero and Childhood Exposure to Parental Smoking to Childhood Cancer: A Possible Link and the Need for Action." *Human Experimental Toxicology,* 1999 Apr.; 18(4): 192–201.

11. Wilkinson, C. E., et al. "Trends in Food and Nutrient Intakes by Adults: NFCS 1977-78, CSFI 1989-1991, and CSFII 1994-95." *Family Economics and Nutrition Review,* 1997 10(4).

12. Haines, P. S., et al. "Trends in Breakfast Consumption of U.S. Adults between 1965 and 1991." American Dietetic Association. 1996 May; 96(5): 464–70.

13. Cnattingius, S., et al. "Pre-pregnancy Weight and the Risk of Adverse Pregnancy Outcomes." *New England Journal of Medicine,* January 15, 1998, 338(3): 147–153.

14. Werler, M., et al. "Prepregnant Weight in Relation to Risk of Neural Tube Defects." *Journal of the American Medical Association,* 275, 14, April 10, 1996: 1089.

Shaw, G. "Risk of Neural Tube Defect Affected Pregnancies among Obese Women." Journal of the American Medical Association, 275, 14, April 10, 1996: 1093.

15. Clark, A. M., et al. "Weight Loss Results in Significant Improvement in Pregnancy and Ovulation Rates in Anovulatory Obese Women." *Human Reproduction,* 1995 Oct. 10(10): 2705–12.

16. Worthington-Roberts, Bonnie, and Sue Williams. *Nutrition in Pregnancy and Lactation,* 6th edition, Brown and Benchmark Publishers, 1997, p. 32.

17. Shen, H. M., et al. "Evaluation of Oxidative DNA Damage in Human Sperm and Its Association with Male Infertility." *Journal of Andrology,* 1999 Nov.–Dec.; 20(6): 718–23.

18. Fraga, C. G., et al. *Mutation Research,* 1996 Apr. 13; 351(2): 199–203.

19. Augood. C. "Smoking and Female Infertility: A Systematic Review and Meta-Analysis." *Human Reproduction,* 1998 Jun.; 13(6): 1532–9.

20. Bolumar, F., et al. "Caffeine Intake and Delayed Conception: A European Multicenter Study on Infertility and Subfecundity." European Study Group on Infertility and Subfecundity. *American Journal of Epidemiology,* 1997 Feb. 15; 145(4): 324–34.

21. Pirke, K., et al. "Dieting Influences the Menstrual Cycle: Vegetarian versus Nonvegetarian Diet." *Fertility and Sterility,* 46, 6, 1986: 1083.

22. Stewart, D. "Reproductive Functions in Eating Disorders." *Annals of Medicine,* 24, 1992: 287.

23. Ibid.

24. Rushton, D. "Ferritin and Fertility." Letter. *The Lancet,* 337, 1991: 1554.

25. Jensen, T. K., et al. "Does Moderate Alcohol Consumption Affect Fertility? Follow Up Study among Couples Planning First Pregnancy." *British Medical Journal,* 1998 Aug. 22; 317(7157): 505–10.

26. Cicero, T. J., et al. "Acute Alcohol Exposure Markedly Influences Male Fertility and Fetal Outcome in the Male Rat." *Life Science* 1994; 55(12): 901–10.

27. Dawson, E., et al. "Effect of Vitamin C Supplementation on Sperm Quality of Heavy Smokers." *Federation of the American Societies for Experimental Biology Journal,* 5, 4, 1991: A915.

Dawson, E. "Effect of Ascorbic Acid on Male Fertility." Annals of the New York Academy of Science, 498, 1987: 312.

28. Werbach, M. *Nutritional Influences on Illness.* 2nd edition. Tarzana, Calif.: Third Line Press, 1993: 376–381.

29. Kemmann, E., et al. "Amenorrhea Associated with Carotenemia." *Journal of the American Medical Association,* 249, 7, 1983: 926.

30. Shortbridge, L. "Advances in the Assessment of the Effect of Environmental and Occupational Toxins on Reproduction." *Journal of Perinatal and Neonatal Nursing,* 3, 4, 1990: 1.

31. Fraga, C. "Ascorbic Acid Protects against Endogenous Oxidative DNA Damage in Human Sperm." Proceedings of the National Academy of Sciences, 88, December 1991: 11003.

32. U.S. Environmental Protection Agency, Office of Water. *Lead in Your Drinking Water,* June 1993, pub # EPA/810-F93-001.

33. Wilson, J. *The Pre-Pregnancy Planner.* Garden City, N.Y.: Doubleday & Co. Inc., 1986: 70.

34. Lindbohm, M. L., et al. "Effects of Paternal Occupational Exposure on Spontaneous Abortions." *American Journal of Public Health,* 81, 1991: 1029.

35. Shortbridge, L. "Advances in the Assessment of the Effect of Environmental and Occupational Toxins on Reproduction."*Journal of Perinatal and Neonatal Nursing,* 3, 4, 1990: 1.

36. *Food-Borne Risks in Pregnancy,* March of Dimes Birth Defects Foundation, 1998, Pub # 09-1305-99 8/99.

37. Center for Disease Control. "Recommendations for the Use of Folic Acid to Reduce the Number of Cases of Spina Bifida and Other Neural Tube Defects." *Morbidity and Mortality Weekly,* 11, 41 (RR-14), September 1992: 1, 3.

38. Ries, C., et al. "Impact of Commercial Eating on Nutrient Adequacy." *Journal of the American Dietetic Association,* 87, 1987: 463.

39. American College of Obstetricians and Gynecologists. *Planning for Pregnancy, Birth, and Beyond.* Washington, D.C.: ACOG, 1990: 10.

Chapter 2

1. International Food Information Council and the American Dietetic Association. "How Are Kids Making Food Choices?" July 1991.

2. Cong, K., et al. "Calcium Supplementation during Pregnancy for Reducing Pregnancy-Induced Hypertension." *Chinese Medical Journal,* 108, 1, January 1995: 57.

3. Committee on Diet and Health, National Research Council. *Diet and Health: Implications for Reducing Chronic Disease Risk.* Washington, D.C.: National Academy Press, 1989: 514–515.

4. Scholl, T.O. "Anemia vs. Iron Deficiency: Increased Risk of Preterm Delivery in a Prospective Study." *American Journal of Clinical Nutrition,* 1992 May; 55 (5): 985–8.

5. Duyff, R. L. *The American Dietetic Association's Complete Food and Nutrition Guide.* Wylie, N.Y.: 1998, page 106.

6. Committee on Diet and Health, National Research Council. *Diet and Health: Implications for Reducing Chronic Disease Risk.* Washington, D.C.: National Academy Press, 1989: 678.

7. Carmichael, S. L., and B. A. Abrams. "Critical Review of the Relationship between Gestational Weight Gain and Preterm Delivery." *Obstetrics and Gynecology,* 1997 May; 89 (5 pt. 2): 865–73.

8. Office of Public Information, University of California-Berkeley. News Release. May 1992.

9. Committee to Study the Prevention of Low Birth Weight, Division of Disease Prevention and Health Promotion, Institute of Medicine. *Preventing Low Birth Weight.* Washington, D.C.: National Academy Press, 1985: 1.

10. Hickey, C., et al. "Relationship of Psychosocial Status to Low Prenatal Weight Gain among Nonobese Black and White Women Delivering at Term." *Obstetrics and Gynecology,* 86, 2, August 1995: 177.

11. Tuthill, D. P., et al. "Maternal Cigarette Smoking and Pregnancy Outcome." *Pædiatric Perinatology and Epidemiology,* 1999 July; 13 (3): 245–53.

12. Lichtenstein, A. H., et al. "Dietary Fat Consumption and Health." *Nutrition Reviews.* 1998 May; 56 (5 pt. 2): S3–19; discussion S19–28.

13. Stender, S., et al. "The Influence of Trans-Fatty Acids on Health: A Report from the Danish Nutrition Council." *Clinical Science* (Colch) 88, 4, April 1995: 375.

14. American Heart Association. *The American Heart Association Diet–An Eating Plan for Healthy Americans.* 1998.

15. NIH Consensus Conference. "NIH Consensus-Development Panel on Optimal Calcium Intake." *Journal of the American Medical Association,* 272, 24, December 28, 1994: 1942.

16. Committee on Diet and Health, National Research Council. *Diet and Health: Implications for Reducing Chronic Disease Risk.* Washington, D.C.: National Academy Press, 1989: 515.

17. Rothman, K. "Teratogenicity of High Vitamin A Intake." *New England Journal of Medicine,* 333, 21, November 1995: 1369.

18. Specker, B. "Do North American Women Need Supplemental Vitamin D during Pregnancy?" *American Journal of Clinical Nutrition,* 59, 2, suppl., February 1994: 484S.

19. Studzinski, G., and D. Moore. "Sunlight–Can It Prevent as well as Cause Cancer?" *Cancer Research,* 55, 18, September 1995: 4014.

20. Bailey, L. "The Role of Folate in Human Nutrition." *Nutrition Today,* September/October 1990: 12.

21. "Knowledge and Use of Folic Acid by Women of Childbearing Age–United States, 1995 and 1998." *Morbidity and Mortality Weekly Report,* 1999 April 30; 48(16): 325–7.

22. Committee on Diet and Health, National Research Council. *Diet and Health: Implications for Reducing Chronic Disease Risk.* Washington, D.C.: National Academy Press, 1989: 71.

23. Jameson, S. "Zinc Status in Pregnancy: The Effect of Zinc Therapy on Perinatal Mortality, Prematurity, and Placental Ablation." *Annals of the New York Academy of Science,* 15, 678, March 1993: 178.

24. Committee on Diet and Halth, National Research Council. *Diet and Health: Implications for Reducing Chronic Disease Risk.* Washington, D.C.: National Academy Press, 1989: 422.

25. Ibid: 73.

26. National Academy of Sciences Report: *Nutrition during Pregnancy:* 15.

27. Ibid: 16, 254.

28. Rothman, K. "Teratogenicity of High Vitamin A Intake.*" New England Journal of Medicine,* 333, 21, November 1995: 1369.

29. Belizan, J., et al. "Calcium Supplementation to Prevent Hypertensive Disorders of Pregnancy." *New England Journal of Medicine,* 325, November 14, 1991: 1399.

Yabes-Almirante, C. "Calcium Supplementation in Pregnancy to Prevent Pregnancy-Induced Hypertension (PIH)." *Journal of Perinatal Medicine,* 1998; 26(5): 347–53.

Crowther, C. A., et al. "Calcium Supplementation in Nulliparous Women for the Prevention of Pregnancy-Induced Hypertension, Preeclampsia and Preterm Birth: An Australian Randomized Trial." FRACOG and the ACT Study Group. *Australia-New Zealand Journal of Obstetrics and Gynæcology,* 1999 Feb.; 39(1): 12–8.

30. Gulson, B. L. "Mobilization of Lead from the Skeleton during the Postnatal Period is Larger than during Pregnancy." *Journal of Laboratory and Clinical Medicine,* 1998 Apr.; 131(4): 324–9.

McGowan, J. A. "Bone: Target and Source of Environmental Pollutant Exposure." *Otolaryngology Head and Neck Surgery,* 1996 Feb.; 114(2): 220–3.

31. Hallberg, L., et al. "Calcium Effect of Different Amounts on Nonheme and Heme Iron Absorption in Humans." *American Journal of Clinical Nutrition,* 53, 1991: 112.

32. Kahn, A. "Prenatal Exposure to Cigarettes in Infants with Obstructive Sleep Apnea." *Pediatrics,* 93, 5, May 1994: 778.

33. Olds, D. "Intellectual Impairment in Children of Women Who Smoke Cigarettes during Pregnancy." *Pediatrics,* 93, 2, February 1994: 221.

34. Kandel, D. B., and J. R. Udry. "Prenatal Effects of Maternal Smoking on Daughters' Smoking: Nicotine or Testosterone Exposure?" *American Journal of Public Health,* 1999 Sep.; 89(9): 1377–83.

Weissman, M. M., et al. "Maternal Smoking during Pregnancy and Psychopathology in Offspring Followed to Adulthood. *Journal of the American Academy of Child and Adolescent Psychiatry,* 1999 Jul.; 38(7): 892–9.

Brennan, P. A., et al. "Maternal Smoking during Pregnancy and Adult Male Criminal Outcomes." *Archives of General Psychiatry,* 1999 Mar.; 56(3): 215–9.

35. Wahlgren, D. R. "Involuntary Smoking and Asthma." *Current Opinions in Pulmonary Medicine,* 2000 Jan.; 6(1): 31–6.

36. Subcommittee on Nutritional Status and Weight Gain during Pregnancy. *Nutrition during Pregnancy.* Washington, D.C.: National Academy Press, 1990: 394.

37. Farley, D. "Dangers of Lead Still Linger." *FDA Consumer,* Jan.–Feb. 1998. 32(1).

38. *Consumer Reports Magazine.* "Lead in Water, Pipe Nightmares.*" Consumer Reports Magazine,* July 1995: 463.

39. Farley, D. "Dangers of Lead Still Linger." *FDA Consumer,* Jan.–Feb. 1998. 32(1).

40. West, J. R. "Fetal Alcohol Syndrome: A Review for Texas Physicians." *Texas Medicine,* 1998 Jul.; 94(7): 61–7.

41. *Diet and Health:* 450.

42. "Update: Trends in Fetal Alcohol Syndrome: United States, 1979-1993." *Morbidity and Mortality Weekly Report,* 1995 Apr. 7; 44(13): 249–51.

43. Ibid.

44. Hinds, T. S., et al. "The Effect of Caffeine on Pregnancy Outcome Variables." *Nutrition Reviews,* 1996 July; 54 (7): 203–7.

45. Jacobson, M., et al. *Safe Food: Eating Wisely in a Risky World.* Los Angeles, Calif.: Living Planet Press, 1991: 45.

46. *The Boston Globe.* December 13, 1989: 1.

47. Sullivan, K. "Maternal Implications of Cocaine Use during Pregnancy." *The Journal of Perinatal and Neonatal Nursing,* 3, 4, 1990: 12.

48. Ibid.

49. Haines, P., et al. "Eating Patterns and Energy and Nutrient Intakes of U.S. Women." *Journal of the American Dietetic Association,* 92, 6, June 1992: 698.

50. Ibid.

Chapter 3

1. Subcommittee on Nutritional Status and Weight Gain during Pregnancy. *Nutrition during Pregnancy.* Washington, D.C.: National Academy Press, 1990: 430.

2. Food and Nutrition Board. *Recommended Dietary Allowances.* Revised 1989. Washington, D.C.: National Academy Press, 1998.

3. National Academy of Sciences. *Nutrition during Pregnancy.* Washington, D.C.: National Academy Press, 1990: 386.

4. Scholl, T. "Low Zinc Intake during Pregnancy: Its Association with Preterm and Very Preterm Delivery." *American Journal of Epidemiology,* 137, 10, May 15, 1993: 1115.

5. Slavin, J. L., et al. "Plausible Mechanisms for the Protectiveness of Whole Grains." *American Journal of Clinical Nutrition,* 1999 Sep.; 70(3 suppl.): 459S–463S.

6. Anderson, J. W., et al. "Effects of Psyllium on Glucose and Serum Lipid Responses in Men with Type II Diabetes and Hypercholesterolemia." *American Journal of Clinical Nutrition,* 1999 Oct.; 70(4): 466–73.

Cohen, L. A. "Dietary Fiber and Breast Cancer." *Anticancer Research,* 1999 Sep.–Oct.; 19(5A): 3685–8.

7. National Center for Nutrition and Dietetics, The American Dietetic Association. "Whole Grain Goodness–Three Are Key." Nutrition Fact Sheet.

8. Committee on Diet and Halth, National Research Council. *Diet and Health: Implications for Reducing Chronic Disease Risk.* Washington, D.C.: National Academy Press, 1989: 678.

9. Aikins, Murphy P. "Alternative Therapies for Nausea and Vomiting of Pregnancy.*" Obstetrics and Gynecology,* 1998 Jan. 91(1): 149–55.

Chapter 4

1. Subcommittee on Nutritional Status and Weight Gain during Pregnancy. *Nutrition during Pregnancy.* Washington, D.C.: National Academy Press, 1990: 12.

2. American Dietetic Association. "Position of the American Dietetic Association: Vegetarian Diets." *Journal of the American Dietetic Association,* 93, 11, November 1993: 1317.

3. Anderson, J., et al. "Meta-Analysis of the Effects of Soy Protein Intake on Serum Cholesterol." *New England Journal of Medicine,* 333, 5, August 3, 1995: 276.

4. Widhalm, K. "Effect of Soy Protein Diet versus Standard Low-Fat, Low-Cholesterol Diet on Lipid and Lipoprotein Levels in Children with Familial or Polygenic Hypercholesteroloemia." *Journal of Pediatrics,* 123, 1, July 1993: 30.

5. Scheiber, M. D., and R. W. Rebar. "Isoflavones and Postmenopausal Bone Health: A Viable Alternative to Estrogen Therapy?" *Menopause,* 1999 Fall; 6(3): 233–41.

6. Food and Nutrition Board. *Recommended Dietary Allowances.* 10th edition. Washington, D.C.: National Academy Press, 1989.

7. Szilagyi, A., et al. "Lactose Handling by Women with Lactose Malabsorption Is Improved during Pregnancy." *Clinical and Investigative Medicine,* 1996 Dec; 19(6): 416–26.

8. Solomons, N., et al. "Dietary Manipulation of Postprandial Colonic Lactose Fermentation: Effect of Solid Foods in a Meal." *American Journal of Clinical Nutrition,* 41, 1985: 199.

9. Lee, C., and C. Hardy. "Cocoa Feeding and Human Lactose Intolerance." *American Journal of Clinical Nutrition,* 49, 5, 1989: 840.

10. Recker, R., et al. "Calcium Absorbability from Milk Products, an Imitation Milk-and-

Calcium Carbonate." *American Journal of Clinical Nutrition,* 47, 1988: 93.

11. Whitney, E., and F. Sizer. *Nutrition: Concepts and Controversies.* Saint Paul, Minn.: West Publishing Company, 1988: 248.

12. CSPI Staff. *Nutrition Action Healthletter,* May 1992: 11.

Chapter 5

1. Food and Nutrition Board, Institute of Medicine. *Dietary Reference Intakes: Recommended Intakes for Individuals,* Washington, D.C.: National Academy of Sciences, 1999.

2. Subcommittee on Nutritional Status and Weight Gain during Pregnancy. *Nutrition during Pregnancy.* Washington, D.C.: National Academy Press, 1990: 265.

3. Wolraich, M. L., et al. "The Effect of Sugar on Behavior or Cognition in Children: A Meta-Analysis." *Journal of the American Medical Association,* 1995 Nov. 22–29; 274(20): 1617–21.

Overgaard, C., and A. Knudsen. "Pain-Relieving Effect of Sucrose in Newborns during Heel Prick." *Biology of the Neonate,* 1999 May; 75(5): 279–84.

4. U.S. Department of Agriculture. *Report of the Dietary Guidelines Committee on the Dietary Guidelines for Americans 2000,* March 2000.

American Dietetic Association. "Position of the American Dietetic Association: Use of Nutritive and Non-Nutritive Sweeteners." *Journal of the American Dietetic Association,* 98, 1998, 580–587.

Chapter 6

1. Key T. J., et al. "Health Benefits of a Vegetarian Diet." *Proceedings of the Nutrition Society,* 1999 May; 58(2): 271–5.

2. Sacks, F. M., et al. "A Dietary Approach to Prevent Hypertension: A Review of the Dietary Approaches to Stop Hypertension (DASH) Study." *Clinics in Cardiology,* 1999 Jul.; 22(7 suppl.): III6–10.)

"Position of the American Dietetic Association: Vegetarian Diets." *Journal of the American Dietetic Association,* 1997; 97: 1317.

3. Ornish, D. "Intensive Lifestyle Changes for Reversal of Coronary Heart Disease." *Journal of the American Medical Association,* 1998 Dec. 16; 280(23): 2001–7.

4. "Position of the American Dietetic Association: Vegetarian Diets." *Journal of the American Dietetic Association,* 1997; 97: 1317.

5. Janelle, K., and S. Barr. "Nutrient Intakes and Eating Behavior Scores of Vegetarian and Nonvegetarian Women." *Journal of the American Dietetic Association,* 95, 2, February 1995: 180.

6. Craig, W. J. "Iron status of Vegetarians." *American Journal of Clinical Nutrition,* 1994 May; 59(5 suppl.): 1233S–1237S.

Food and Nutrition Board. *Recommended Dietary Allowances,* Revised 1989. Washington, D.C.: National Academy Press, 1998.

7. "Position of the American Dietetic Association: Vegetarian Diets." *Journal of the American Dietetic Association,* 1997; 97: 1317.

8. Messina, Mark and Virginia. *The Dietitian's Guide to Vegetarian Diets.* Gaithersburg, Md.: Aspen Publishers, 1996. 110–112.

9. "Position of the American Dietetic Association: Vegetarian Diets." *Journal of the American Dietetic Association,* 1997; 97: 1317.

10. Glerup, H., et al. "Commonly Recommended Daily Intake of Vitamin D Is Not Sufficient if Sunlight Exposure Is Limited." *Journal of Internal Medicine,* 2000 Feb.; 247(2): 260–8.

11. Freeland-Graves, J., et al. "Zinc Status of Vegetarians." *Journal of the American Dietetic Association,* 80, 12, December 1980: 655.

12. Messina, Mark and Virginia. *The Dietitian's Guide to Vegetarian Diets.* Gaithersburg, Md.: Aspen Publishers, 1996. 28.

13. "Position of the American Dietetic Association: Vegetarian Diets." *Journal of the American Dietetic Association,* 1997; 97: 1317.

Chapter 7

1. Rosenn, B., et al. "Glycemic Thresholds for Spontaneous Abortion and Congenital Malformations in Insulin-Dependent Diabetes Mellitus." *Obstetrics and Gynecology,* 84, 4 October 1994: 515–20.

2. American Diabetes Association. Clinical Practice Recommendations. *Diabetes Care,* 23, (Suppl. 1), January 2000.

3. American Diabetes Association. *Diabetes and Pregnancy: What to Expect.* American Diabetes Association, 1989: 15.

4. Remsberg, K. E., et al. "Diabetes in Pregnancy and Cesarean Delivery." *Diabetes Care,* 22, 9, September 1999: 1561–7.

Berkowitz, G. S., et al. "Risk Factors for Preterm Birth Subtypes." *Epidemiology,* 9, 3 May 1998: 279–85.

American Diabetes Association. "Proceedings of the Fourth Annual Workshop Conference on Gestational Diabetes." *Diabetes Care,* 21 (Suppl. 2), August 1998.

Sibai, B. M., et al. "Risks of Pre-eclampsia and Adverse Neonatal Outcomes among Women with Pregestational Diabetes Mellitus." *American Journal of Obstetrics and Gynecology,* 182, 2, February 2000: 364–9.

5. American College of Obstetricians and Gynecologists. *Planning for Pregnancy, Birth, and Beyond.* Washington, D.C.: ACOG, 1990: 133.

6. American Diabetes Association. "Proceedings of the Fourth Annual Workshop Conference on Gestational Diabetes." *Diabetes Care,* 21 (Suppl. 2), August 1998.

7. American Diabetes Association. "Position Statement of the American Diabetes Association on Preconception Care of Women with Diabetes." American Diabetes Clinical Practice Recommendations. *Diabetes Care,* 21 (Suppl. 1), 1998.

8. California Department of Health Services. California Diabetes and Pregnancy Program: Sweet Success Guidelines for Care, 1999.

9. Krall, L., and R. S. Beaser. *Joslin Diabetes Manual.* 12th edition. Philadelphia, Pa.: Lea and Febiger, 1989: 236.

10. Ruggiero, L., et al. "Impact of Social Support and Stress on Compliance in Women with Gestational Diabetes Mellitus." *Diabetes Care,* 13, 1990: 441.

11. American Diabetes Association. "Why Worry About Gestational Diabetes?" in Diabetes Info [on-line publication]. Alexandria, Va.: 1999 [cited 31 March 2000 from www.diabetes.org].

12. Finney, L. S., and J. M. Gonzalez-Campoy. "Dietary Chromium and Diabetes: Is There a Relationship?" *Clinical Diabetes,* 15, 1 January/February 1997.

13. Ibid: 16.

14. Ibid: 14–15.

15. Langer, O., et al. "Intensified versus Conventional Management of Gestational Diabetes." *American Journal of Obstetrics and Gynecology,* 170, 4, April 1994: 1036.

16. American Diabetes Association. "Proceedings of the Fourth Annual Workshop Conference on Gestational Diabetes." *Diabetes Care,* 21 (Suppl. 2), August 1998.

17. King, H. "Epidemiology of Glucose Intolerance and Gestational Diabetes in Women of Childbearing Age." Proceedings of the Fourth Annual Workshop Conference on Gestational Diabetes. *Diabetes Care,* 21 (Suppl 2), August 1998.

18. American Diabetes Association. "Clinical Practice Recommendations 1998." *Diabetes Care,* 21 (Suppl. 1), 1998.

19. American Diabetes Association. *Gestational Diabetes and Pregnancy: What to Expect.* Alexandria, Va.: American Diabetes Association Inc., 1989: 13.

20. *Sweet Success Diabetes and Pregnancy Program Guidelines for Care.* Sacramento, Calif.: State of California Department of Health Services, Maternal and Child Health, 1992.

21. Spears, B. Telephone interview. April 1992.

22. Jovanovic-Peterson, L., and C. Peterson. "Is Exercise Safe or Useful for Gestational Diabetic Women?" *Diabetes,* 40, Suppl. 2: 179.

23. Jovanovic-Peterson, L. *Managing Your Gestational Diabetes.* Minneapolis, Minn.: Chronimed Publishing Inc., 1994: 55–56.

24. Powers, M. "Guidelines for Making Food Adjustments for Exercise for People," "Nutrition Guide for Professionals," and "Diabetic Education and Meal Planning." American Dietetic Association and American Diabetes Association, 1988, 41.

25. American Dietetic Association. "Position of The American Dietetic Association: Use of Nutritive and Nonnutritive Sweeteners." *Journal of the American Dietetic Association,* 98, 1998: 580–587.

26. Ibid.

27. Ibid.

28. *Chemical Cuisine: CSPI's Guide to Food Additives.* Center for Science in the Public Interest, 2000.

California Diabetes and Pregnancy Program Sweet Success Guidelines for Care. California Department of Health Services, 1999.

29. *Chemical Cuisine: CSPI's Guide to Food Additives.* Center for Science in the Public Interest, 2000.

30. Huggins, C. E. "Natural Sweetener Not Yet Ready for FDA Approval." In Reuters Health Information [online publication]. New York: 27 March 2000 [cited 3 April 2000 from www.reutershealth.com].

31. DiGiacomo, J. E., and W. W. Hay, Jr. "Fetal Glucose Metabolism and Oxygen Consumption during Sustained Hypoglycemia." *Metabolism,* 39, 2, February 1990: 193.

32. Stenninger, E., et al. "Long-Term Neurological Dysfunction and Neonatal Hypoglycemia after Diabetic Pregnancy." *Archives of Diseases in Children: Fetal and Neonatal Edition,* 1998 Nov; 79(3): F174–9.

33. American Diabetes Association. "Clinical Practice Recommendations: Position Statement on Gestational Diabetes Mellitus." *Diabetes Care,* Volume 21, Supplement 1. 1998.

34. U.S. Department of Health and Human Services. *Working Group Report on High Blood Pressure in Pregnancy, High Blood Pressure Education Program.* Washington, D.C.: NIH Publication 91-3029, 1991.

35. Ibid: 6.

Eskenazl, B., et al. "A Multivariate Analysis of Risk Factors for Preeclampsia." *Journal of the American Medical Association,* 266, 2, July 10, 1991: 237.

36. Villar, J., and J. Repke. "Calcium Supplementation May Reduce Preterm Delivery in High Risk Populations." *American Journal of Obstetrics and Gynecology,* 1124, 1990: 103.

Cong, K., et al. "Calcium Supplementation during Pregnancy for Reducing Pregnancy-Induced Hypertension." *Chinese Medical Journal,* 108, 1, January 1995: 57.

37. Marcoux, S., et al. "Job Strain and Pregnancy-Induced Hypertension." *Epidemiology,* 1999 Jul.; 10(4): 376–82.

38. U.S. Department of Health and Human Services. *Working Group Report on High Blood Pressure in Pregnancy.* Washington, D.C.: NIH Publication: 14.

39. Ibid: 2–3.

40. Ibid: 29.

41. Ibid: 6.

42. National Vital Statistics Report, Births: Final Data for 1997. 47,18, April 1999.

Brown, J. "Nutrition and Multifetal Pregnancy." *Journal of the American Dietetic Association,* 100, 3, March 2000.

43. National Vital Statistics Report, Births: Final Data for 1997. 47,18, April 1999.

44. Brown, J. "Nutrition and Multifetal Pregnancy." *Journal of the American Dietetic Association,* 100, 3, March 2000.

45. Subcommittee on Nutritional Status and Weight Gain during Pregnancy. *Nutrition during Pregnancy.* Washington, D.C.: National Academy Press, 1990: 12.

46. Pederson, A. L. "Weight Gain Patterns during Twin Gestation." *Jounal of the American Dietetic Association,* 89, 5, May 1989: 642.

47. Luke, B., et al. "The Importance of Early Weight Gain in the Intrauterine Growth and Birth Weight of Twins." *American Journal of Obstetrics and Gynecology,* 1998 Nov.; 179(5): 1155–61.

48. Lantz, M. E., et al. "Maternal Weight Gain Patterns and Birth Weight Outcome in Twin Gestation." *Obstetrics and Gynecology,* 1996 Apr.; 87(4): 551–6.

49. Smith, L. G. Jr. "Calcium Homeostasis in Pregnant Women Receiving Long-Term Magnesium Sulfate Therapy for Preterm Labor." *American Journal of Obstetrics and Gynecology,* 1992 Jul.; 167(1): 45–51.

50. Levav, A. L., et al. "Long-Term Magnesium Sulfate Tocolysis and Maternal Osteoporosis in a Triplet Pregnancy: A Case Report." *American Journal of Perinatology,* 1998 Jan.; 15(1): 43–6.

51. Okah, F. A. "Bone Turnover and Mineral Metabolism in the Last Trimester of Pregnancy: Effect of Multiple Gestation." *Obstetrics and Gynecology,* 1996 Aug.; 88(2): 168–73.

52. Foreman-van Drongelen, M. M., et al. "Essential Fatty Acid Status Measured in Umbilical Vessel Walls of Infants Born after a Multiple Pregnancy." *Early Human Development,* 1996 Nov. 21; 46(3): 205–15.

Zeijdner, E. E., et al. "Essential Fatty Acid Status in Plasma Phospholipids of Mother and Neonate after Multiple Pregnancy." *Prostaglandins Leukotrienes and Essential Fatty Acids,* 1997 May; 56(5): 395–401.

53. Ollis, T. E., et al. "Australian Food Sources and Intakes of Omega-6 and Omega-3 Polyunsaturated Fatty Acids." *Annals of Nutrition and Metabolism,* 1999 Nov.; 43(6): 346–355.

54. Luke, B., et al. "Improving Outcomes in Twin Pregnancies: Obstetric, Neonatal and Healthcare Cost Implications." *American Journal of Obstetrics and Gynecology,* in press.

55. Dubois, S., et al. "Twin Pregnancy: The Impact of the Higgins Nutrition Intervention Program on Maternal and Neonatal Outcomes." *American Journal of Clinical Nutrition,* 53, 1991: 1397.

56. Cambell, D., et al. "Maternal Nutrition in Twin Pregnancy." *Acta Genetica Gemellologica,* 32, 1982: 221.

57. Cnattingius, S., et al. "Delayed Childbearing and Risk of Adverse Perinatal Outcome: A Population-Based Study." *Journal of the American Medical Association,* 1992 Aug. 19; 268(7): 886–90.

58. Cnattingius, S., et al. "Do Delayed Childbearers Face Increased Risks of Adverse Pregnancy Outcomes after the First Birth?" *Obstetrics and Gynecology,* 1993 Apr.; 81(4): 512–6.

59. Van Katwijk, C., and L. L. Peeters. "Clinical Aspects of Pregnancy after the Age of 35 Years: A Review of the Literature." *Human Reproductive Update,* 1998 Mar.-Apr.; 4(2): 185–94.

60. Cnattingius, S., et al. "Obstacles to Reducing Cesarean Rates in a Low-Cesarean Setting: The Effect of Maternal Age, Height, and Weight." *Obstetrics and Gynecology,* 1998 Oct.; 92(4 Pt. 1): 501–6.

61. Gilbert, W. M., et al. "Childbearing beyond Age 40: Pregnancy Outcome in 24,032 Cases." *Obstetrics and Gynecology,* 1999 Jan.; 93(1): 9–14.

62. Worthington-Roberts, S., and S. R. Williams. *Nutrition in Pregnancy and Lactation,* 6th edition. Dubuque, Iowa: Times Mirror Higher Education Group, Inc., 1997. 33–34.

63. Prysak, M., et al. "Pregnancy Outcome in Nulliparous Women 35 Years and Older." *Obstetrics and Gynecology,* 1995 Jan.; 85(1): 65–70.

64. National Vital Statistics Report. Births: Final Data for 1997. Volume 47, Number 18, April 1999.

65. Scholl, T., et al. "Maternal Growth during Pregnancy and the Competition for Nutrients." *American Journal of Clinical Nutrition,* 60, August 1994: 183.

66. Hediger, M. L., et al. "Implications of the Camden Study of Adolescent Pregnancy: Interactions among Maternal Growth, Nutritional Status, and Body Composition." *Annals of the New York Academy of Science,* 1997 May 28; 817: 281–91.

67. Munoz, K. A., et al. "Food Intakes of U.S. Children and Adolescents Compared with Recommendations." *Pediatrics,* 1997 Sep.; 100 (3 Pt. 1): 323–9.

68. Krebs-Smith, S. M., et al. "Fruit and Vegetable Intakes of Children and Adolescents in the United States." *Archives of Pediatric and Adolescent Medicine,* 1996 Jan.; 150(1): 81–6.

69. Guthrie, J. F., and J. F. Morton. "Food Sources of Added Sweeteners in the Diets of Americans." *Journal of the American Dietetic Association,* January 2000, 100(1): 43–51, quiz 49–50.

70. "Guidelines for School Health Programs to Promote Lifelong Healthy Eating." *Morbidity and Mortality Weekly Report,* June 14, 1996. Volume 45, Number RR-9.

71. American Academy of Pediatrics Committee on Adolescence. "Adolescent Pregnancy: Current Trends and Issues 1998." *Pediatrics,* Volume 103(2) February 1999. 516–520.

72. Casanueva, E., et al. "Weight Gain during Pregnancy in Adolescents: Evaluation of a Non-Nutritional Intervention." *Reviews of Investigative Clinics,* 1994 Mar.–Apr.; 46(2): 157–61.

73. Ibid.

74. Desjardins, E., and D. Hardwick. "How Many Visits by Health Professionals Are Needed to Make a Difference in Low Birth Weight? A Dose-Response Study of the Toronto Healthiest Babies Possible Program." *Canadian Journal of Public Health,* 1999 July–August; 90(4): 224–8.

75. Lenders, C. M., et al. "Effect of High Sugar Intake by Low-Income Pregnant Adolescents on Infant Birth Weight." *Journal of Adolescent Health,* 1994 Nov.; 15(7): 596–602.

76. Subcommittee on Nutritional Status and Weight Gain during Pregnancy. *Nutrition during Pregnancy.* Washington, D.C.: National Academy Press, 1990: 10.

77. Hediger, M., et al. "Patterns of Weight Gain in Adolescent Pregnancy: Effects on Birth Weight and Preterm Delivery.*" Obstetrics and Gynecology,* 74, 1, July 1989: 6.

78. Rees, J. M., et al. "Weight Gain in Adolescents during Pregnancy: Rate Related to Birth-Weight Outcome." *American Journal of Clinical Nutrition,* 1992 Nov.; 56(5): 868–73.

79. Scholl, T. O., et. al. "Low Zinc Intake during Pregnancy: Its Association with Preterm and Very Preterm Delivery." *American Journal of Epidemiology,* 1993 May 15; 137(10): 1115–24.

80. Goldenberg, R. L. "The Effect of Zinc Supplementation on Pregnancy Outcome." *Journal of the American Medical Association,* 1995 Aug. 9; 274(6): 463–8.

81. Worthington-Roberts, B. S., and S. R. Williams. *Nutrition in Pregnancy and Lactation,* 6th edition. Dubuque, Iowa: Times Mirror Higher Education Group, Inc., 1997.

Chapter 8

1. Lanting, C., et al. "Neurological Differences between Nine-Year-Old Children Fed Breast Milk or Formula Milk as Babies." *The Lancet,* 344, 1994: 1319.

Cunnane, S. C., et al. "Breast-Fed Infants Achieve a Higher Rate of Brain and Whole Body Docosahexaenoate Accumulation than Formula-Fed Infants Not Consuming Dietary Docosahexaenoate." *Lipids,* 35, 1, January 2000: 105–11.

2. Gordon, A. E., et al. "The Protective Effect of Breast Feeding in Relation to Sudden Infant Death Syndrome (SIDS): III. Detection of IgA Antibodies in Human Milk That Bind to Bacterial Toxins Implicated in SIDS." *FEMS Immunology and Medical Microbiology,* 1999, Aug. 1; 25(1-2): 175–82.

3. American Academy of Pediatrics, Work Group on Breastfeeding. Policy Statement: "Breastfeeding and the Use of Human Milk." *Pediatrics,* 100, 6, December 1997: 1035–1039.

4. Potischman, N., and R. Troisi. "In-Utero and Early Life Exposures in Relation to Risk of Breast Cancer." *Cancer Causes Control,* 1999, Dec.; 10(6): 561–73.

Newcomb, P. A., et al. "Lactation in Relation to Postmenopausal Breast Cancer." *American Journal of Epidemiology,* 1999 Jul., 15; 150(2): 174–82.

Labbok, M. H. "Health Sequelae of Breastfeeding for the Mother." *Clinics in Perinatology,* 262, 2, viii–ix June 1999; 491–503.

5. American Academy of Pediatrics, Work Group on Breastfeeding. Policy Statement: "Breastfeeding and the Use of Human Milk." *Pediatrics,* 100, 6, December 1997: 1035–1039.

Labbok, M. H. "Health Sequelae of Breastfeeding for the Mother." *Clinics in Perinatology,* 26, 2, viii–ix , June 1999; 491–503.

6. U.S. Department of Health and Human Services. *Healthy People 2000 Progress Review: Maternal and Infant Health.* May 5, 1999.

7. Crase, B. Personal communication. May 1996, 1992.

8. Ibid.

9. Ibid.

10. Krebs, N., M.D. Presentation; Colorado Dietetic Association Annual Meeting. May 14, 1992.

11. Nafziger, S., M.D. Reprinted with permission of author from *Community Network Newsletter,* 1st quarter, 1992; Pueblo, Colo.

12. Modified from the Colorado Breast-Feeding Task Force.

13. Schanler, R. J. "Pediatricians' Practices and Attitudes Regarding Breastfeeding Promotion." *Pediatrics,* Volume 103, Number 3, March 1999, e35.

14. Colorado Breast-Feeding Task Force.

15. Krebs, N. Personal communication. June 1992.

16. Modified from the Colorado Breast-Feeding Task Force.

17. Subcommittee on Nutritional Status during Lactation, et al. *Nutrition during Lactation.* Washington, D.C.: National Academy Press, 1990: 74.

18. Dewey, K. G. "Energy and Protein Requirements during Lactation." *Annual Review of Nutrition,* 17, 1997: 19–36.

19. Strode, M. A., et al. "Effects of Short-Term Caloric Restriction on Lactational Performance in Well-Nourished Women." *Acta Pædiatrica Scandinavica,* 75, 1986: 222.

Butte, N., et al. "Effect of Maternal Diet and Body Composition on Lactational Performance." *American Journal of Clinical Nutrition,* 39, February 1984: 296.

20. Food and Nutrition Board. *Recommended Dietary Allowances.* 10th edition. Washington, D.C.: National Academy Press, 1989.

21. Subcommittee on Nutritional Status during Lactation, et al. *Nutrition during Lactation.* Washington, D.C.: National Academy Press, 1990: 219.

22. Gulson, B. L., et al. "Impact of Diet on Lead in Blood and Urine in Female Adults and Relevance to Mobilization of Lead from Bone Stores." *Environmental Health Perspectives,* 107, 4, April 1999: 257–63.
Gulson, B. L., et al. "Relationships of Lead in Breast Milk to Lead in Blood, Urine, and Diet of the Infant and Mother." *Environmental Health Perspectives,* 106, 10, October 1998: 667–74.

23. Food and Nutrition Board. "Dietary Reference Intakes: Recommended Intakes for Individuals." Washington, D.C.: National Academy Press, 1999.

24. Sanders, T. A. "Essential Fatty Acid Requirements in Pregnancy, Lactation, and Infancy." *American Journal of Clinical Nutrition,* 70, 3 Suppl, September, 1999: 55s-59s.

25. Marcus, P. M., et al. "Adolescent Reproductive Events and Subsequent Breast Cancer." *American Journal of Public Health,* 89, 8, August 1999: 1244–7.

26. Schanler, R. J., and S. A. Atkinson. "Effects of Nutrients in Human Milk on the Recipient Premature Infant." *Journal of Mammary Gland Biology and Neoplasia,* 1999 Jul.; 4(3): 297–307.

27. Hattevig, G., et al. "Effects of Maternal Dietary Avoidance during Lactation on Allergy in Children at 10 Years of Age." *Acta Pædiatrica,* 1999 Jan.; 88(1): 7–12.

28. Chandra, R. K., et al. "Five-Year Follow-Up of High-Risk Infants with Family History of Allergy Who Were Exclusively Breast-Fed or Fed Partial Whey Hydrolysate, Soy, and Conventional Cow's Milk Formulas." *Journal of Pediatric Gastroenterology Nutrition,* 24, 4, April 1997: 380–8.

29. Subcommittee on Nutritional Status during Lactation, et al. *Nutrition during Lactation.* Washington, D.C.: National Academy Press, 1990: 168.

30. Ibid: 14.

31. Schanler, R. J., and S. A. Atkinson. "Effects of Nutrients in Human Milk on the Recipient Premature Infant." *Journal of Mammary Gland Biology and Neoplasia,* 1999 Jul.; 4(3): 297–307.

32. Lucas, A., et al. "Breast Milk and Subsequent Intelligence Quotient." *The Lancet,* 339, 1992: 261.

33. Little, R., et al. "Maternal Alcohol Use during Breastfeeding and Infant Mental and Motor Development at One Year." *New England Journal of Medicine,* 321, 7, August 1989: 425.

34. Mennella, J. "The Transfer of Alcohol to Human Milk." *New England Journal of Medicine,* 325, 14, October 1991: 981.

35. Mennella, J. A., and C. J. Gerrish. "Effects of Exposure to Alcohol in Mother's Milk on Infant Sleep." *Pediatrics,* 101, 5, E2, May 1998.

36. Subcommittee on Nutritional Status during Lactation, et al. *Nutrition during Lactation.* Washington, D.C.: National Academy Press, 1990: 177.

37. Von Kries, et al. "Breastfeeding and Obesity; A Cross-Sectional Study." *British Medical Journal,* 319, 7203, July 1999: 147–150.

38. McCrory, M. A., et al. "Randomized Trial of the Short-Term Effects of Dieting Compared with Dieting plus Aerobic Exercise on Lactation Performance." *American Journal of Clinical Nutrition,* 69, 5, May 1999: 959–67.
Lovelady, C. A. "The Effect of Weight Loss in Overweight Lactating Women on the Growth of Their Infants." *New England Journal of Medicine,* 342, 2000: 449-53.

39. Merchant, K., et al. "Maternal and Fetal Responses to the Stresses of Lactation Concurrent with Pregnancy and Short Recuperative Intervals." *American Journal of Clinical Nutrition,* 52, 1990: 280.

40. Melton, L. J., III, et al. "Influence of Breastfeeding and Other Reproductive Factors on Bone Mass Later in Life." *Osteoporosis International,* 3, 2, March 1993: 76–83.
Lopez, J. M., et al. "Bone Turnover and Density in Healthy Women During Breastfeeding and After Weaning." *Osteoporosis International,* 6, 2, 1996: 153–154.

41. Villalpando, S., and M. del Prado. "Interrelation Among Dietary Energy and Fat Intakes, Maternal Body Fatness and Milk Total Lipid in Humans." *Journal of Mammary Gland Biology and Neoplasia,* 4, 3, July 1999: 285–295.

Piccianoo, M. F., et al. "Human Milk: Nutritional Aspects of a Dynamic Food." *Biology of the Neonate,* 74, 2, 1998: 84–93.

Innis, S. M., and D. J. King. "Trans Fatty Acids in Human Milk Are Inversely Associated with Concentration of Essential c0s-n-6 and n-3 Fatty Acids in Plasma Lipids of Breastfed Infants." *American Journal of Clinical Nutrition,* 70, 3, September 1999: 383–390.

Hayat, L., et al. "Fatty Acid Composition of Human Milk in Kuwait Mothers."

42. Worthington-Roberts, B., and S. R. Williams. *Nutrition in Pregnancy and Lactation,* 6th edition. Dubuque, Iowa: Brown and Benchmark Publishers, 1997.

43. Patandin, S. "Effects of Environmental Exposure to Polychlorinated Biphenyls and Dioxins on Cognitive Abilities in Dutch Children at 42 Months of Age." *Journal of Pediatrics,* 134, 1, January 1999: 33–41.

44. Crase, B. Personal communication. May 1992.

45. Rogan, W. J., et al. "Pollutants in Breast Milk." *Archives in Pediatric and Adolescent Medicine,* 150, 9, September 1996: 981–90.

46. La Leche League International Staff. *The Womanly Art of Breastfeeding.* 4th revised edition. Franklin Park, Ill.: La Leche League International, 1987: 348.

47. Nafziger, S., M.D. Personal communication. June 1992.

48. Dewey, K. G., et al. "A Randomized Study of the Effects of Aerobic Exercise by Lactating Women on Breast-Milk Volume and Composition." *New England Journal of Medicine,* 330, 7, February 1994: 449–53.

49. Food and Nutrition Board. *Dietary Reference Intakes: Recommended Intakes for Individuals.* National Academy Press, 1999.

50. Potischman, N., and R. Troisi. "In-Utero and Early Life Exposures in Relation to Risk of Breast Cancer." *Cancer Causes Control,* 1999, Dec.; 10(6): 561–73.

Newcomb, P. A., et al. "Lactation in Relation to Postmenopausal Breast Cancer." *American Journal of Epidemiology,* 1999 Jul., 15; 150(2): 174–82.

Labbok, M. H. "Health Sequelae of Breastfeeding for the Mother." *Clinics in Perinatology,* 262, 2, viii–ix June 1999; 491–503.

51. Freudenheim, J., et al. "Exposure to Breast Milk in Infancy and the Risk of Breast Cancer." *Epidemiology,* 5, 1994: 324.

52. Committee on Nutrition. "Iron-Fortified Infant Formulas." *Pediatrics,* 84, 6, December 1989: 114.

53. American Academy of Pediatrics. "Infant Feeding Practices and Their Possible Relationship to the Etiology of Diabetes Mellitus." *Pediatrics,* 94, 5, November 1994: 752.

54. Shannon, M., and J. Graef. "Hazards of Lead in Infant Formula." Letter. *New England Journal of Medicine,* 326, 2, January 9, 1992: 137.

Chapter 9

1. Gerlin, A. "Workplace Nursing Becoming a Benefit." *The Wall Street Journal,* December 29, 1994.

2. Brownell, K. D. "The Central Role of Lifestyle Change in Long-Term Weight Management." *Clinical Cornerstone,* 2, 3, 1999: 43–51.

3. Wing, R. R., and R. W. Jeffery. "Benefits of Recruiting Participants with Friends and Increasing Social Support for Weight Loss and Maintenance." *Consulting Clinical Psychology,* 67, 1, February 1999, 132–8.

4. Williams, G. C., et al. "Motivational Predictors of Weight Loss and Weight-loss Maintenance." *Journal of Personal Social Psychology,* 70, 1, January 1996: 115–26.

5. Brownell, K. D. "The Central Role of Lifestyle Change in Long-Term Weight Management." *Clinical Cornerstone,* 2, 3, 1999: 43–51.

6. International Food and Information Council. *Food Insight: Current Topics in Food Safety and Nutrition,* March/April 1992.

7. Greene, G., et al. "Postpartum Weight Change: How Much of the Weight Gained in Pregnancy Will Be Lost after Delivery." *Obstetrics and Gynecology,* 71, 5, May 1988: 701.

8. Fuentes-Afflick, E., and N. A. Hessol. "Interpregnancy Interval and the Risk of Premature Infants." *Obstetrics and Gynecology,* 95, 3, March 2000: 383–90.

Chapter 10

1. American College of Obstetricians and Gynecologists. *Planning for Pregnancy, Birth, and Beyond.* Washington, D.C.: ACOG, 1990: 77, 82.

2. Jovanovic-Peterson, L., and C. Peterson. "Is Exercise Safe or Useful for Gestational Diabetic Women?" *Diabetes,* 40, suppl. 2, December 1991: 179.

3. American College of Obstetricians and Gynecologists. *Exercise during Pregnancy and the Postnatal Period.* ACOG Home Exercise Programs. Washington, D.C.: ©1985. Reprinted with permission.

4. Ibid.

5. Grediagin, A., et al. "Exercise Treatment Does Not Effect Body Composition Change in Untrained Moderately Overfat Women." *Journal of the American Dietetic Association,* 95, 6, June 1995: 661.

6. American College of Obstetricians and Gynecologists. *ACOG Guide to Planning for Pregnancy, Birth, and Beyond.* Washington, D.C.: ACOG ©1990. Reprinted with permission.

Chapter 11
1. The Food and Drug Administration. "The New Food Label." *FDA Backgrounder,* April 1994.

2. Ibid.

3. *Consumer Reports on Health,* March 1992: 18.

4. Whitmire, D. Telephone interview. June 1992.

5. Food Marketing Institute. *Food Safety and the Microwave: A Consumer Guide to Food Quality and Safe Handling.*

6. Sharara, F. I., et al. "Environmental Toxicants and Female Reproduction." *Fertility and Sterility,* 70(4) Oct. 1998: 613–22.

7. Groth, Edward III, and Mark Silbergeld. *Report to the FDA with Results of Recent Tests Conducted by Consumers Union.* June 1998.

8. Groth, Edward III, Project Director. *Do You Know What You're Eating? An Analysis of U.S. Government Data on Pesticide Residues in Foods,* Consumers Union, February 1999.

9. U.S. Department of Agriculture, Agriculture Marketing Service. *National Organic Program Proposed Rule,* December 1997.

10. Jacobson, M., et al. *Safe Food: Eating Wisely in a Risky World.* Los Angeles, Calif.: Living Planet Press, 1991: 72.

11. Reprinted from *Safe Food,* © 1991, available for $9.95 at CSPI, 1875 Connecticut Ave. NW #300, Washington, DC 20009.

12. Dairy Industry Coalition. "Facts about BST and Milk Safety."

13. Daughaday, W. H., and D. M. Barbano. "Bovine Somatotropin Supplementation of Dairy Cows: Is the Milk Safe?" *Journal of the American Medical Association,* 264, 8, 1990: 1003.

14. Kendall, P. Telephone interview. June 1992.

15. National Pork Producers Council. *Today's Pork in Foodservice,* 1988: 6.

16. Wilson, L. "Producing Leaner Beef More Efficiently." Presentation at Pennsylvania State University, 1989.

17. Texas A & M University. *Growth Promoting Hormones: A Scientific Review,* January 1989.

18. EPA Fact Sheet. *Polychlorinated Dibenzo-p-dioxins and Related Compounds Update: Impact on Fish Advisories,* September 1999.
    EPA Fact Sheet. *PCB Update: Impact on Fish Advisories,* September 1999.

19. EPA Fact Sheet. *Mercury Update: Impact on Fish Advisories,* September 1999.

20. Connor, W. E. "Impact of Omega 3 Fatty Acids in Health and Disease." *American Journal of Clinical Nutrition,* 71, (1 Suppl.): 171s–175s.
    Carlson, S. E. "Long-Chain Polyunsaturated Fatty Acids and Development of Human Infants." *Acta Pædiatrica,* 88, 430: 72–77.

21. National Fisheries Institute. *Omega 3 Content of Fish and Shellfish.*

22. Ollis, T. E., et al. "Australian Food Sources and Intakes of Omega-6 and Omega-3 Polyunsaturated Fatty Acids." *Annals of Nutrition and Metabolism,* 1999 Nov.; 43(6): 346–355.

23. Makrides, M., and R. A. Gibson. "Long-Chain Polyunsaturated Fatty Acid Requirements During Pregnancy and Lactation." *American Journal of Clinical Nutrition,* 71, (1 Suppl.): 1308s–311s.

24. Vanderbeek, C. Telephone interview. May 1996.

25. *Consumer Reports Magazine,* 57, 2, February 1992: 106.
    Harsila, J. Telephone interview. May 1992.
    Jacobson, M., et al. *Safe Food: Eating Wisely in a Risky World.* Los Angeles, Calif.: Living Planet Press, 1991: 13.

26. U.S. Department of Agriculture, Food Safety and Inspection Service. *Focus on Beef: From Farm to Table,* revised May 1998.
    U. S. Department of Agriculture and Food Safety and Inspection Service. *Minimum Internal Temperatures: Use a Meat Thermometer,* June 1997.

Chapter 15
1. American Dry Bean Board. *Good Health Is Habit-Forming: Commit to the Bean Routine.*

Recommended Resources

As you may know, there are many, many good books about health and nutrition. I had a hard time picking only a few.

Prepregnancy Planning

Lauersen, Niels H., M.D., and Colette Bouchez. *Getting Pregnant: What Couples Need to Know Right Now.* Fireside.

Sussman, John R., M.D., and B. Blake Levitt. *Before You Conceive: The Complete Prepregnancy Guide.* Bantam.

Tannenhaus, Norra. *Pre-Conceptions: What You Can Do Before Pregnancy to Help You Have a Healthy Baby.* Contemporary Books.

Pregnancy

Bard, Maureen. *Getting Organized for Your New Baby.* Meadowbrook.

Brott, Armin A., and Jennifer Ash. *The Expectant Father: Facts, Tips, and Advice for Dads-to-Be.* Abbeville Press.

Curtis, Glade B., M.D. *Your Pregnancy Week by Week* and *Your Pregnancy After 30.* Fisher Books.

Erick, Miriam. *No More Morning Sickness: A Survival Guide for Pregnant Women.* Plume. *Take Two Crackers and Call Me in the Morning: A Real-Life Guide to Surviving Morning Sickness.* Grinnen-Barrett.

Graham, Janis. *Your Pregnancy Companion.* Pocket Books.

Hotchner, Tracy. *Pregnancy Pure and Simple.* Avon Books.

Nilsson, Lennart. *A Child Is Born.* Dell.

Noble, Elizabeth. *Essential Exercises for the Childbearing Year.* New Life Images.

Sears, William, M.D., and Martha Sears. *The Birth Book.* Little, Brown.

Shapiro, Howard, M.D. *The Pregnancy Book for Today's Woman.* HarperCollins.

Simkin, Penny, Janet Whalley, and Ann Keppler. *Pregnancy, Childbirth, and the Newborn.* Meadowbrook.

Spencer, Paula, et al. Parenting *Guide to Pregnancy and Childbirth.* Ballantine Books.

Stone, Joanne, M.D., Keith Eddleman, M.D., and Mary Murray. *Pregnancy for Dummies.* IDG Books.

Stoppard, Miriam, M.D. *New Pregnancy and Birth Book.* Ballantine Books.

Baby Names

Lansky, Bruce. *The Very Best Baby Name Book.* Meadowbrook.

High-Risk Pregnancy/Birth

Rich, Laurie. *When Pregnancy Isn't Perfect.* Larata Press.

Diabetes and Gestational Diabetes

American Diabetes Association. *Diabetes: What to Expect* and *Gestational Diabetes: What to Expect.* The American Diabetes Association.

Cryer, Philip. *American Diabetes Association Complete Guide to Diabetes: The Ultimate Home Diabetes Reference.* Bantam Books.

Franz, Marion. *Exchanges for All Occasions.* International Diabetes Center.

Hayes, Marcia, Jane Stephenson, and Jackie Boucher. *No Fuss Diabetes Recipes for 1 or 2.* Chronimed Publishing.

Hess, Mary Abbott. *The Art of Cooking for the Diabetic.* Signet.

Jovanovic-Peterson, Lois, M.D., with Morton Stone. *Managing Your Gestational Diabetes: A Guide for You and Your Baby's Good Health.* Chronimed Publishing.

Marks, Betty. *The Microwave Diabetes Cookbook.* Surrey Books.

Palumbo, P.J., M.D., and Joyce Daly Margie. *The All-In-One Diabetic Cookbook.* New American Library.

Polin, Bonnie Sanders, and Frances Towner Giedt. *The Joslin Diabetes Gourmet Cookbook.* Bantam Books.

Multiple Births

Agnew, Connie, et al. *Twins! Expert Advice from Two Practicing Physicians on Pregnancy, Birth, and the First Year of Life with Twins.* HarperCollins.

Baglivi Tinglof, Christina. *Double Duty: The Parents' Guide to Raising Twins, from Pregnancy through the School Years.* Contemporary Books.

Luke, Barbara and Tamara Eberlein. *When You're Expecting Twins, Triplets or Quads: The Complete Resource.* HarperCollins.

Noble, Elizabeth. *Having Twins: A Parent's Guide to Pregnancy, Birth, and Early Childhood.* Houghton Mifflin.

Rothbart, Betty. *Multiple Blessings: From Pregnancy through Childhood, a Guide for Parents of Twins, Triplets, or More.* Hearst Books.

Prematurity
Tracy, Amy and Dianne Maroney. *Your Premature Baby and Child: Helpful Answers and Advice for Parents.* Berkley Publishing Group.

Teen Pregnancy
Arthur, Shirley. *Surviving Teen Pregnancy: Your Choices, Dreams, and Decisions.* Morning Glory Press.

Hammerslough, Jane. *Everything You Need to Know about Teen Motherhood.* Rosen Publishing Group.

Lindsay, Jeanne Warren. *School-Age Parents: The Challenge of Three Generation Living,* and *Teens Parenting: Your Pregnancy and Newborn Journey,* and *Your Baby's First Year.* Morning Glory Press.

Infertility
Aronson, Diane and Resolve (organization). *Resolving Infertility: Understanding the Options and Choosing Solutions When You Want to Have a Baby.* HarperCollins.

Levitt, B. Blake. *50 Essential Things to Do When the Doctor Says It's Infertility.* Plume.

Miller, Manya Deleon, and Ronald Clisham. *The Complete Fertility Organizer: A Guidebook and Record-Keeper for Women.* John Wiley and Sons.

Raab, Diana. *Getting Pregnant and Staying Pregnant: Overcoming Infertility and Managing Your High-Risk Pregnancy.* Hunter House.

Rosenberg, Helane S., and Yakov M. Epstein. *Getting Pregnant When You Thought You Couldn't.* Warner Books.

Rosenthal, M. Sara. *The Fertility Sourcebook: Everything You Need to Know.* Lowell House.

Stone, Frances and Philip. *Pennies from Heaven: 101 Meditations for Couples Trying to Get Pregnant.* Penguin.

Weschler, Toni. *Taking Charge of Your Fertility.* Harper Perennial.

Breastfeeding
Behan, Eileen. *Eat Well, Lose Weight While Breastfeeding.* Villard Books.

Gotsch, Gwen and Judy Torgus. *The Womanly Art of Breastfeeding.* Plume.

Gotsch, Gwen. *Breast Feeding Your Premature Baby.* La Leche League International.

Gromada, Karen Kerkhoff. *Mothering Multiples: Breastfeeding and Caring for Twins or More.* La Leche League International.

Huggins, Kathleen. *The Nursing Mother's Companion.* 4th Edition. Harvard Common Press.

Moran, Elaine. *Bon Appetit, Baby! The Breastfeeding Kit.* Treasure Chest Books.

Pryor, Gale. *Nursing Mother, Working Mother: The Essential Guide for Breastfeeding and Staying Close to Your Baby After You Return to Work.* Harvard Common Press.

Sears, William. *The Breastfeeding Book.* Little, Brown.

Parenthood
Black Fatherhood: The Guide to Male Parenting. Impact! Publications.

Brazelton, T. Berry, M.D. *Touchpoints: Your Child's Emotional and Behavioral Development.* Perseus Press.

Cline, Foster W., and Jim Fay. *Parenting with Love and Logic: Teaching Children Responsibility.* Navpress.

Crary, Elizabeth. *Without Spanking or Spoiling: A Practical Approach to Toddler and Preschool Guidance.* Parenting Press.

Einzig, Mitchell J., M.D., ed. *Baby and Child Emergency First Aid Handbook.* Meadowbrook.

Eisenberg, Arlene, et al. *What to Expect the First Year.* Workman Publishing.

Hart, Terril H., M.D., ed. *The Parent's Guide to Baby and Child Medical Care.* Meadowbrook.

Hunter, Brenda. *Home by Choice.* Multnomah Books.

Huntley, Becky. *The Sleep Book for Tired Parents.* Parenting Press.

Johnson, Spencer, M.D. *The One Minute Mother.* William Morrow.

Kelly, Paula, M.D., ed. *First-Year Baby Care.* Meadowbrook.

Lague, Louise. *The Working Mom's Book of Hints, Tips, and Everyday Wisdom.* Petersons Guides.

Lansky, Vicki. *Getting Your Child to Sleep...and Back to Sleep: Tips for Parents of Infants, Toddlers, and Preschoolers.* Book Peddlers. *Practical Parenting Tips.* Meadowbrook.

Saavedra, Beth Wilson. *Meditations for New Mothers.* Workman Publishing.

Any books by parenting experts Penelope Leach, T. Berry Brazelton, or William Sears.

Baby Products

Fields, Denise and Alan. *Baby Bargains*. Windsor Peak Press.

Jones, Sandy, and the editors of Consumer Reports. *Guide to Baby Products, 6th Edition*. Consumer Reports Books.

Pregnancy and Parenting Books with a Touch of Humor

Atalla, Bill. *Thirteen Months of Pregnancy: A Guide for the Pregnant Father*. Oddly Enough.

Bernard, Susan. *The Mommy Guide: Real-Life Advice and Tips from Over 250 Moms and Other Experts*. NTC Publishing.

Glick, Eunice. *Expect the Unexpected When You're Expecting!* HarperTrade.

Gookin, Sandra Hardin and Dan, eds. *Parenting for Dummies*. IDG Books.

Hill, Thomas. *What to Expect When Your Wife Is Expanding*. Andrews McMeel Publishing.

Justice, Jeff. *The Pregnant Husband's Handbook*. Strawberry Patch.

Justice, Jeff, and Diane Pfeifer. *You Know You're a New Parent When...*. Strawberry Patch.

Lovine, Vicki. *The Girlfriends' Guide to Pregnancy: Or Everything Your Doctor Won't Tell You*. Pocket Books.

Feeding Your Infant and Child

Lansky, Vicki. *Feed Me! I'm Yours*. Meadowbrook.

Nissenberg, Sandra, et al. *How Should I Feed My Child? From Pregnancy to Preschool*. John Wiley and Sons.

Satter, Ellyn. *Child of Mine: Feeding with Love and Good Sense* and *How to Get Your Kid to Eat...But Not Too Much*. Bull Publishing.

Swinney, Bridget. *Healthy Food for Healthy Kids*. Meadowbrook.

General Nutrition

Donkersloot, Mary. *The Fast-Food Diet: Quick and Healthy Eating at Home and on the Go*. Fireside.

Duyff, Roberta Larson. *The American Dietetic Association's Complete Food and Nutrition Guide*. John Wiley and Sons.

Evers, Connie L. *How to Teach Nutrition to Kids*. 24 Carrot Press.

Finn, Susan, and Linda Stern Kass. *The Real Life Nutrition Book: Making the Right Choices Without Changing Your Life-Style*. Penguin Books.

Lambert-Lagacé, Louise. *The Nutrition Challenge for Women*. Bell Publishing.

Tribole, Evelyn. *Eating on the Run*. Human Kinetics Publishing. *Stealth Health: How to Sneak Nutrition Painlessly into Your Diet*. Penguin.

Warshaw, Hope. *The Restaurant Companion: A Guide to Healthier Eating Out*. Surrey Books.

Cookbooks

General-Healthy

The American Diabetes Association and the American Dietetic Association Family Cookbook. Simon & Schuster.

Colorado Dietetic Assocation staff. *Simply Colorado: Nutritious Recipes for Busy People*. Colorado Dietetic Association.

Cull, Julie Metcalf. *The Quality Time Family Cookbook*. Chronimed Publishing.

Fletcher, Anne. *Eating Thin for Life: Food Secrets and Recipes from People Who Have Lost Weight and Kept It Off*. Houghton Mifflin.

Gadia, Madhu. *Lite and Luscious Cuisine of India*. Piquant Publishing.

Mycoskie, Pam. *Butter Busters: The Cookbook*. Warner Books.

Oxmoor House. *Cooking Light Cookbook Series*. Oxmoor House.

Ponichtera, Brenda. *Quick & Healthy Recipes and Ideas*. ScaleDown Publishing.

Smith, M.J. *366 Low-Fat Brand-Name Recipes in Minutes!* John Wiley and Sons.

Tribole, Evelyn. *Healthy Homestyle Cooking*. Rodale Press. *Healthy Homestyle Desserts*. Viking.

Seafood

Hansen, Evie and Cindy Snyder. *Seafood Twice a Week*. National Seafood Educators.

Harsila, Janis, and Evie Hansen. *Light-Hearted Seafood: Tasty, Quick, Healthy*. National Seafood Educators.

Ver Ploeg, Marcie, et al. *Seafood Cooking for Dummies*. IDG Books.

Vegetarian

Callan, Ginny. *Beyond the Moon Cookbook*. Harper Perennial.

Crocker, Betty. *Betty Crocker's Vegetarian Cooking.* Simon and Schuster.

Elliot, Rose. *The Vegetarian Mother and Baby Book.* Pantheon Books.

Havala, Suzanne. *Simple, Lowfat and Vegetarian.* Vegetarian Resource Group. *Being Vegetarian.* John Wiley and Sons.

Hinman, Bobbie, and Millie Snyder. *Lean and Luscious and Meatless.* Prima Communications.

Katzen, Mollie. *Moosewood Cookbook,* and *The Enchanted Broccoli Forest,* and *Still Life with Menu Cookbook.* Ten Speed Press.

Kirchner, Bharti. *Vegetarian Burgers.* HarperCollins.

Lakhani, Mrs. *Indian Recipes for a Healthy Heart.* Fahil Publishers.

Mangum, Karen. *Life's Simple Pleasures.* Harvest Press. *Vegetarian Pleasure Revised.* Millenium Group.

Robertson, Laurel, et al. *The New Laurel's Kitchen.* Ten Speed Press.

Wasserman, Debra. *Meatless Meals for Working People* and *Simply Vegan.* Vegetarian Resource Group.

Weight Control/Weight Maintenance/Low-Fat Eating

Bailey, Covert. *The Ultimate Fit or Fat* and *Smart Exercise.* Houghton Mifflin.

Berry, Frank, and Bridget Swinney. *Make the Change for a Healthy Heart.* Fall River Press.

Connor, Sonja, and William Connor, M.D. *The New American Diet.* Fireside.

Ferguson, Cassandra and James, M.D. *Habits Not Diets.* Bell Publishing.

Fletcher, Anne. *Thin For Life.* Houghton Mifflin.

Goor, Ron and Nancy. *Choose to Lose.* Houghton Mifflin.

Katahn, Martin and Jamie Pope. *The T-Factor 2000 Fat Gram Counter.* R.S. Means.

Lund, JoAnna. *Healthy Exchanges Cookbook.* Putnam.

McDougall, Mary and John, M.D. *The McDougall Program for Maximum Weight Loss.* Plume.

Moquette-Magee, Elaine. *Fight Fat and Win!* Chronimed Publishing.

Nash, Joyce. *Maximize Your Body Potential.* Bull Publishing.

Pope, Jamie. *The Last Five Pounds.* Pocket Books.

Stevens, Tree. *Living and Loving Low Fat.* Northwest.

Tribole, Evelyn, and Elyse Resch. *Intuitive Eating.* St. Martin's Press.

Ulene, Art. *Lose Weight with Dr. Art Ulene.* Ulysses Press.

Waterhouse, Debra. *Outsmarting the Female Fat Cell.* Warner Books.

Other Resources

American Dietetic Association Consumer Nutrition Hotline, 800-366-1655, www.eatright.org.

Confinement Line: a support network for women on bed rest, 703-941-7183.

Consumer Product Safety Commission, 800-638-2772.

National Organization of Mothers of Twins Clubs, 877-540-2200.

Sidelines: support for those experiencing a high-risk pregnancy, www.sidelines.org.

Triplet Connection, 209-474-0885.

Twin Services (counseling and referrals), 510-524-0863.

Vegetarian Resource Group, 410-366-8343, www.vrg.org.

Newsletters and Magazines

American Health Magazine.

Cooking Light Magazine.

Diet and Nutrition Letter, Tufts University.

Environmental Nutrition, The Professional Newsletter of Diet, Nutrition, and Health.

Health Magazine.

Nutrition Action Health Letter, Center for Science in the Public Interest, Washington, D.C.

Vegetarian Journal, Vegetarian Resource Group.

Wellness Letter, University of California, Berkeley.

Index

Abdomen, tightening, 179
Acesulfame K (sweetener),
    125
Additives, food, 203–5
Alcohol use
    avoiding, 11
    birth defects and, 5, 42
    breastfeeding and, 169
    infertility and, 10
    unknown pregnancy and,
        15
Alitame (sweetener), 125
American Diabetes
    Association, 108
Allergies, food, 168
Amenorrhea, 10
Ames, Bruce, 11
Anemia, 33
    fatigue and, 59
    low-birth-weight baby and,
        19
    preventing, 72–74
Ankle swelling, 87
Antimicrobials, 204
Antioxidants, 204
Artificial flavoring, 204
Artificial sweeteners,
    124–25, 203
Ascorbic acid, 33
Asian convenience foods,
    241
Aspartame (sweetener),
    124–25
Aspirin, 11, 44, 165

Baby
    birth weight, 17–18. See
        also Low birth weight
    diabetes, influence on,
        112–13, 115–16, 126–27

high blood pressure, risks
    to, 129
influence of pregnancy
    over age 35 on, 145
smoking, risks to, 39
teen pregnancy, influence
    on, 148–49
See also Breastfeeding;
    Fetal growth
Backache, 87, 195
Bacteria, food-borne, 13,
    210–11, 221, 223–24
Beans, 101. See also Beans in
    Recipe Index
Bed rest
    eating while on, 140–41
    entertainment during,
        142–43
    exercise and, 143, 195
    need for, 128, 131–32
    setting up room for, 140
    survival tips, 143–44
Beef, safety risks, 219–21. See
    also Beef in Recipe Index
Beer, 169
Before-Baby Eating Plan, 8,
    11
Best-for-Baby Breastfeeding
    Eating Plan, 161–62
Beta-carotene, 31
Beverages, 257
    caffeine content, 42–44
    calcium content, 70
    high-energy drink, 86
    milk, 70–72
    See also Fluids; Water
Biotin, 29
Birth control pills, 14–15
Birth defects
    alcohol use and, 5, 42

folate and, 33
food safety and, 225
poor nutrition and, 5, 7
preexisting diabetes and, 5
vitamin C and, 11
vitamin supplements and,
    12, 37
Birth weight, 17–18
Blood glucose. See Blood
    sugar
Blood pressure. See High
    blood pressure
Blood sugar
    controlling, 108, 122
    high, 111, 127
    low, 110–11, 112–13, 123,
        126
    monitoring, 113, 121
    testing for diabetes with,
        116–17
    See also Diabetes
Bonding and bottlefeeding,
    174
Bottlefeeding, 173–174
Breakfast
    benefits of, 184–85
    blender, 261
    fast-food, 251
    ideas for, 291–92
    recipes, 296–98, 310
Breast cancer, 173
Breast changes, 60
Breastfeeding
    alcohol use and, 169
    allergies and, 168
    benefits, 153–54
    breast cancer and, 173
    caffeine and, 168
    decision about, 152
    drugs and, 165

environmental contaminants and, 170–71
fat and, 170
fathers and, 157–58
food poisoning and, 172
gassy foods and, 167
in hospital, 159–60
multiple births and, 165–66
nutrition during, 161–65
obstacles to, 154–57
osteoporosis and, 170
for premature infants, 166–67, 168
preparing for, 158–59
problems with, 151–52
questions about, 167–73
seeking help with, 157, smoking and, 169
teen pregnancy and, 166
vegetarian eating and, 166, 172
weight loss during, 169–70
working and, 156–57, 177–78
Budget, eating on, 205–8
Buying food. See Shopping for food

Caffeine
breastfeeding and, 168
effect of, 42–43
food/beverage sources, 43
infertility and, 9
limiting, 12, 13–14
Calcium
breastfeeding needs for, 163–64
in chocolate milk, 71
in fast foods, 250
food/beverage sources, 30, 70, 71, 164
functions, 30
lactose intolerance and, 69–70

managing blood pressure and, 130
multiple births and, 135
need for, 19, 68
in prenatal vitamins, 72
sneaking into diet, 68–72
supplements, 38–39
teen pregnancy and, 149
third-trimester needs, 83
vegetarian eating and, 94–95
Calories
adding to diet, 138
amount needed for pregnancy, 113, 237
amount needed for breastfeeding, 162
Campylobacterosis, 221, 223
Cancer, breast, 173
Carbohydrates, 118–19
Carrots and infertility, 10
Cereals, vitamin-fortified, 94
Chickenpox, 41
Chocolate milk, 71–72
Choline, 30
Chromium, 35, 66, 115
Chronic high blood pressure, 130
Chronic hypertension, 129
Cigarettes. See Smoking cigarettes
Cobalamin, 30
Cocaine, 44
Coloring agents, 204
Company's Coming! Menus, 293–94
Complete proteins, 66, 67
Complimentary proteins, 98
Confinement Line, the, 108
Connor, Sonja, 26–27
Constipation, 77–78
Convenience foods
adding extras to, 238
cost, 207

menus, 236–42
shopping for, 235
sodium in, 236
vegetarian, 102–3
for whole family, 238
See also Fast foods
Cooking. See Food preparation
Copper, 34–35
Counseling, prepregnancy, 3–4, 17
Crase, Betty, 154, 171
Cravings for food, 59–60
Crawford, Michael, 5, 7
Crohn's disease, 153
Curing agents, 204
Cytomegalovirus (CMV), 41

Dairy products, 69–72, 77, 217–19
Dehydration, 112
Delivery. See Labor and delivery
Desserts, 75, 256. See also Desserts in Recipe Index
Diabetes
controlling, 15, 108–10, 113–14, 117–18
coping with, 114–15
eating plan for, 118–22
effect on baby, 5, 112–13
effect on mother, 110–11
exercise and, 122–23
food exchanges, 258
labor and delivery with, 114
questions on, 126–28
recipe variations, 258–59
risk factors, 116
testing for, 116–17
using sweeteners for, 123–26
vegetarian eating and, 104

Diet
  baby's birth weight and,
    17–18
  breastfeeding and, 170–72
  evaluating, 64–66, 83–84
  for multiple births preg-
    nancy, 135–39
  survey on pregnant
    women's, 6–7
  ten steps to a healthy,
    18–20
  weight loss, 8, 181–84
  See also Vegetarian eating
Dietary Reference Intake
  (DRI), 7, 29, 83
Diet foods, 125–26
Don't Feel Like Cooking
  Menus, 259–60
Don't Feel Like Cooking or
  Eating Menu, 260
Don't Feel Like Eating
  Menus, 259
Drugs
  avoiding, 11, 44
  breastfeeding and, 165
  found in animal meat, 219

Eating disorders, 10
Eating Expectantly Eating
  Plan, 55–56
  for teens, 147–48
  for vegetarians, 96–98
Eating habits. *See* Diet
Eating out
  choosing wisely, 246–49
  fast foods, 14, 61, 101–2,
    249–56
  food safety and, 211–12
  healthy entrees for,
    247–48
  healthy menus for, 248–49
  vegetarian style, 100–102
  See also Fast foods

Eating Plan
  Before-Baby, 8, 11
  breastfeeding, 161–62
  diabetic, 118–22
  Eating Expectantly, 8,
    55–56, 96–98, 147–48
  teen pregnancy, 147–48
  Thrive on Five, 74–75
Eclampsia, 128
E. coli bacteria, 219
Edema, 87
Eggs, 28
  food safety for, 218–19
  protein from, 51
  storage, 220, 221
  See also Eggs *in Recipe Index*
Emotions, dealing with,
  107–8
Emulsifiers, 204
Energy
  keeping up, tips on, 86–87
  protein and, 51
  weight gain and, 82
Environmental contaminants
  avoiding, 11–12
  breastfeeding and, 170–71
  in fish/seafood, 224
  pesticides, 213, 214, 216
  in workplace, 12–13
Equal, 258–59
Erick, Miriam, 56, 57
Essential fats. *See* Fat
Estrogen, 219–21
Exchanges, food
  diabetic, 120
  vegetarian foods, 105
Exercise
  back strengthening, 195
  benefits, 187–88
  breastfeeding and, 172
  diabetes and, 114, 122–23
  during bed rest, 143, 195
  energy and, 87

fitting into busy lifestyle,
    191–92
  guidelines on, 188–91
  infertility and, 11
  limiting, 190–91
  need for, 19–20
  postpartum, 192–94
  videos, 194
  weight loss and, 181
Fast food
  avoiding, 61
  nutritious choices on, 14,
    249–50
  healthy menus, 250–56
  vegetarian, 101–2
Fat
  breastfeeding and, 170
  multiple births and,
    136–37
  Omega-3, 26, 83, 223,
    225–26
  Omega-6, 26, 137
  substitutes, 204
  suggested menus for,
    27–28
  vegetarian eating and, 96,
    104–5, 166
  watching types and
    amounts of, 25–27
  weight gain and, 21
Fathers
  breastfeeding and, 157–58
  pregnancy planning and,
    11
Fatigue, 59, 86–87, 194
Feel Full Meals, 326–27
Feel Great Menu, 261
Feel Like Staying in Bed but
  Can't Menu, 260–61
Fetal Alcohol Effect (FAE),
  42
Fetal Alcohol Syndrome
  (FAS), 42

Fetal growth
  first, 49–50
  hypoglycemia and, 126
  second, 63–64
  third, 81–82
Fiber
  diabetes, controlling with, 113
  focus on, 53, 55
  food sources, 54
  in whole grains, 10, 19
Figs, 53
First trimester, 49–62
  body changes during, 58–61
  fetal growth during, 49–50
  fiber intake during, 53–55
  menus, 61–62, 259–61
  morning sickness during, 56–58
  nutrient needs during, 52
  protein needs during, 50–52
  recipes, 265–89
  snack ideas for, 262
  weight gain during, 50
Fish and seafood, 171–72
  buying, 226–27
  cooking, 228–29
  environmental contaminants in, 224–25
  food safety for, 223–29
  fresh caught, 171–72
  Omega-3 fatty acids in, 83, 225–26
  storage, 222, 227–28
  See also Fish and Seafood in Recipe Index
Fitness. See Exercise
Flavor enhancers, 204
Flavoring agents, 204
Fluids
  after labor, 176
  breastfeeding and, 163

morning sickness and, 57–58
  need for, 20, 112
Fluoride, 35
Folate (folic acid)
  in fast foods, 253
  in first trimester, 52
  food sources, 14, 32, 165
  importance of, 4–5, 13, 32–33
  multivitamin supplements and, 37
Food additives, 203–5
Food cravings and aversions, 59–60
Food exchanges
  diabetic, 120
  vegetarian foods, 105
Food Guide Pyramid, 18–19, 91–92
Food labels, 123–24, 201–5
Food planning. See Menus; Shopping for food
Food poisoning, 172
Food preparation
  beans, 303
  food safety for, 210–11, 212–14, 216–17, 219, 228–29, 232
  keeping vitamins in vegetables, 209–10
  kitchen tools for, 208–9
  last-minute, 242, 244
  quick and easy, 242–43, 245–46
  seafood, 228–29
Food safety
  bacteria, 13, 210–11, 221, 223–24
  buying organic, 214–15
  eating food, 218
  eating out, 211–12
  environmental contaminants and, 213–14, 224–26

kitchen sanitation, 211, 231–32
  microwaving, 212–13
  preparing foods, 212, 213–14, 216–17, 219, 228–29, 232
  reports on, 229–30
  shopping for food, 215–16, 218, 226–27, 230–31
Food storage
  dairy products, 217
  eggs, 220, 221
  food safety for, 227–28, 233
  meat, 220, 221
  poultry, 220, 221
  seafood, 222, 227–28
  using plastic for, 213
Formula feeding, 152, 173–74
Frozen foods. See Convenience foods
Fruits
  adding to meals, 74–75
  food safety and, 215–17
  pesticides and, 214
  as snacks, 76
  See also Fruits in Recipe Index

Gas-causing foods, 167
Genetic counseling, 4
German measles, 41
Gestational diabetes, 7
  after pregnancy, 127
  effects on baby, 115–16
  effects on mother, 115
  managing, 117–18
  risk factors, 116
  testing for, 116–17
  vegetarian eating and, 104
Glucose, 35, 115, 116–17. See also Blood sugar
Grains, 10, 14, 19. See also Grains in Recipe Index

Health-care workers, 109, 155
Health claims on labels, 202–3
Heartburn, 88
Hemorrhoids, 78
Hepatitis B, 41
Herbal teas, 44
Higgins Nutrition Intervention Program, 137–38
High-carbohydrate foods, 76–77
High blood pressure, 128–32
High blood sugar, 111, 127
High-risk pregnancies
  diabetic eating and exercise plan for, 118–26
  emotions during, 107–8
  gestational diabetes, 7, 104, 115–18
  high blood pressure, 128–33
  multiple births, 133–44
  preexisting diabetes, 108–15
  pregnancy past age 35, 15, 35, 144–45
  support for, 108
  teen pregnancy, 145–49
HIV (Human immunodeficiency virus), 41
Hormones in animal products, 219–20
Hospital
  breastfeeding in, 155, 159–60
  eating vegetarian in, 105
Hot baths, 12
Human parvovirus B19, 42
Hungry Appetite Menus, 292–93
Hyperglycemia, 111, 127
Hypertension, 129
Hypoglycemia, 110–11, 112–13, 126

I Could Cook All Day Menus, 293
Illness during pregnancy, 41–42, 111–12
Incomplete proteins, 66, 67
Infertility, 8–11
Insulin
  adjusting dosage, 109–10, 115
  exercise and, 122–23
  resistance to, 110
  See also Diabetes
Iodine, 35
Iron
  breastfeeding and, 172
  calcium taken with, 38–39
  food sources, 33, 72, 73
  found in fast-foods, 251
  increasing absorption of, 73–74
  infertility and, 10
  multiple births and, 135–36, 138–39
  need for, 5, 19, 33, 72
  preventing anemia, 59
  second trimester, intake during, 66
  teen pregnancy and, 149
  vegetarian eating and, 94

Johnston, Richard B., 42

Kegel exercises, 59, 179
Ketoacidosis, 110
Ketones, 51
Kitchen
  stocking, 199–201
  tools for, 208–9
  See also Food preparation; Food safety
Krebs, Nancy, 159–60

Labor and delivery
  eating after, 104, 105
  high blood pressure after, 132

with diabetes, 114
  See also Postpartum
Lacto-ovo vegetarian, 92–93, 97–98
Lactose intolerance, 69–71
Lead, 231
  avoiding, 11–12, 173–74
  calcium intake and, 38
  exposure to, 40–41
Leftovers, 207–8, 323–25
Linoleic acid, 26, 96, 137
Listeria monocytegenes, 13, 225
Lochia, 178–79
Low birth weight
  anemia and, 19
  caffeine and, 43
  multiple births and, 133–34
  poor nutrition and, 7
  teen pregnancy and, 148–49
Low blood sugar, 110–11, 112–13, 123, 126
Low-calorie convenience foods, 236–37
Low-fat food
  chips, 76
  substitutions, 183
  menu, 27–28
Luke, Barbara, 134

Magnesium, 30–31, 165
Manganese, 35, 52
Margarine, 26
Material Safety Data Sheet (MSDS), 12–13
Meal planning
  for breastfeeding, 161–62
  for a budget, 205–8
  diabetic, 119–21
  food labels, reading, 201–5
  See also Kitchen; Menus; Shopping for food

Meals
    for company, 293–94
    for cooking a lot, 293
    for cooking less, 259–60
    Eating Expectantly, 55–56,
        96–98, 147–48
    feel full, 326–27
    for a hungry appetite,
        292–93
    light, 259
    in minutes, 325–26
    traveling and, 45–46
    using leftovers, 323–25
    See also Convenience
        foods; Menus
Meals in Minutes Menus,
    325–26
Meat
    food safety and, 13,
        219–21, 223
    in multiple births diet, 138
    nutrient content, 36
    thorough cooking of, 212
Menus
    breakfast, 261, 291–92
    convenience food, 239–42
    cutting fat, 27–28
    first-trimester, 56, 61–62,
        259–61
    first week with baby, 176
    healthy fast-food, 250–56
    in restaurants, healthy,
        248–49
    second-trimester, 79,
        292–94
    third-trimester, 89, 323–27
    using leftovers, 323–25
    vegetarian, 97–98, 327–32
Mercury, 224
Microwave cooking, 212–13,
    229
Milk, 70–72
Minerals
    Biotin, 29

breastfeeding and, 163,
    164–65, 172, 173
Chromium, 35, 66
Copper, 34–35
first-trimester needs, 52
Fluoride, 35
Iodine, 35
Magnesium, 30–31, 165
Manganese, 35, 52
Molybdenum, 35
Pantothenic acid, 29
Phosphorus, 30, 125–26
Potassium, 34, 66
second-trimester needs, 66
Selenium, 10, 35
Sodium, 34, 130, 236
third-trimester needs, 83,
    84–85
See also Calcium; Folate;
    Iron; Zinc
Molybdenum, 35
Morning sickness, 52, 56–58,
    61
Multiple birth pregnancy
    baby's birth weight in,
        133–34
    bed rest for, 140–44
    breastfeeding and, 165–66
    diet for, 135–38
    resources for parents, 139
    weight gain and, 138–39

Nafziger, Steven, 172
Nausea, 52, 56–58, 61
Neural tube defects, 4–5, 12,
    37
Niacin, 29
Nursing. See Breastfeeding
Nut products, 216

Omega-3 fatty acids, 26, 83,
    136–37, 223, 225–26
Omega-6 fatty acids, 26, 137
Organic foods, 214–15

Osteoporosis, 170
Overweight women, 8, 9

Pantothenic acid, 29
Pelvic tilt, 195
Persistent organic pollutants
    (POPs), 224
Pesticides, 213, 214, 216. See
    also Environmental conta-
    minants
Phosphorus, 30, 125–26
Pizzas, 243
Polyols, 124
Pork, 219–21. See also Pork in
    Recipe Index
Postpartum
    body changes during,
        178–79
    eating during, 175–76
    exercise during, 188–90,
        192–94
    preparing for next preg-
        nancy, 186
    returning to work, 177–78
    weight loss during, 179–84
    what to expect, 175–76
Potassium, 34, 66
Poultry, 221, 223. See also
    Poultry in Recipe Index
Preeclampsia, 23, 128, 132
Preexisting diabetes
    birth defects and, 5
    effect on mother, 110–11
    labor and delivery with,
        114
    managing, 108–10, 113–14
    sick day rules for, 111–12
Pregnancy
    changing mindset for, 28
    counseling before, 3–4
    illness during, 41–42
    nutrition before, 4–8
    planning for healthy, 6–7,
        11–13, 17–20
    positives of, 46–47

preparing for next, 186
See also First trimester;
High-risk pregnancies;
Labor and delivery;
Postpartum; Second
trimester; Third
trimester
Pregnancy-induced hyper-
tension (PIH), 128–30
Premature infants, 166–67,
168. *See also* Low birth
weight
Prenatal vitamins, 36–37
breastfeeding and, 164
calcium in, 72
Prepregnancy counseling,
3–4
Preservatives, 204
Produce. *See* Fruits; Vegetables
Protein
breastfeeding needs for,
162–63
complementary, 98
first-trimester needs for,
50–52
food sources, 36, 51, 67
snacks high in, 77
vegetarian eating and, 96
Pyridoxine, 32

Quiz
how's your diet?, 64–66,
83–84
prepregnancy, 6–7
weight gain, 23

Recommended Daily
Allowance (RDA), 29
Rest, 128, 131–32, 140–44,
195
Restaurants. *See* Eating out;
Fast food
Retin-A, 31
Riboflavin, 29
Rubella, 41

Saccharin, 124
Salad bars, 247, 249
Salads, main dish, 246. *See
also* Salads *in Recipe Index*
Salmonella bacteria, 221,
223
Sandwiches, 243, 245
Sauna, 12
Seafood. *See* Fish and
seafood
Second trimester, 63–79
baby growth during,
63–64
body changes during,
77–79
breakfast ideas, 291–92
calcium intake during,
68–72
evaluating diet for, 64–66
iron intake during, 72–74
menus, 79, 292–94
nutrient needs during, 66
protein needs during, 66
recipes, 295–322
snack ideas for, 261–63
soy intake during, 68
weight gain during, 64
Selenium, 10, 35
Shopping for food
on a budget, 205–7
for convenience foods,
235
for dairy products, 218
food safety and, 215–16,
231
for produce, 215–16
for seafood, 226–27
for vegetarian eating,
98–100
Sick-day rules, 111–12
Sleeplessness, 88
Smoking cigarettes
breastfeeding and, 169
harm of, 7, 25, 39
infertility and, 9

Snacks
bed rest, 141
Best Bite, 327
controlling diabetes with,
113
diabetic diet and, 121–22
figs, 53
healthy, 75–77
high-energy, 263
ideas for, 261–62
Sodium, 34, 130, 236
Soy, 68
Spears, Bev, 119
Stevia (sweetener), 125
Storing food. *See* Food stor-
age
Stress, 12, 78–79
Sucralose, 125
Sucrose, 123–24
Sudden infant death syn-
drome (SIDS), 153
Sugar, 85–86, 127–28. *See
also* Sweeteners
Sugar alcohols, 124
Supplements, vitamin, 12,
36–39, 137
Sweeteners, 123–26, 203,
204
Swelling, ankle, 87

Tea, herbal, 44
Teen pregnancy
breastfeeding and, 166
eating plan for, 147–48
getting help for, 146
nutrient needs for, 149
weight gain during,
148–49
Teeth and gum changes,
60–61
Textured vegetable protein
(TVP), 68
Thiamin, 29

Third trimester, 81–89
  baby growth during, 81–82
  body changes during, 87–88
  energy, keeping up, 86–87
  menus, 89, 323–27
  nutrient needs during, 83–85
  recipes, 333–70
  snack ideas for, 262–63
  weight gain during, 82–83
Thrive on Five, 74–75
Tocopherol, 34
Tofu, 68. *See also* Tofu *in Recipe Index*
Toxemia, 128
Toxoplasmosis, 13, 42, 225
Trans-fatty acids, 26
Travel during pregnancy, 45–46
Trichinosis, 219
Triplets. *See* Multiple birth pregnancy
Twins. *See* Multiple birth pregnancy
Type II diabetes, 116. *See also* Preexisting diabetes

Underweight women, 8, 9
Urinary tract infection, 115
Urination, frequent, 58–59
Uterus, after birth, 178

Vaginal discharge, 77, 178–79
Vegan diet, 92–93, 97, 166
Vegetables
  adding to meals, 74–75
  food safety and, 215–17
  keeping vitamins in, 209–10
  pesticides and, 214
  as snacks, 76
  See also Vegetable Side Dishes *in Recipe Index*

Vegetarian eating
  after labor, 104
  benefits, 92
  breastfeeding and, 166, 172
  convenience foods, 102–3
  eating out, 100–102
  food exchanges for, 105
  infertility and, 9
  levels of, 92–93
  menus, 96–98, 327–32
  nutrient needs during pregnancy and, 93–96
  rise of, 91–92
  shopping for, 98–100
  weight loss through, 183–84
  See also Vegetarian Dishes *in Recipe Index*
Videos, exercise, 194
Vitamin A, 31, 52
Vitamin B$_1$, 29
Vitamin B$_2$, 29
Vitamin B$_3$, 29
Vitamin B$_6$, 32
  food sources, 84, 165
  in fast foods, 254
  third-trimester needs, 83, 84
  vegetarian eating and, 95
Vitamin B$_{12}$, 30, 94, 172
Vitamin C, 33
  birth defects and, 11
  during second trimester, 66
  food sources, 33
  functions, 33
  in fast foods, 255
  infertility and, 10
Vitamin D, 31–32
  multiple births and, 136
  vegetarian eating and, 95
Vitamin E, 34
Vitamin K, 31

Vitamins
  breastfeeding and, 163, 164, 173
  cooking vegetables to retain, 209–10
  first-trimester needs, 52
  second-trimester needs, 66
  supplements, 12, 36–39, 137
  third-trimester needs, 83–85
  vegetarian diet and, 93–96
  See also names of individual vitamins

Water
  lead in, 40, 173–74, 231
  as nutrient, 52
Websites
  breastfeeding, 167
  diabetes, 108, 116
  fast foods, 256
  fish and wildlife advisories, 224
  food additives, 205
  food safety, 230
  food-borne illnesses, 225
  infant feeding, 174
  multiple births, 139
  pregnancy, 79
  sweeteners, 123
  vegetarian resources, 102
Weight
  ideal, 22
  infertility and, 9
  See also Weight gain; Weight loss
Weight gain
  avoiding too much, 24
  excessive and fast, 23
  first-trimester, 50
  lack of, 24–25
  monitoring, 22–23
  and multiple births, 134–35, 138–39

recommended, 20–22, 50, 135
second-trimester, 64
teen pregnancy and, 147, 148–49
third-trimester, 82–83
Weight loss
breastfeeding and, 162, 169–70
diabetic diet and, 121
infertility and, 8, 9
influence on baby, 5

postpartum, 179–86
vitamin/mineral loss and, 8
Whole grains, 10, 19. *See also* Grains *in Recipe Index*
Wilson, Lowell L., 219
Work
breastfeeding and, 156–57, 177–78
environmental contaminants at, 12–13

Zinc, 33
breast-feeding vegetarians and, 172
food sources, 85, 164
in fast foods, 252
infertility and, 10
teen pregnancy and, 149
third-trimester needs, 83, 84–85
vegetarian eating and, 95

Recipe Index

Beans

Aspen Black Bean Soup, 337
Basic Black Beans, 303
Bean and Corn Bread Bake, 348
Beans 101, 304
Black Bean and Corn Salad, 270
Black Bean Enchilada Casserole, 349
Bridget's Garden Salad, 271
Colorado Stuffed Peppers, 354
Hoppin' John, 357
Lentil Soup, 338
Minute Minestrone, 300
Vegetarian Chili, 340

Beef

Sesame Beef, 361
Spanish Steak Roll with Sautéed Vegetables, 315
Stuffed Eggplant Creole, 316

Beverages

High-Energy Drink, 86

Breads and Muffins

Apple-Date Bran Muffins, 278
Bean and Corn Bread Bake, 348
French French Toast, 296
Pumpkin Muffins, 279
Strawberry Bread, 280
Thrive-on-Five Bread, 281

Cakes and Pies

See Desserts

Cheese

Boursin Cheese Spread, 334
Caramel Dip, 335
Cheese-Topped Orange Roughy, 351
Country Brunch Casserole, 355
Creamy Pesto Pasta, 309
Delightful Spinach, 266
Rocky Mountain Quesadillas, 277
Salmon Pâté, 267
Spinach-Stuffed Shells, 362

Chicken

Apricot-Glazed Chicken, 347
Chicken and Shrimp with Fruit Salsa, 352–53

Creole

Stuffed Eggplant Creole, 316

Desserts

Berry Mousse Parfait, 319
Crepes, 310–311
Favorite Snack Cake, 367
Fruit Crisp, 368
Fruit Pizza for a Crowd, 369
Mocha Java Cake, 320
Peach Pops, 284
Pumpkin Roll, 321
Quick and Easy Blueberry Cobbler, 322
Sunshine Sorbet, 370
Tropical Pudding, 288

Dips and Spreads

Basic Black Beans, 303
Boursin Cheese Spread, 334
Caramel Dip, 335

Delightful Spinach, 266
Salmon Pâté, 267

Eggs

Broccoli Quiche, 350
French French Toast, 296
Mock Egg Foo Yung, 358

Fish and Seafood

Cheese-Topped Orange Roughy, 351
Chicken and Shrimp with Fruit Salsa, 352–53
Crab Marinara, 356
Quick Grilled Fish, 360
Salmon en Papillote, 314
Salmon Pâté, 267
Stuffed Eggplant Creole, 316

Fondue

Company Fondue, 308

Fruits

Apple Pie à la Mode Shake, 282
Apple-Date Bran Muffins, 278
Banana-Orange Flip, 283
Berry Mousse Parfait, 319
Chicken-and-Spinach Salad, 272
Favorite Snack Cake, 367
Fruit Crisp, 368
Pancakes with Raspberry Sauce, 297
Peach Pops, 284
Piña Colada Frappé, 286
Quick and Easy Blueberry Cobbler, 322
Raspberry Surprise Shake, 287

Salsa, 352
Strawberry Bread, 280
Sunshine Sorbet, 370
Tangy Salad, 302
Tropical Pudding, 288
Very Berry Shake, 289

Grains
Bulgur-and-Veggie Mix, 341
Colorado Stuffed Peppers, 354
Hoppin' John, 357
Mushroom-and-Barley Soup, 301
Oat-Nut Burgers, 359
See also Breads and Muffins

Lamb
Leg of Lamb, 313

Mexican Dishes
Black Bean Enchilada Casserole, 349
Mexican Kale-and-Pork Soup, 339
Rocky Mountain Quesadillas, 277
Vegetarian Breakfast Tacos, 366

Muffins
See Breads and Muffins

Nuts
Oat-Nut Burgers, 359

Pancakes
Crepe Dinner, 310–11
Pancakes with Raspberry Sauce, 297
Quick and Healthier Pancakes, 298

Pasta
Crab Marinara, 356
Creamy Pesto Pasta, 309
Pasta with Quick Alfredo Sauce, 276
Spinach-Stuffed Shells, 362

Peanut Butter
Peanut-Butter-Chocolate Shake, 285

Pork
Basic Black Beans, 303
Country Brunch Casserole, 355
Greek Island Pita Pockets, 312
Hoppin' John, 357
Mexican Kale-and-Pork Soup, 339

Poultry
Chicken Roll-Ups, 307
Chicken-and-Spinach Salad, 272
Turkey Pot Pie, 317
Turkey with Hoisin Sauce, 318

Salads
Asian Salad, 269
Black Bean and Corn Salad, 270
Bridget's Garden Salad, 271
Chicken-and-Spinach Salad, 272
Tangy Salad, 302

Salsa
Fruit Salsa, 352

Sauces
Company Fondue, 308
Cream Sauce, 275

Dijon Sauces, 308, 336
Hoisin Sauce, 318
Horseradish Mayonnaise Sauce, 308
Pasta with Quick Alfredo Sauce, 276
Raspberry Sauce, 297
Roasted Red Pepper Sauce, 364
Sesame Beef Sauce, 361
Sweet and Sour Sauce, 308
Yogurt Sauces, 270, 312

Shakes
Apple Pie à la Mode Shake, 282
Banana-Orange Flip, 283
Peanut-Butter-Chocolate Shake, 285
Piña Colada Frappé, 286
Raspberry Surprise Shake, 287
Very Berry Shake, 289

Snacks
Baked Tortilla Chips, 270
Berry Mousse Parfait, 319
Carrots Antibes, 273
Favorite Snack Cake, 367
Rocky Mountain Quesadillas, 277

Soups
Aspen Black Bean Soup, 337
Basic Black Bean, 303
Creamy Asparagus Soup, 268
Leek-and-Potato Soup, 299
Lentil Soup, 338
Mexican Kale-and-Pork Soup, 339
Minute Minestrone, 300
Mushroom-and-Barley Soup, 301

Tofu

Mock Egg Foo Yung, 358
Stuffed Eggplant Creole, 316
Tofu Loaf, 363
Vegetable-and-Tofu Stir-Fry, 365

Turkey

Turkey Pot Pie, 317
Turkey with Hoisin Sauce, 318

Veal

Veal Piccata with Roasted Red Pepper Sauce, 364

Vegetable Side Dishes

Bulgur-and-Veggie Mix, 341
Carrots Antibes, 273
Delightful Spinach, 266

Easy Microwave Potatoes, 342
Kids' Carrots, 343
Oven-Fried Zucchini Sticks, 274
Potatoes Marie Louise, 305
Ratatouille, 344
Roasted New Potatoes/Home Fries, 345
Spring Vegetables in Cream Sauce, 275
Thanksgiving Sweet Potatoes, 306
Vegetables in Vinaigrette, 346

Vegetarian Dishes

Bean and Corn Bread Bake, 348
Black Bean Enchilada

Casserole, 349
Broccoli Quiche, 350
Colorado Stuffed Peppers, 354
Creamy Pesto Pasta, 309
Crepe Dinner, 310–11
Minute Minestrone, 300
Mock Egg Foo Yung, 358
Oat-Nut Burgers, 359
Pasta with Quick Alfredo Sauce, 276
Ratatouille, 344
Spinach-Stuffed Shells, 362
Tofu Loaf, 363
Vegetable-and-Tofu Stir-Fry, 365
Vegetarian Breakfast Tacos, 366
Vegetarian Chili, 340

Notes

Notes

Notes

Notes

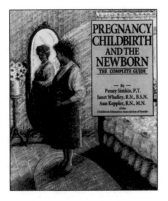

Pregnancy, Childbirth, and the Newborn

by Simkin, Whalley, and Keppler

More complete and up-to-date than any other pregnancy guide, this remarkable book is the bible for childbirth educators from coast to coast. Called "excellent" by the *American Journal of Nursing*.

Order #1169

Getting Organized for Your New Baby

by Maureen Bard

This revised and expanded favorite will ensure that when baby is ready to come–the parents are ready to go! Here is an essential planning tool to help prepare parents for pregnancy, birth, and baby's first few months. It provides checklists, how-to hints, forms, charts, and bibliographies to make it easy for parents to get scheduled, budgeted, and prioritized.

Order #1229

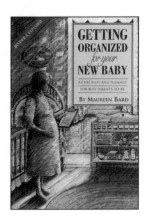

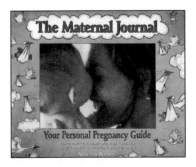

The Maternal Journal

by Matthew Bennett

This colorful, photo-filled pregnancy planner/calendar is a quick and delightful way for expectant mothers to learn what to expect and do during the nine months of pregnancy and first three months of parenthood.

Order #3171

The Very Best Baby Name Book in the Whole Wide World

by Bruce Lansky

This book is the very best way to help you name your baby. It contains more than 30,000 popular and unusual names from around the world, complete with origins, famous namesakes, and variations.

Order #1030

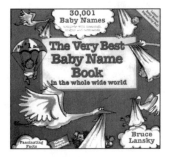

Look for Meadowbrook Press books where you buy books. You may also order books by using the form printed below.

Order Form

Quantity	Title	Author	Order No.	Unit Cost (U.S. $)	Total
	35,000+ Baby Names	Lansky, B.	1225	$5.95	
	Baby & Child Emergency First-Aid Handbook	Einzig/Hart	1381	$8.00	
	Baby & Child Medical Care	Hart, T.	1159	$9.00	
	Baby Names around the World	Lansky, B.	1235	$13.00	
	Baby Name Survey Book	Lansky/Sinrod	1270	$9.00	
	Baby Play & Learn	Warner, P.	1275	$9.00	
	Best Baby Name Book	Lansky, B.	1029	$5.00	
	Best Baby Shower Book	Cooke, C.	1239	$7.00	
	Discipline without Shouting or Spanking	Wyckoff/Unell	1079	$6.00	
	Familiarity Breeds Children	Lansky, B.	4015	$7.00	
	Feed Me! I'm Yours	Lansky, V.	1109	$9.00	
	First-Year Baby Care	Kelly, P.	1119	$10.00	
	Gentle Discipline	Lighter, D.	1085	$6.00	
	Getting Organized for Your New Baby	Bard, M.	1229	$9.00	
	Grandma Knows Best	McBride, M.	4009	$7.00	
	Healthy Food for Healthy Kids	Swinney, B.	1129	$12.00	
	Joy of Grandparenting	Sherins/Hollerman	3502	$7.00	
	Joy of Parenthood	Blaustone, J.	3500	$7.00	
	Maternal Journal	Bennett, M.	3171	$10.00	
	Practical Parenting Tips	Lansky, V.	1180	$8.00	
	Pregnancy, Childbirth, and the Newborn	Simkin/Whalley/Keppler	1169	$12.00	
	Very Best Baby Name Book	Lansky, B.	1030	$8.00	
	When You Were a Baby	Haley, A.	1391	$8.00	
				Subtotal	
			Shipping and Handling		
			MN residents add 6.5% sales tax		
				Total	

YES! Please send me the books indicated above. Add $2.00 shipping and handling for the first book with a retail price up to $9.99 or $3.00 for the first book with a retail price over $9.99. Add $1.00 shipping and handling for each additional book. All orders must be prepaid. Most orders are shipped within 2 days by U.S. Mail (7–9 delivery days). Rush shipping is available for an extra charge. Overseas postage will be billed. **Quantity discounts available upon request.**

Send book(s) to:

Name _____

Address _____

City _____ State _____ Zip _____

Telephone (_____)_____

Payment via:

☐ Check or money order payable to Meadowbrook Press (No cash or C.O.D.s please.)

☐ Visa (for orders over $10.00 only)   ☐ MasterCard (for orders over $10.00 only)

Account #_____

Signature _____ Exp. Date _____

A FREE Meadowbrook catalog is available upon request.
You can also phone us for orders of $10.00 or more at 800-338-2232.

Mail to: Meadowbrook Press
5451 Smetana Drive, Minnetonka, Minnesota 55343

Phone 952-930-1100   Toll-Free 800-338-2232   Fax 952-930-1940
For more information visit our website: www.meadowbrookpress.com